# DIFFERENT
## BODIES

---

# DIFFERENT
## DIETS

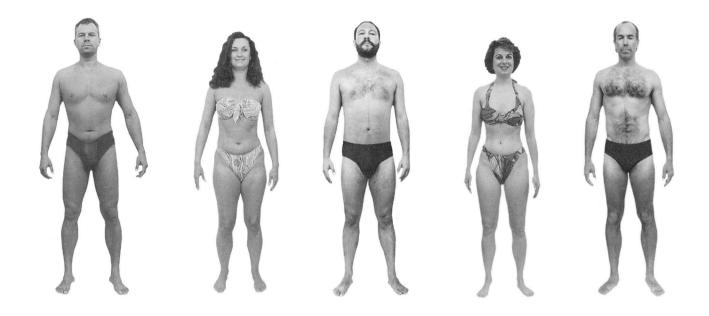

# Carolyn Mein, D.C.

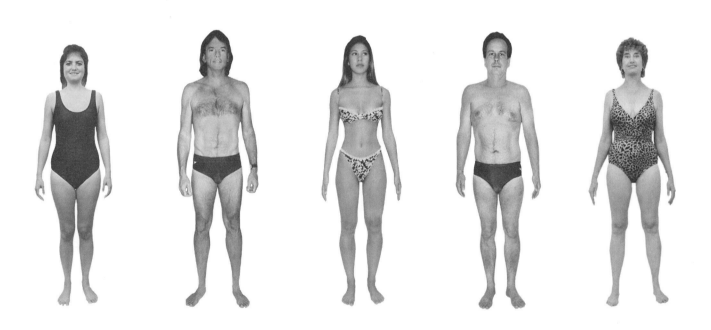

# DIFFERENT
# BODIES

## The Revolutionary
## 25 Body Type System

# DIFFERENT
# DIETS

ReganBooks  *An Imprint of* HarperCollins*Publishers*

This book is written as a source of information only. The information contained in this book should by no means be considered a substitute for the advice of a qualified medical professional, who should always be consulted before beginning any new diet, exercise, or other health program.

All efforts have been made to ensure the accuracy of the information contained in this book as of the date published. The author and the publisher expressly disclaim responsibility for any adverse effects arising from the use or application of the information contained herein.

FIRST EDITION

Printed on acid-free paper

*Designed by Kate Nichols*

Library of Congress Cataloging-in-Publication Data

Mein, Carolyn L.
Different bodies, different diets / Carolyn Mein.— 1st ed.
p. cm.
Includes index.
ISBN 0-06-039390-4
1. Chiropractic. 2. Women—Nutrition. 3. Somatotypes. I. Title.

RZ242 .M448 2001
613.2'082—dc21
00-051790

01 02 03 04 05 QW 10 9 8 7 6 5 4 3 2 1

To all our wonderful patients,
friends, participants, and everyone
who has ever searched for their ideal diet,
or looked to better understand themselves.

And to our parents:

Nadine A. Mein
Orville E. Mein

# Acknowledgments

I would like to express my gratitude to everyone who has helped me in this endeavor. Special thanks to everyone who was photographed as part of this project, especially to those whose photos are in the book.

Most important, my deep, heartfelt gratitude and appreciation to all my special patients and friends who so freely shared with me their experiences and insights during the developing and refining of the diets, menus, and psychological profiles. I am particularly grateful to those who so willingly revealed themselves and shared their personal awareness by answering my seemingly endless questions. For without them this work would never have been possible. I would like to specifically acknowledge:

George Goodheart, D.C., for developing muscle testing as an accurate means of communicating with the intelligence of the body

Elliot Abravanel, M.D., for his *Dr. Abravanel's Body Type and Lifetime Nutritional Plan,* which opened the door for my research

Anthony Liu for his graphic design and visionary artwork, as well as for doing the computer scanning and layout work for all the photographs

Carol Kemp for her observant eye in helping me identify the distinguishing characteristics of the body types; for her assistance with: the diet, photo selection, layout, captions, and questionnaires; and for her support throughout this undertaking

Nadine Mein, my mother, for her untiring patience and perseverance in typing and checking various sections of the book for accuracy and completeness

Theresa Foy DiGeronimo for simplifying and organizing this material

My office staff—Renee Marsh, Gerri McCaffrey, Elaine Hoover, D.C., Terri Lew, Nancy Alaura, Amanda Stevenson, L.Ac., and Kathy Gunningham—for their dedication in taking photos, interviewing participants, and organizing data

Wayne Mein, my brother, for his many hours of dedicated assistance with typing and photos

Juawayne Kettler, developer of Blisswork, for the use of her studio during photography sessions and for her support and enthusiastic recommendation of the Body Type Diet to her many students

Maureen Regan, my agent, for performing many valuable services in bringing this project to light, without her support and professional guidance, the road to publication would have been a perilous and difficult one

The team at ReganBooks and HarperCollins, who did an outstanding job for me. First and foremost, I want to thank Judith Regan for believing in my book from the start, and second, many thanks to Doug Corcoran, Renee Iwaszkiewicz, Kurt Andrews, Cassie Jones, Joyce Wong, Lucy Albanese, Shelby Meizlik, and Carl Raymond for their expertise and enthusiasm.

My appreciation to all the participants who, after applying the diet designed for their type, provided me with valuable feedback and menu ideas.

My thanks and love to all of you!

# Contents

**Part 2**
**The 25 Body Types: Profiles and Diets**

# Introduction

How many different diets have you tried in an attempt to gain health, increase energy, or lose weight? The reality is that each of the many diets out there is valuable for someone. But which ones are right for you? How do you decide? In a single day, we are faced with a multitude of decisions regarding what to eat. Unfortunately, the contradictions about what foods are best are astounding and confusing. We are offered contradictory information regarding even the most essential nutrients like fat, carbohydrates, protein, and water, just to name a few. The question is, Which parts of the information are right or wrong for you?

With degrees in chiropractic, acupuncture, clinical nutrition, bio-nutrition, and applied kinesiology, I searched for a way to answer that question and was unable to find one system or diet that worked for everyone. About sixteen years ago, following my own dietary challenges, I was introduced to a book that explained why this was so. The book, *Dr. Abravanel's Body Type and Lifetime Nutritional Plan* by Elliot D. Abravanel, M.D., and Elizabeth A. King, was based on Dr. Henry G. Bieler's research on the control of the body by the dominant glands and their regulatory factors. The premise was that dietary requirements are different for different people because of the differences in their dominant glandular systems.

Dr. Bieler worked extensively with two types and introduced a third. Dr. Abravanel explored the third and included a fourth for women. As I worked with Abravanel's typing system, I found the same thing I found with every other typing system—some people seemed to be a blend of more than one type. Intrigued by the idea of an accurate body typing system that would not leave some people "in-between" types, I began discovering the missing types.

Today I am satisfied that there are only 25 types. To make sure all the body types were identified, I offered free body typing sessions to the general public for three years. I typed everyone in my practice and worked extensively with each individual's diet. I also went to Japan specifically to see if there were cultural differences in body type. I found the same 25 types in the Asian population as I did in the Western world. Everyone I have evaluated has been one of the 25 types.

The results of this work are offered to you in this book. They finally answer questions like:

- What is my ideal weight?
- What foods should I eat and when is the best time to eat them?

► What type of exercise is best and most effective for me?
► Why do diets work for some people and not for others?
► How much fat am I really supposed to eat?
► Why do certain foods cause me to be tired, bloated, or irritable?

By answering these questions, my new body typing program will allow you to create your ideal body and ensure your maximum performance.

## The Basis of Body Typing

The basis of the 25 Body Type System is that every person has a dominant gland, organ, or system (referred to simply as the dominant gland). It is present at birth and remains dominant throughout one's life. This dominant gland is what determines certain physical characteristics and psychological traits of a particular body type. Each type has its own unique psychological profile, dietary guidelines, and recommended types of exercise.

## Weight Loss and Weight Gain

The Body Type Diet is a system for weight loss through health. There is no deprivation, no portion control, and no suffering. The key is to bring your body back into balance by eating what supports your body and avoiding foods that cause your body stress. The benefits of having your body in balance are vitality, stamina, maximum energy, and reaching your ideal weight, whether through weight loss or weight gain.

## Achieving Balance and Health

This is not a program that requires huge amounts of "willpower." There are over 450 foods to choose from every day, and the foods are divided into three categories: Ultra-Support Foods, Basic Support Foods, and Stressful Foods. Approximately 90 percent of the foods are included in the Ultra-Support and Basic Support categories, leaving a mere 10 percent in the Stressful Foods category. (Stressful Foods should not be consumed more than once a month.)

## Psychological Profile

Your type-related psychological profile will provide you with insights allowing for greater self-understanding as well as compassion and expanded awareness of the strengths and challenges of others. The knowledge and perception of deep-seated tendencies, concerns, and motivations can offer you a greater sense of direction and acceptance of yourself and those around you.

## Body-Typing Family and Friends

When you are finished body-typing yourself, you'll find you can't resist body-typing your family, friends, and coworkers. You'll also be able to use the psychological profiles to enhance your relationships in your family and career. Body-typing those you live and work closely with will give you knowledge that will enable you to support their strengths, understand their motivations, and gain a greater understanding of the areas in which they are challenged.

This book is designed to provide all the tools necessary for you and your loved ones to live a healthy and exuberant life. Have fun and enjoy the process!

# PART 1

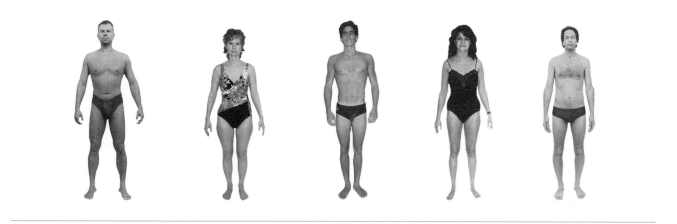

# Identifying and Understanding
# Your Body Type

# CHAPTER 1

# What Are Body Types?

Why are there so many commercial diets on the market? If even one of them really worked for all people, that's the only one we'd all need! But obviously, there is no such thing as a one-diet-fits-all program. We have seen liquid diets, protein diets, low-carb diets, high-carb diets, all-fruit diets, water/fast diets, diets sponsored by Weight Watchers, Jenny Craig, and Overeaters Anonymous. Some of these work for some people, some work for a short time, and some fail miserably. The reason for the disappointing results is simple: We are all different. Our bodies are different; our nutritional needs are different; and our dietary requirements are very different.

So the bottom line is this: To find and maintain your ideal body weight and live with maximum vitality and energy, you need a diet that is carefully tailored to your particular body type—a diet that caters to your natural cravings and needs; a diet you can live with forever. That's exactly what you'll find in the Body Type Diet program.

## Introducing the Body Type Diet

This book is about a program of weight control and health that restores the body's natural balance through an understanding of individual body types. After years of researching this subject, I have identified 25 specific body types based on dominant glands, organs, and body systems. (See the photos illustrating all 25 on pages 8 to 11.) I am confident that identifying your body type and learning how to feed it will allow you to easily obtain your perfect body weight and optimum health.

Knowing your body type is like having an owner's manual for your body. When you buy a BMW, you don't get a manual for a Fiat—although both are cars, each has unique requirements to ensure maximum performance. Imagine how annoyed you'd be if a car dealer insisted that you didn't need the manual published for your new BMW, because "all cars are really pretty much the same." Well, that's what you've been told all these years about diet plans—that all people's dietary needs are pretty much the same. Body typing says loud and clear: They are not!

We all have bodies, but they come in different "models" or "body types." Figuring out your body type provides the "manual" that enables you to create your ideal body and ensure your maximum performance. In the chapters of this book you will find that each of

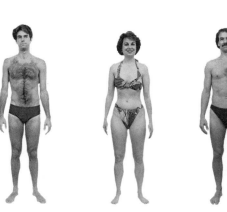

the 25 different body types has its own unique psychological profile, dietary guidelines, weight-loss and weight-gain guide, and recommended types of exercise.

It's important to focus on your unique diet and health needs because the action of the dominant gland in your body can deplete the nutrients needed for high-performance functioning of your specific body type. Certain foods stimulate and weaken your dominant gland; other foods support or rebuild it. The Body Type Diet guides you to the foods that keep your body type strong. This is a system for weight control through health. The key is to bring your body back into balance by eating what supports your body and avoiding foods that cause your body stress.

The collection of photos on the following pages will give you an overview of the name and appearance of each of the 25 body types for males and females. In Chapter 2 you'll learn how to identify your specific body type.

## The Advantages of Body Typing

By identifying your body type, you gain specific knowledge of and insight into many areas of diet that control your personal requirements for lifelong health and vitality. Through body typing you'll learn:

- ▶ What foods your body requires to maintain, gain, or lose weight
- ▶ How much fat and protein your body needs
- ▶ The best time of day to eat certain foods
- ▶ Why you have certain food cravings and how to get rid of them
- ▶ What types of exercise are most effective for you
- ▶ What your ideal yet realistic body type looks and feels like
- ▶ What foods your particular body type needs to gain vitality, stamina, and maximum energy
- ▶ How to get healthy and stay healthy
- ▶ What motivates you, challenges you, and aids your emotional and spiritual growth

This is a long list of advantages that can be yours when you use the Body Type Diet program to nurture both the physical and psychological aspects of your dietary needs.

## Successful Weight Control with Body Typing

One of the first indications that your body is under excessive stress is an imbalance in your weight. While weight gain is generally the most common symptom of the body being out of balance, so is weight loss.

Maintaining your ideal weight and energy level is the goal of this program; that goal is achieved through an individualized diet that's just right for your body type. (From here on, the word *diet* means "the consumption of foods chosen to support your body.") The easiest way to manage your weight is by changing your diet to include the foods your body needs most and eliminate those that are stressful.

Even minor dietary changes geared to support your dominant gland can have amazing results—you often don't have to do very much before you see a difference. By simply creating more variety in your weekly menus, or by eating certain foods at specific times of the day, you will be able to increase your health and sense of well-being as well as attain and maintain your proper weight.

Often people with long histories of yo-yo dieting or those who have battled weight all their lives (including those who were "born heavy" or started the battle in their teens) have finally been able to rid themselves of unwanted pounds and inches by sticking to a diet plan that is tailor-made for their body type. And what they really appreciate with this body typing program is that they can keep the weight off!

Darlene is a typical example of how the Body Type Diet can change someone's life. Darlene had battled a weight problem since her teens. Her thick waist and heavy thighs prompted her to try every diet that came along. She was thoroughly familiar with the grapefruit diet, Slim Fast, Dexatrim, and on and on. She had even resorted to trying a tablespoon of vinegar every day to see if that could possibly help. Exercise didn't work either. She had tried to exhaustion every routine that promised her a slender waist.

When she came to me, Darlene was five feet two inches and weighed 173 pounds. Her body type was Pancreas, and her weight gain was due to her overstressed dominant gland. I also discovered that everything she had been doing to lose weight was counterproductive for her body type. I outlined a dietary plan that would be nutritionally supportive and would help her lose the excess pounds.

After only six months of following her eating plan, Darlene had lost 38 pounds. When she began to follow the diet that was right for her body type, she lost weight easily and consistently. Darlene was finally able to stop struggling with weight and begin enjoying a healthy life with increased vitality, self-esteem, and energy.

Because your body type is something that you are born with, it contains the blueprint for how you gain weight and what you must do to take it off. When you understand your body's specific needs, it helps eliminate any guilt you might feel when you avoid the diets that are working for your friends and relatives. You know what your particular body needs!

## It's More than Diet and Exercise

Many people achieve their ideal weight through diet and exercise, and you know that they intend to keep that weight off forever. Yet a year later, many of them are once again overweight. Why is it so hard to maintain a healthy weight? The answer is very basic and simple: While weight loss is typically addressed from the physical aspect, true dietary success cannot be maintained without addressing the total person. Body typing addresses achieving and maintaining your ideal weight using all the necessary components: physical, emotional, mental, and spiritual.

### The Physical Aspect

The physical aspect of weight loss involves diet and exercise, as well as general health. Weight gain or loss is often the first indication your body is out of balance. Hormonal changes and stress are commonly known to increase the need for nutrients, especially essential fatty acids and certain amino acids. To get the nutrients your body needs from your diet, you need to eat the foods that supply the nutrients you need at times when your body can best assimilate them. Your body type diet tells you which foods to emphasize and provides the guidelines you need. There is no deprivation, no portion control, and no suffering. This is a program that offers each body type an abundance of delicious foods along with exercise options that bring weight control through good health rather than deprivation.

### The Emotional Aspect

The emotional aspect can be just as important as the physical in achieving and maintaining ideal weight.

Each body type has a specific learning lesson. To face the truth is the lesson for the Pancreas body type who has an inborn fear of betrayal. For the Stomach body type who feels safe by controlling their world, the lesson is to allow change.

When we think of the emotional aspect of weight, we usually think of using food to nurture ourselves or to stuff unpleasant emotions. While this is one aspect, there is more. Unresolved emotional stress can be as subtle as a lifelong pattern we have simply accepted and felt powerless to change. Since life is about growth and our bodies eventually reflect our emotional states, sooner or later, we are forced to face ourselves. Each body type profile describes how characteristic traits are expressed negatively, or "at worst," and positively, or "at best," providing a way of identifying emotional patterns.

Simply being aware of deep-seated emotional patterns is not enough to clear them. Emotions are like water and need to be free to move, thus allowing us to experience both sides of the feeling. Most of us are aware of the negative side of an emotion, such as control, but how many of us know the positive side? We know all too well how it feels to be controlled by someone else, what it takes to control our environment, and the fear of losing control. So, is the opposite of control being out of control? No, it is balance. That's nice, but how do you get there? I wrote *Releasing Emotional Patterns with Essential Oils* to show both sides of an emotion and to provide a way of quickly and efficiently clearing emotional patterns. While clearing emotional patterns is important for everyone, for some body types it is essential to achieving and maintaining ideal weight.

To determine if you are using food as an emotional buffer, ask yourself:

- ▶ Are you overeating to fill that hollow space inside?
- ▶ Do you use food, especially sweets, to reward yourself?
- ▶ Is food, particularly salty or fatty snacks, a necessary part of any social event?
- ▶ Do you nurture yourself with food?
- ▶ Do you use excess weight as a buffer?

If you answer yes, frequently, to any of these questions, body typing will help you check for an underlying emotional component that may be sabotaging your efforts to control your weight.

## 25 BODY TYPES

The basis of the 25 Body Type System is that every person has a dominant gland, organ, or system. It is present at birth and remains dominant throughout one's life. This dominant gland is what determines certain physical characteristics and psychological traits.

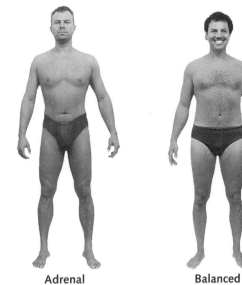
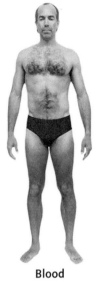

**Adrenal**

**Balanced**

**Blood**

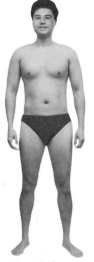
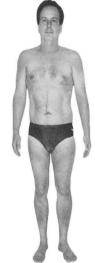
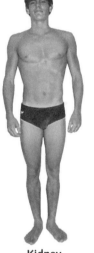
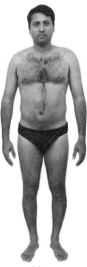
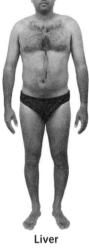

**Hypothalamus**

**Intestinal**

**Kidney**

**Liver**

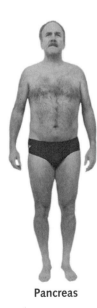
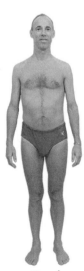
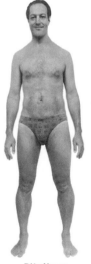
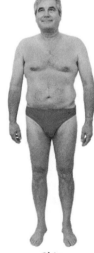
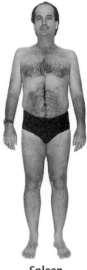

**Pancreas**

**Pineal**

**Pituitary**

**Skin**

**Spleen**

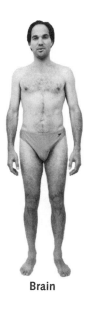

Brain

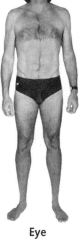

Eye

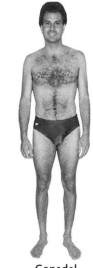

Gallbladder

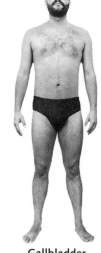

Gonadal

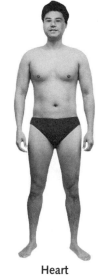

Heart

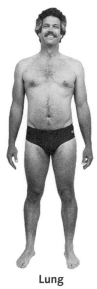

Lung

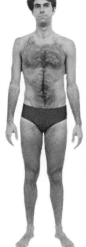

Lymph

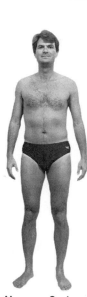

Medulla

Nervous System

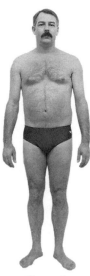

Stomach

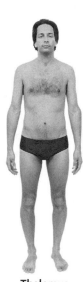

Thalamus

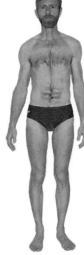

Thymus

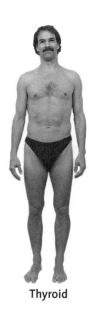

Thyroid

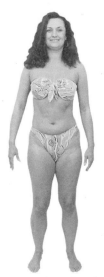

Adrenal

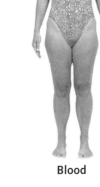

Balanced

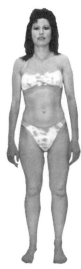

Blood

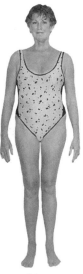

Brain

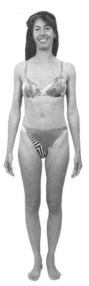

Hypothalmus

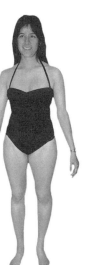

Intestinal

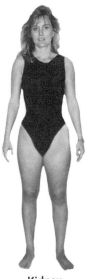

Kidney

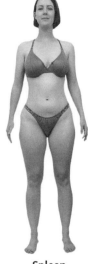

Liver

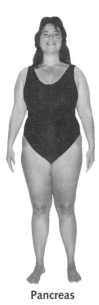

Pancreas

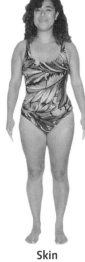

Pineal

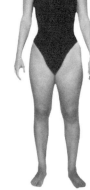

Pituitary

Skin

Spleen

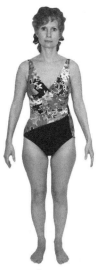

Eye

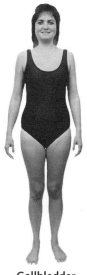

Gallbladder

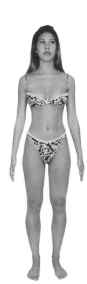

Gonadal

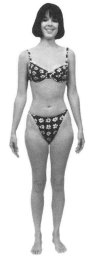

Heart

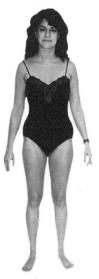

Lung

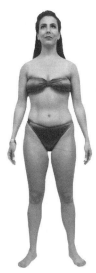

Lymph

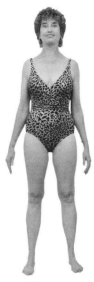

Medulla

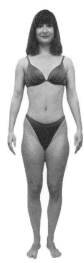

Nervous System

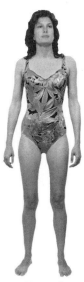

Stomach

Thalamus

Thymus

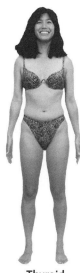

Thyroid

## The Mental Aspect

The mental aspect involves focus. Where you focus your attention during dieting can determine success or failure. Body typing will help you focus on results, goals, and outcomes rather than solely on food. (If you focus your attention solely on food, you spend more time thinking about food and therefore more time wanting and eating food.) Use visualization to see yourself reaching your goal and enjoying the benefits of good health and focus on the positives, not any perceived negatives of changing your eating patterns.

The mental aspect also focuses attention on your passions. Your body type psychological profile (explained below) explores areas of passion that are common to those with your body type. When you use this information as a tool to explore your passions and focus on expressing them in your life, you will not use unfulfilled passions as an emotional excuse to turn to food.

## The Spiritual Aspect

The spiritual aspect involves intuition—that indefinable inkling that makes you sense "I had a feeling I needed to do that." Body typing will encourage you to pay more attention to your intuition and let it play a role in achieving and maintaining your ideal weight. On some level, you already know what you need to eat and when you need to eat it. Body typing will help you bring out the inner voice that will enable you to reach your ideal weight and keep it forever.

## The Psychological Side of Body Typing

Each body type has a distinct physical appearance that sets it off from the others, but each also has distinct psychological aspects. The information you'll gain from the psychological profile in the chapter about your body type will give you insights into your basic nature. These insights will allow you to look at your personal challenges from a new perspective. You'll see yourself at your best and at your worst, and you'll learn to use this knowledge of deep-seated tendencies to gain a greater sense of direction and an acceptance of who you really are. Your psychological profile will also supply you with the map you need to seek a path around the roadblocks that have kept you from attaining your ideal weight and physical health in the past.

Once you have learned how to body-type yourself, it's fascinating to do the same for your family, friends, and coworkers. When you identify the body types of others, you can use their psychological profiles to gain a greater understanding of their strengths, challenges, and motivations. This awareness will enhance your relationships with your family and coworkers.

## "If I Follow the Diet, What Can I Expect?"

Stand before a full-length mirror in your underwear or a bathing suit. Turn and observe yourself carefully from all angles: front, back, and side views. Where do you appear to have excess weight? Is there a look of disproportion, a heaviness in some areas, while others seem just right? Or maybe you need to put on a little weight in certain parts of your body?

The weight you carry on your body is a good reflection of how your system uses the food you eat. Eating the foods that are right for your particular body type at the times of the day when they are most effective for your system will enable you to give your body just what it needs. This conscious eating will cause your body to lose unnecessary weight so that your system can function properly without the mental and physical stress of dieting. And if you want to gain weight, it will be much easier because you will know what to eat as well as the times of the day when your system will get the best results from your food intake.

Eating for your body type is different from the usual weight-loss diets because you are now supplying your system with foods that are supportive of it. Weight-loss diets usually stress deprivation of some kind, which often causes a rebound effect when you go off the diet. Eating the right foods for your body type allows you to reach and then maintain your correct body weight. This in itself is a step toward optimal health.

Without regard to weight loss or gain, there are other comments I hear from patients who have begun to follow the special diets for their body types. Most often I hear "I feel better!" Many tell me that they have a higher energy level and that they no longer feel hungry between meals. Some are better able to avoid the sweets and caffeine that they were dependent on for that little boost that got them through the day. Often they are able to accomplish much more because of better endurance, and they have more energy at the end of the day.

What it really comes down to is this: If you follow the eating regimen tailored to your particular body type, you will be using food the way nature, or your special nature, meant you to. When you support your body with the diet plan best suited for it, you can achieve an optimal state of physical health and well-being.

You must eat in order to live, so why not eat those foods that enliven you, unlocking the stores of energy and vitality that you may never have known before? At the same time, you can maintain that energy flow as it constantly replenishes and rebuilds your system.

Overall, body typing is a researched and tested method of identifying a person's unique dietary needs. It gives you the knowledge and hands-on tools you need to feed both your body and soul for the ultimate in health and well-being. The next chapter will take you step-by-step through the body type identification process. In just a few minutes you will uncover the secret that has sabotaged your past dieting efforts and that will open the door to a whole new you.

# CHAPTER 2

# What Is Your Body Type?

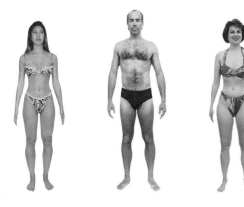

Are you a Heart body type or a Liver type? An Eye type or a Brain type? That's what you will find out in this chapter. Your body type is determined by your dominant gland. This gland greatly influences your general appearance, including your body shape and structure, as well as your weight gain pattern and metabolism. The process of identifying your body type is a search for this gland that controls your health and weight.

Your body type can be found among the 25 distinct body types described in this chapter. The methods of determining a female or male body type are explained step-by-step to make it easy for you to identify your particular type. Then, once you know your body type, you can go to Part 2, where the body types are listed in alphabetical order. Here you will find the psychological profile and dietary profile that will help you achieve the mental and physical balance you need to obtain and keep vital health and ideal weight.

## A Four-Step Method to Identify Your Body Type

Following this four-step process can identify all body types:

1. **Physical characteristics.** Physical characteristics, such as weight gain areas and waist types for women and torso shape and muscular appearance for men, are important because they provide obvious clues to your dominant gland. As you follow the instructions for identifying your physical characteristics, you'll find that some physical traits are so distinctive that their presence alone can be enough to identify a type, while other traits are more subtle or are identifiable by a composite of common features. Identifying your dominant physical characteristics will narrow your possibilities down to a handful of body types. Step 2 will help you reduce this list even more.

2. **Photo ID.** This step will show you photographs of women and men who represent each body type. The photos illustrate the identifying physical characteristics, while the accompanying text describes other distinguishing features. Often you will know your type for sure at this point. But as you look at the photos, remember that the physical characteristics are guides, not absolutes. Don't rule out a type just because you don't have 100 percent of the possible characteristics. If the photos do not help you zero in on the one type

that is absolutely you, you'll move to the third step of the identification process.

**3. Psychological identity.** In addition to the physical characteristics, certain psychological tendencies are more pronounced in certain body types, and this can help you better define your own body type. The "essence" and "aspects" of each body type will give you psychological information that when added to your physical information will help you come up with your personal body type.

**4. Confirmation.** To confirm which body type is you exactly, you can peek ahead to the psychological profiles in each body type chapter in Part 2. This will give you more information that will definitely nail down your type. Some people are so surprised to find their every move described on these pages that they wonder if I've been riding around in their back pocket for the last twenty years!

## STEP 1: Physical Characteristics

### Identifying Female Body Types

As a woman, your first clue to determining your body type, or dominant gland, is your weight-gain pattern. Where do you gain weight first? What area of your body poses the greatest challenge when you try to lose weight or maintain your figure? Your dominant gland corresponds to this particular area.

### Weight-Gain Pattern

Look at the three photos below. Do you tend to gain weight in your upper body? Entire body? Or lower body?

Once you've identified your weight-gain pattern, you can begin to narrow down the list of possible body types. The following lists tell you which body types are commonly found among each of the three weight-gain patterns.

*Upper Body Weight-Gain Pattern:* Adrenal, Brain, Intestinal, Liver, Pancreas, Skin, or Stomach
*Entire Body Weight-Gain Pattern:* Adrenal, Intestinal, Nervous System, Pituitary, Skin, or Stomach
*Lower Body Weight-Gain Pattern:* The lower body is where most women gain weight, so this group con-

NOTE: You will notice that some body types appear on more than one list. This is because certain types can have more than one weight-gain pattern. While your weight-gain pattern can change during your lifetime, your body type remains the same. The goal is to find the pattern you were born with.

**Upper body gain** refers to the torso, particularly across your back. The first sign is that your bras get too tight or blouses start to gap and won't stay buttoned.

**Entire body gain** is when it's hard to say where you gain—it's all over, with no particular spot especially noticeable. Because your weight gain is so even, you can carry large amounts of weight without it being too apparent.

**Lower body gain** includes the waist, lower abdomen, upper hips, lower hips, buttocks, and thighs. Not all of these areas will necessarily be a problem. You will usually notice weight gain first in either the lower abdomen or buttocks; thighs may or may not be involved.

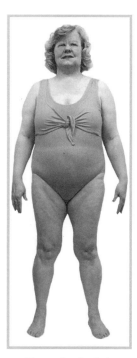
**Upper Body Gain**

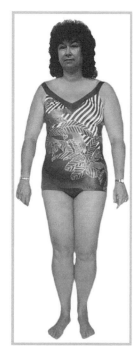
**Entire Body Gain**

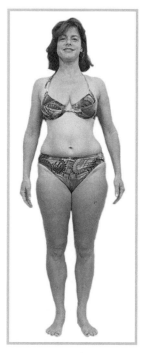
**Lower Body Gain**

tains the greatest number of body types. But this long list can be broken down further by determining exactly where the lower body weight occurs. Use the following photos and descriptions as your guide.

*Time to Jump Ahead* Now it's time to jump ahead to Step 2: Photo ID on page 19 if you find that your weight-gain pattern is in the:

- ▶ Upper body
- ▶ Entire body
- ▶ Lower body in the buttocks and thighs or in the lower abdomen

In the Photo ID section you will see four pictures of each body type along with information about associated personality characteristics, distinguishing physical features, and weight-gain patterns. Examine the photos and facts for each of the body types your weight-gain pattern says you might be. Some women can find their personal body type with great certainty right here, but most still have several possibilities to choose from.

Then it's time to move on to Step 3: Psychological Identity on page 70. Here you can examine the essence and aspect of each of the types you think you might be. This information may be all you need to separate the types and find the one that matches you. However, if you are still uncertain, see Step 4: Confirmation on page 75. This is one more optional step that some people find very helpful in making their final decision.

*Not So Fast—Lower Abdomen and Thighs!* If your weight-gain pattern is in the lower abdomen and thighs, your list of possible body types is still quite long and you need to do a little more narrowing down before you can move to the Photo ID step. Take a look at the shape of your waist and compare it with the photos on page 17. Your waist shape will help you narrow down the list of possible body types to explore in steps 2 and 3.

If your waist is either straight or well defined, you're ready to move on to Step 2: Photo ID, page 19. Look through the pictures and read the captions for each of the suggested body types. If you need a little more information, move to Step 3: Psychological Identity, page 70.

However, if your waist is defined, the list of possible body types is awfully long to use the Photo ID

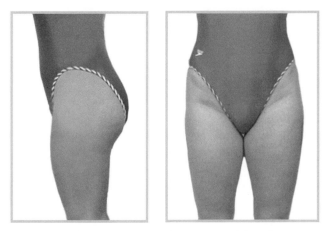

**Buttocks and Thighs:** Balanced, Eye, Gonadal, Kidney, Lymph, Pineal.

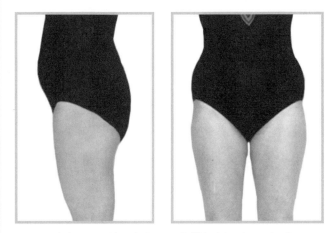

**Lower Abdomen:** Blood, Brain, Gallbladder, Intestinal, Lung, Pancreas.

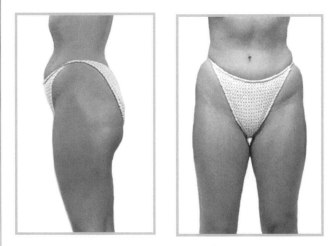

**Lower Abdomen and Thighs:** Adrenal, Balanced, Blood, Eye, Heart, Hypothalamus, Kidney, Lymph, Medulla, Nervous System, Pancreas, Pineal, Skin, Spleen, Stomach, Thalamus, Thymus, Thyroid.

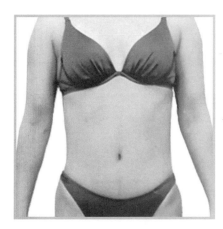

**Straight:** Adrenal, Blood, Eye, Hypothalamus, Medulla, Nervous System, Skin, Stomach, Thymus.

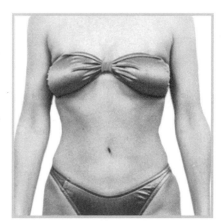

**Defined:** Balanced, Blood, Eye, Heart, Hypothalamus, Kidney, Lymph, Medulla, Nervous System, Pancreas, Pineal, Skin, Spleen, Stomach, Thalamus, Thymus, Thyroid.

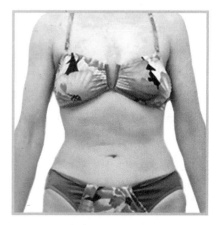

**Well Defined:** Eye, Heart, Kidney, Pancreas, Spleen, Thyroid.

comparison method of step 2. It might be easier for you to jump ahead to Step 3: Psychological Identity on page 70. Reading this information may make it easy for you to cross out types that don't fit who you are. Then, with your shorter list, you can go back to the photos in step 2 and zero in on the body type that best describes you.

## Identifying Male Body Types

For men, body types are distinguished by two main physical characteristics: (1) torso shape and (2) muscle definition. Use the photos and descriptions below to select the torso shape and muscular appearance that most closely resemble your own.

### Torso Shape

The physical characteristics of a man's torso fall within a range, so you may feel you stand between two shapes. Look at your basic shape, regardless of current weight, and select the description that most closely resembles you. If you are not sure, choose average.

### Muscular Appearance

Muscular appearance has nothing to do with muscle tone, or how much you exercise. It has to do with how solid or soft your musculature generally appears to be. Some types have a soft layer of fat under the skin covering the muscle. This minimizes muscle definition, so they look soft regardless of how much they work out.

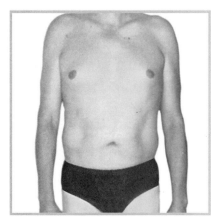

A **thick torso** appears straight. It's easy to put on weight in the chest and across the back.

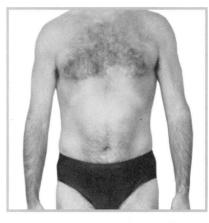

An **average torso** is proportional to the rest of the body. Weight gain tends to be in the abdomen and around the waist.

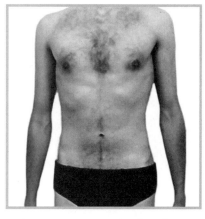

A **thin torso** appears slender. The problem is often one of needing to gain weight rather than lose it.

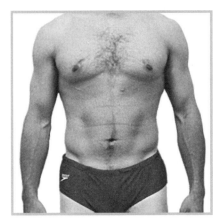

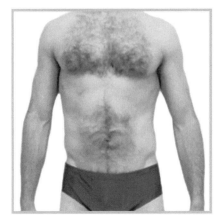

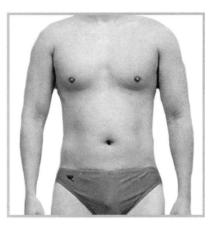

A **well-defined body** looks firm regardless of exercise. It's easy to achieve muscle definition with a basic workout program.

An **average body** responds to exercise and can achieve muscle definition with a basic to advanced program. However, it takes a reasonable amount of time and effort.

A **soft layer body** will have great difficulty achieving muscle definition, no matter how hard this type works out in the gym.

| | Thick Torso | Average Torso | Thin Torso |
|---|---|---|---|
| Well-Defined Body | Adrenal | Adrenal<br>Kidney<br>Lymph<br>Nervous System<br>Thalamus<br>Thymus<br>Thyroid | Kidney<br>Nervous System<br>Thalamus<br>Thymus<br>Thyroid |
| Average Body | Adrenal<br>Brain<br>Heart<br>Hypothalamus<br>Intestinal<br>Pancreas<br>Liver<br>Skin<br>Spleen<br>Stomach | Adrenal<br>Balanced<br>Blood<br>Brain<br>Eye<br>Gonadal<br>Heart<br>Kidney<br>Lung<br>Medulla<br>Nervous System<br>Pineal<br>Pituitary<br>Skin<br>Thalamus<br>Thymus<br>Thyroid | Eye<br>Kidney<br>Nervous System<br>Pineal<br>Thalamus<br>Thymus<br>Thyroid |
| Soft Layer Body | Gallbladder<br>Heart<br>Intestinal<br>Pancreas<br>Skin<br>Spleen | Eye<br>Gallbladder<br>Heart<br>Pituitary | Eye |

## Body Type Matchup

Use the chart on page 18 to match your torso type with your muscle definition type. Where the two meet, you'll find the dominant glands that determine your possible body types.

## Narrowing the Field

You can see from the chart that if you have a well-defined body with a thick torso, you are an Adrenal body type. If you have a soft layer body and a thin torso, you're definitely an Eye body type. In the other cases, however, you have narrowed down the field of 25 to a more manageable group, but you'll need to use Step 2: Photo ID and Step 3: Psychological Identity to find your unique type. If you are in tune with your body and can clearly visualize it, go to the following Photo ID section to look up each possible body type in your category and select the one that best fits you. (Remember that the physical characteristics are guides, not absolutes, so don't rule out a type just because you don't have 100 percent of all the possible characteristics.) If you'd rather, you can skip to Step 3: Psychological Identity on page 70 and narrow down your choices based on the essence and aspects of your personality. Either way, your goal is to find the one body type that best describes you physically and psychologically and that determines the ideal lifestyle and diet for you. If you have narrowed the field, but still are trying to decide between two similar types, you can go to step 4 and compare the psychological profiles.

## STEP 2: Photo ID

The following photos identify the physical characteristics of the 25 male and female body types. The text that accompanies each photo grouping gives you information about personality characteristics, distinguishing features, and weight-gain patterns.

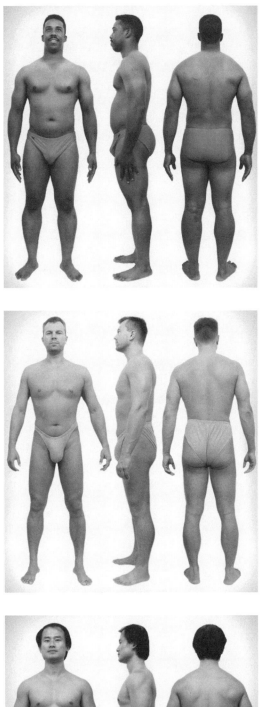

## ADRENAL MALE AND FEMALE

### Physical/Mental

#### Personality Characteristics

Personality tends to be expressed in one of two ways:

- ▸ Distinguished by their high energy, physical strength, and endurance
- ▸ Forceful and dynamic, they easily make their presence known
- ▸ By nature, outgoing, and charismatic
- ▸ Women are often gregarious and vivacious

### Adrenal Male

#### Distinguishing Physical Features

- ▸ Strong, stocky appearance
- ▸ Classic football linebacker
- ▸ Well-defined-to-average, heavy musculature throughout torso, arms, thighs, and calves
- ▸ Wide, sturdy, grounded stance

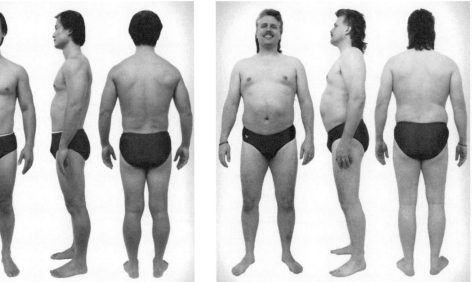

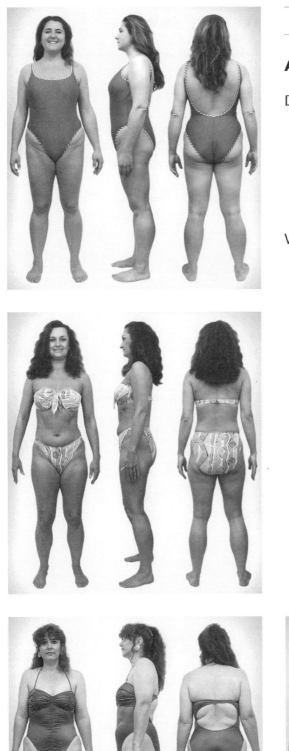

## Adrenal Female

### Distinguishing Physical Features

- ► Boyish figure with straight, poorly defined waist
- ► Dense, solid musculature
- ► Wide, sturdy, grounded stance
- ► Excess weight easy to gain and often fluctuates, according to emotional state

### Weight-Gain Pattern

- ► Initial gain in abdomen; waist; upper, middle, and entire back; upper hips; upper arms; breasts; upper two-thirds to entire thighs; and face
- ► Alternative weight-gain pattern limits: in thighs to upper inner, with predominant gain in upper body

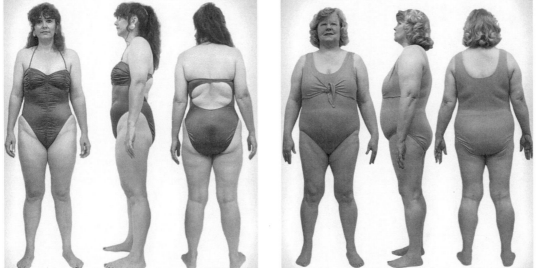

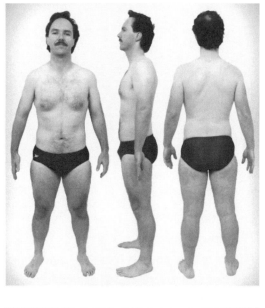

## BALANCED MALE AND FEMALE

### Spiritual/Mental

Personality Characteristics

- ► Precise analytical mind coupled with a gentle demeanor
- ► Balance of work and play essential
- ► Music or creativity an intrinsic part of life
- ► Wide variety of capabilities
- ► Basic nature gentle, playful, and adventurous

### Balanced Male

Distinguishing Physical Features

- ► Often long-waisted, with long torso and short legs, or short torso with long legs
- ► May have wide hips
- ► Height: average to very tall
- ► Physical characteristics show strong secondary gland influence

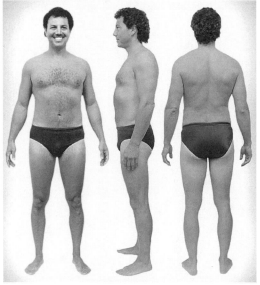

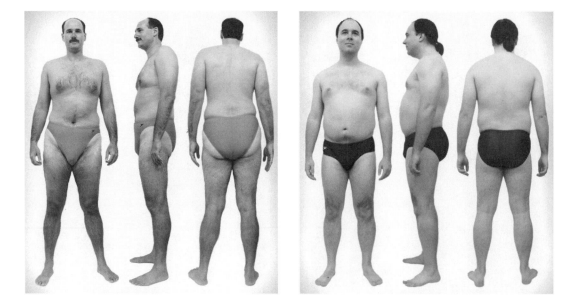

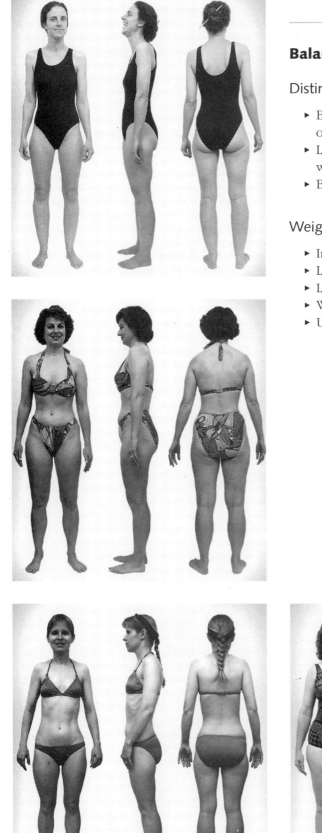

## Balanced Female

### Distinguishing Physical Features

▸ Buttocks somewhat flat, due to blending into upper and outer thighs, creating a rather droopy appearance

▸ Long-waisted with short to average legs, or short-waisted with long legs

▸ Bright, sparkling eyes especially when smiling

### Weight-Gain Pattern

▸ Initial weight gain in entire upper two-thirds of thighs

▸ Lower buttocks

▸ Lower abdomen

▸ Waist

▸ Upper and/or lower hips

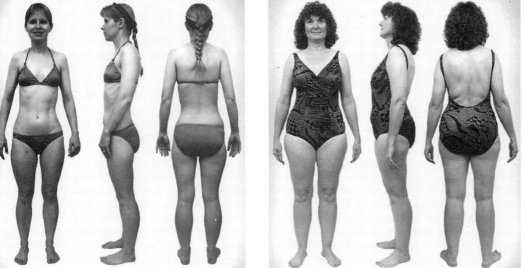

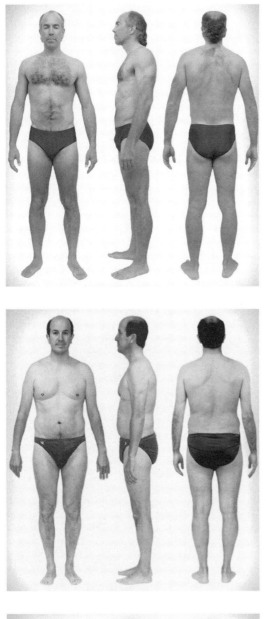

## BLOOD MALE AND FEMALE

### Physical/Emotional

Personality Characteristics

- ▸ Go to great lengths to maintain harmony
- ▸ Social and environmental harmony essential to health and well-being

### Blood Male

Distinguishing Physical Features

- ▸ High forehead, often with receding hairline
- ▸ Average, proportionate torso with average body musculature
- ▸ Height: short to tall
- ▸ May have long arms
- ▸ Buttocks relatively flat to rounded

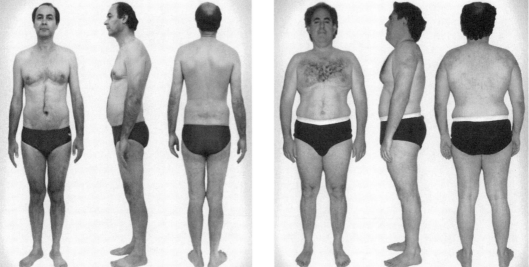

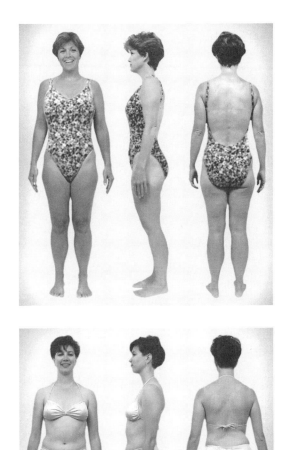

## Blood Female

### Distinguishing Physical Features

▶ Expressive, receptive eyes that immediately draw attention to face
▶ Often have low forehead
▶ Lower back curvature average to swayed
▶ Buttocks relatively flat to rounded
▶ Straight or defined waist, often short-waisted
▶ Average, elongated musculature with little definition

### Weight-Gain Pattern

▶ Initial gain in lower abdomen
▶ Upper hips
▶ Waist
▶ Upper inner to outer two-thirds of thighs

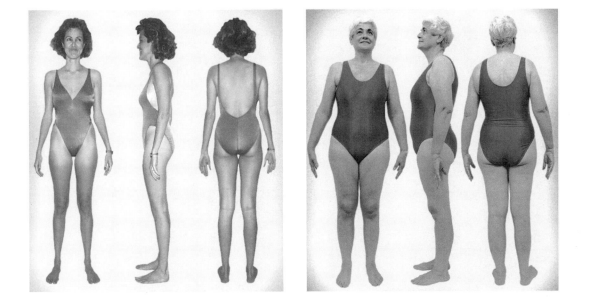

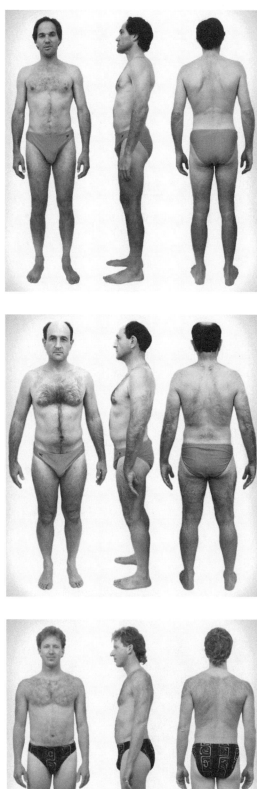

## BRAIN MALE AND FEMALE

### Spiritual/Mental

Personality Characteristics

▸ Known for intensely gathering information
▸ Precise in speech and actions
▸ Strong desire to do things right

### Brain Male

Distinguishing Physical Features

▸ Average, proportionate torso
▸ Average musculature
▸ Dominant forehead, often high
▸ Magnetic face with deep, piercing, or compelling eyes
▸ Height: short to tall
Alternative appearance:
▸ Thick, straight torso with thick, solid musculature

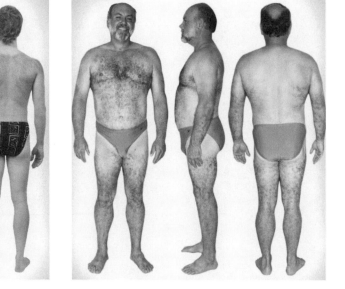

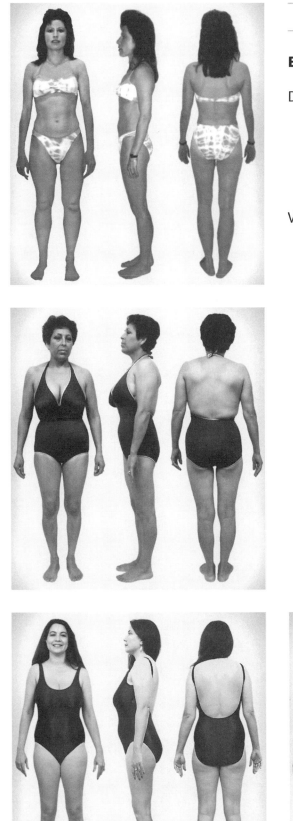

## Brain Female

### Distinguishing Physical Features

- ▶ Dominant forehead, often high
- ▶ Frequently have dominant striking face with piercing or commanding eyes
- ▶ Usually endowed with large breasts

### Weight-Gain Pattern

- ▶ Initial gain in breasts
- ▶ Upper hips
- ▶ Waist
- ▶ Lower abdomen
- ▶ Possibly upper inner thighs
- ▶ May have difficulty gaining or maintaining weight

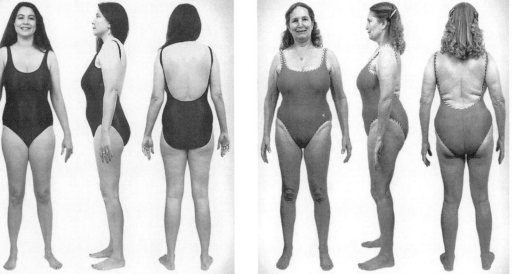

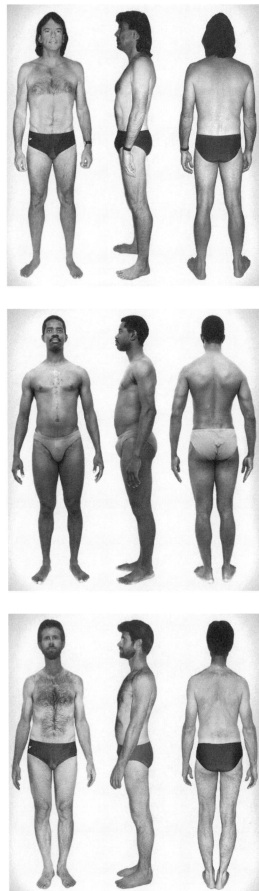

## EYE MALE AND FEMALE

### Spiritual/Mental

Personality Characteristics

- ► Vision is dominant sense and is reflected in excellent eyesight and/or ability to see, recognize, or observe what others don't notice
- ► Visualize what they want to manifest and make it happen

### Eye Male

Distinguishing Physical Features

- ► Eyes dominant or hooded
- ► Layer of fat in upper body, giving a soft appearance (unless extensively exercised)
- ► May have tendency toward bowlegs
- ► Thin to average torso
- ► Musculature average to soft layer

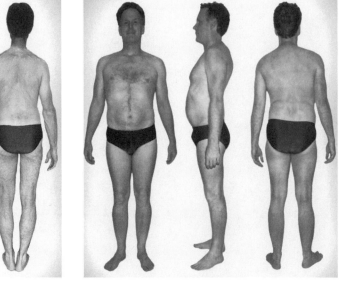

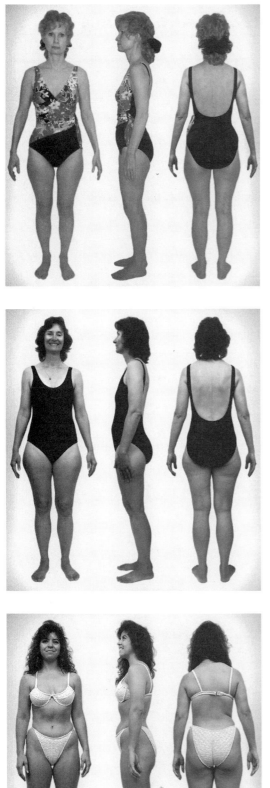

## Eye Female

### Distinguishing Physical Features

- ▶ Characteristic protrusion on upper third of outer thighs
- ▶ Eyes dominant or hooded
- ▶ Body may be at least a full size smaller above the waist than below
- ▶ Often have broad, square palms with short fingers
- ▶ Waist straight to well-defined

### Weight-Gain Pattern

- ▶ Initial gain on upper third of outer thighs
- ▶ Upper inner thighs
- ▶ Lower abdomen
- ▶ Lower buttocks

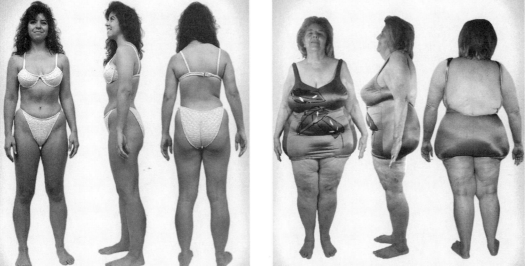

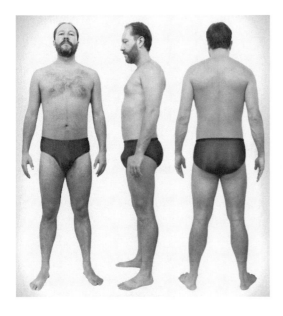

## GALLBLADDER MALE AND FEMALE

### Physical/Emotional

Personality Characteristics

- ► Practical, helpful, down-to-earth
- ► Consistent, reliable, and dependable
- ► Often timid or reserved, preferring to work behind the scenes
- ► Satisfaction comes from making themselves useful to those around them

### Gallbladder Male

Distinguishing Physical Features

- ► Average to thick, strong, stocky torso
- ► Soft layer covering abdomen, making muscle definition there difficult to attain
- ► Buttocks generally rounded
- ► Height: short to average

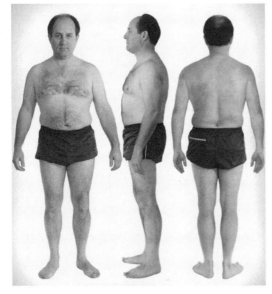

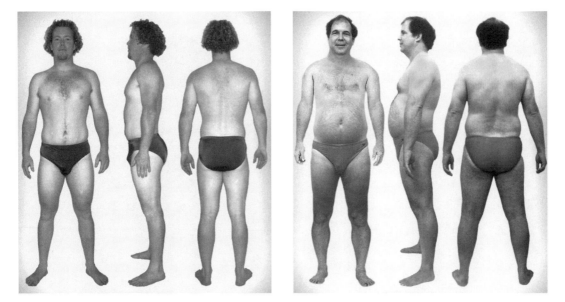

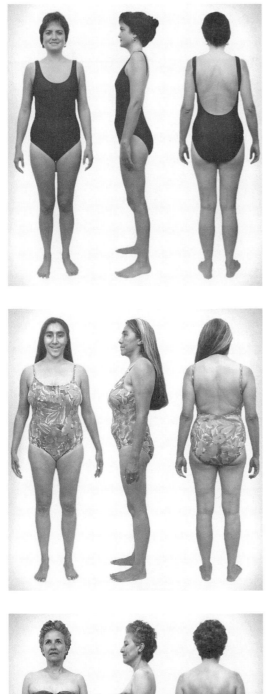

## Gallbladder Female

### Distinguishing Physical Features

▶ Solid torso with most of weight gain in lower abdomen
▶ Slender legs with little or no weight gain in thighs except upper inner
▶ May have small, deep-set eyes

### Weight-Gain Pattern

▶ Initial weight-gain in lower abdomen
▶ Waist
▶ Upper hips
▶ Little or no gain in thighs, legs, lower hips, and buttocks

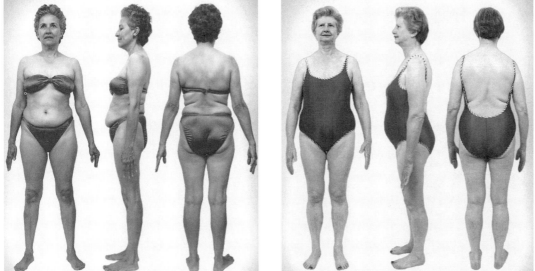

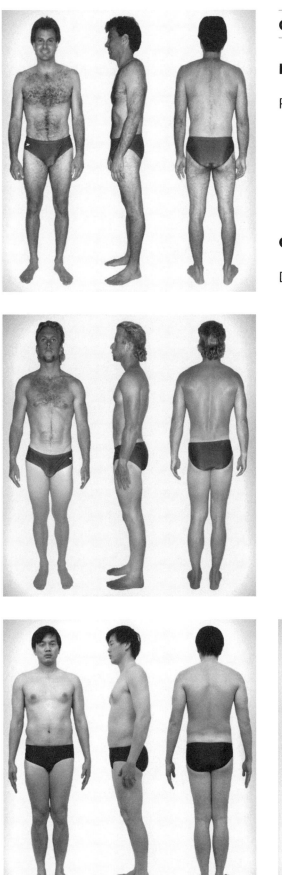

# GONADAL MALE AND FEMALE

## Physical/Emotional

### Personality Characteristics

▶ When stressed, often lose mental clarity and will look for and do "no brainer" jobs
▶ More people- than task-oriented
▶ Thrive on substantial human contact
▶ Generally light and playful

## Gonadal Male

### Distinguishing Physical Features

▶ Typically have swayback with prominent buttocks, although may have straight to average lower back curvature with relatively flat to prominent buttocks
▶ Average body musculature and torso
▶ Well-proportioned body

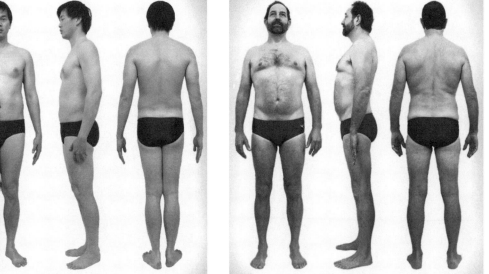

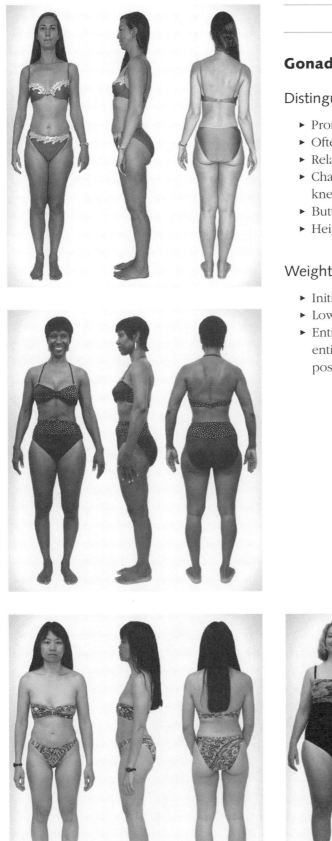

## Gonadal Female

### Distinguishing Physical Features

- ▶ Prominent muscular buttocks
- ▶ Often swaybacked
- ▶ Relatively flat stomach
- ▶ Characteristic muscular thighs that appear developed to the knees
- ▶ Buttocks prominent to rounded
- ▶ Height: petite to average

### Weight-Gain Pattern

- ▶ Initial gain in buttocks
- ▶ Lower hips
- ▶ Entire thighs, with main protrusion on upper outer third and entire inner thighs continuing to knees, inner knees, and possibly waist

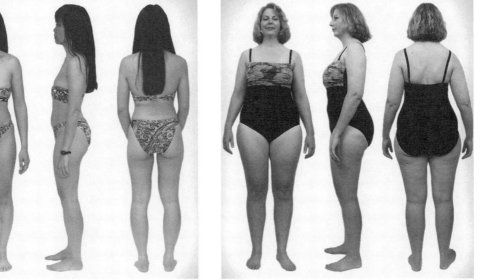

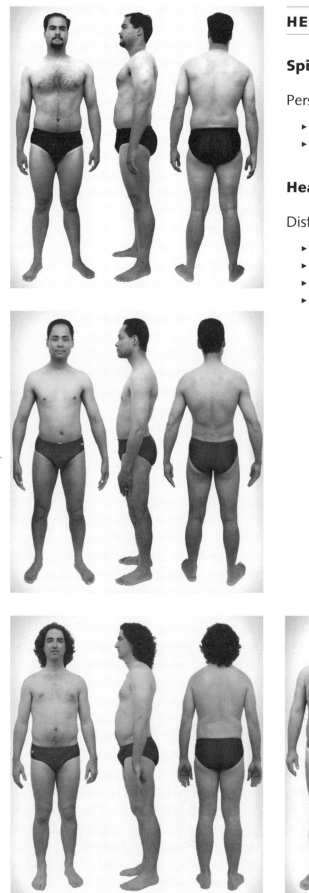

## HEART MALE AND FEMALE

### Spiritual/Emotional

Personality Characteristics

▸ Bring their own rhythm or music to their environment
▸ Readily influence others' moods

### Heart Male

Distinguishing Physical Features

▸ Often remind others of a teddy bear they want to hug
▸ Average, proportionate to thick straight torso
▸ Muscle definition difficult to attain
▸ Height: average to tall

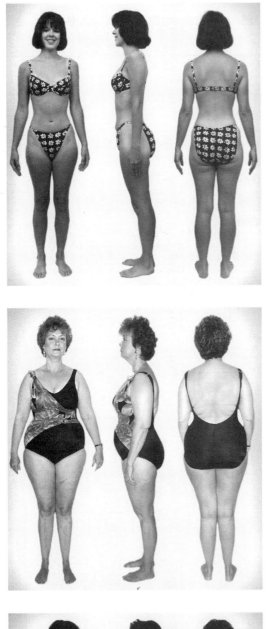

## Heart Female

### Distinguishing Physical Features

- ▶ Soft, round, heart-shaped face
- ▶ Firm, shapely, rounded to prominent buttocks
- ▶ Layer of softness covering muscle, resulting in little definition
- ▶ Often at least a full size smaller above waist than below
- ▶ Height: petite to average

### Weight-Gain Pattern

- ▶ Initial gain in lower abdomen
- ▶ Entire upper two-thirds of thighs, including upper inner thighs, inner knees, waist, middle back, and upper hips
- ▶ Alternative pattern: lower abdomen, lower hips, and thighs

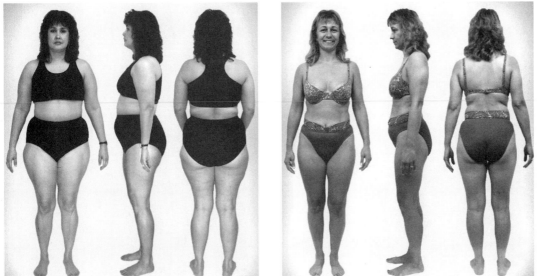

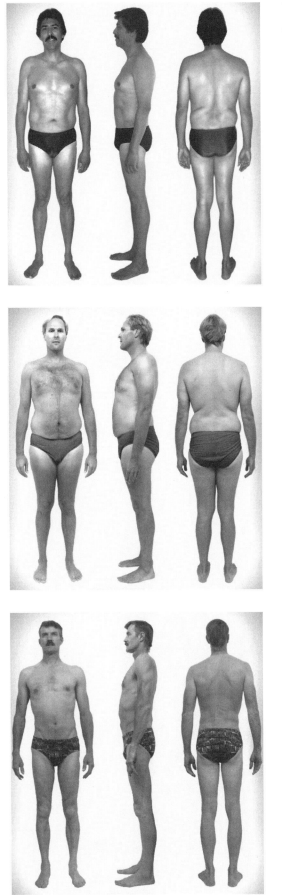

## HYPOTHALAMUS MALE AND FEMALE

### Spiritual/Mental

Personality Characteristics

- ▸ Characterized by extremes
- ▸ Become completely immersed in a project, then transfer all their energy to something else
- ▸ Seem to go through phases

### Hypothalamus Male

Distinguishing Physical Features

- ▸ Dominant chest
- ▸ Thick, straight torso
- ▸ Average, solid musculature
- ▸ Smaller lower body
- ▸ Thin to average thighs and calves
- ▸ Height: average to very tall

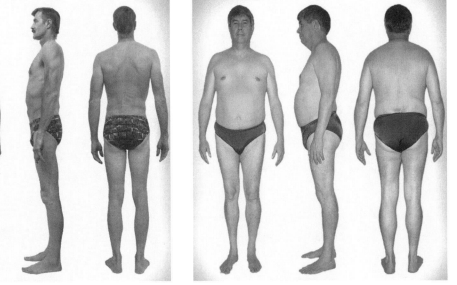

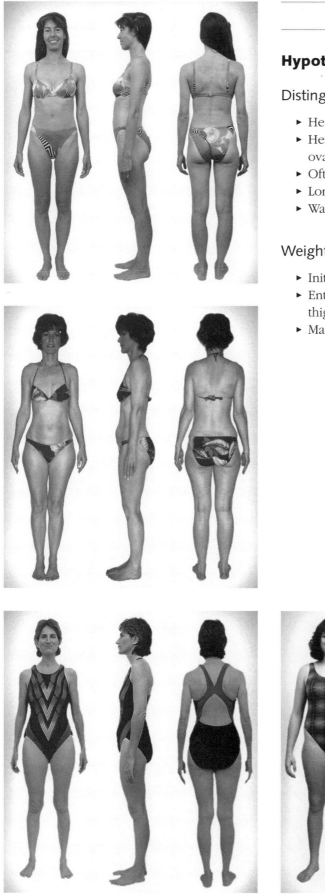

## Hypothalamus Female

### Distinguishing Physical Features

- ► Height: average to very tall
- ► Head small to average, with long, narrow, rectangular, or oval face
- ► Often have wistful, distant look in eyes
- ► Long, slender torso
- ► Waist straight to defined, average to long

### Weight-Gain Pattern

- ► Initial gain in lower abdomen
- ► Entire upper two-thirds of thighs, including upper inner thighs, buttocks, upper hips, and waist
- ► May have difficulty gaining or maintaining weight

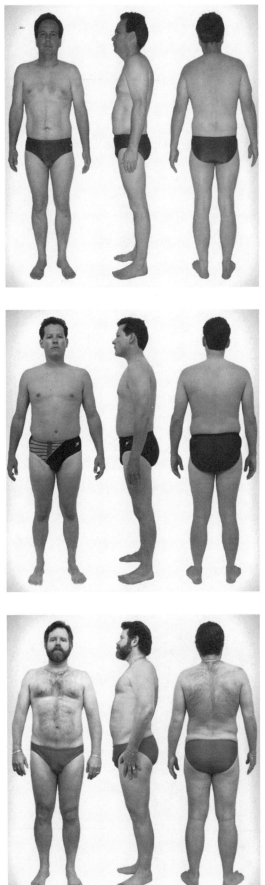

## INTESTINAL MALE AND FEMALE

### Spiritual/Emotional

Personality Characteristics

- ► Emotionally sensitive, but generally don't trust their emotions
- ► Approach life with openness, then let go of what isn't appropriate
- ► Need new experiences to grow mentally, emotionally, or spiritually (or will expand physically)

### Intestinal Male

Distinguishing Physical Features

- ► Thick, straight torso
- ► Soft, spongy layer of fat just beneath skin covers muscle, minimizes muscle definition
- ► Frequently have muscle weakness under chin which eventually results in double chin
- ► Height: average to very tall

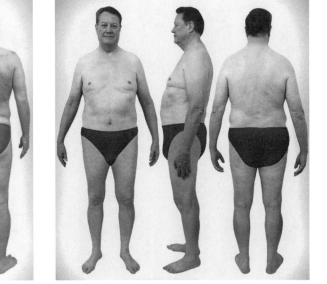

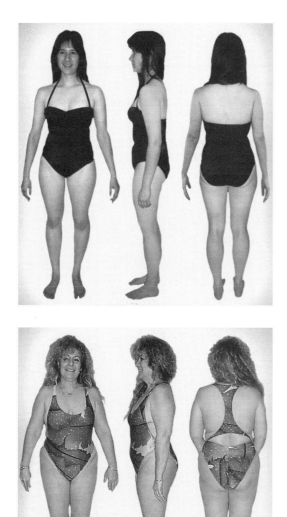

## Intestinal Female

### Distinguishing Physical Features

▶ Solid body with layer of softness covering muscle, reducing muscle definition
▶ Often have muscle weakness under chin that gives rise to double chin
▶ Bone structure small to medium
▶ Height ranges from petite to very tall
▶ Breasts: average to large
▶ Buttocks relatively flat to rounded
▶ Lower back curvature straight to average
▶ Average to short-waisted

### Weight-Gain Pattern

▶ Weight accumulates primarily over intestinal region—more in front than in back of body
▶ Initial gain in lower to entire abdomen
▶ Waist
▶ Upper hips
▶ Inner knees
▶ Entire inner and possibly entire upper two-thirds of thighs
▶ May gain initially in breasts
▶ Capable of carrying large amounts of weight

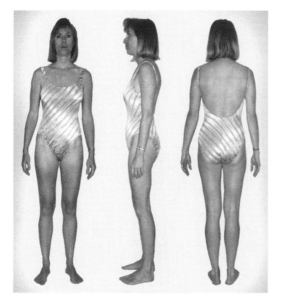

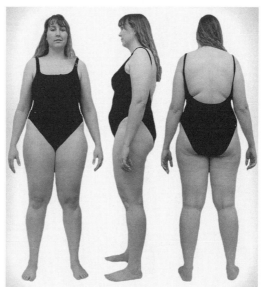

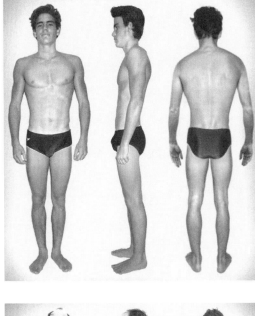

## KIDNEY MALE AND FEMALE

### Physical/Emotional

Personality Characteristics

▸ Tend to procrastinate but force themselves to excel when under pressure of deadlines, time, or performance

### Kidney Male

Distinguishing Physical Features

▸ Typically have markedly broad shoulders and long, slender torso
▸ Long, oval face with V-shaped chin and high forehead
▸ Often striking or energetic eyes
▸ Musculature: average to well-defined
▸ Torso: thin to average
▸ Height: average to tall

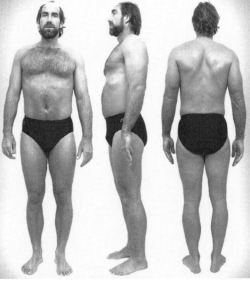

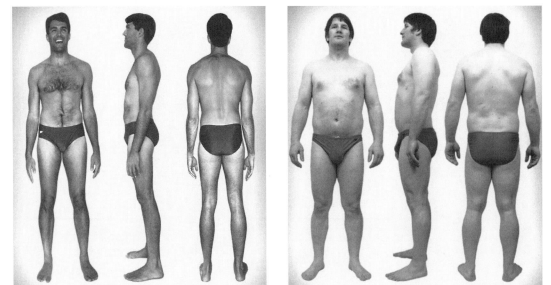

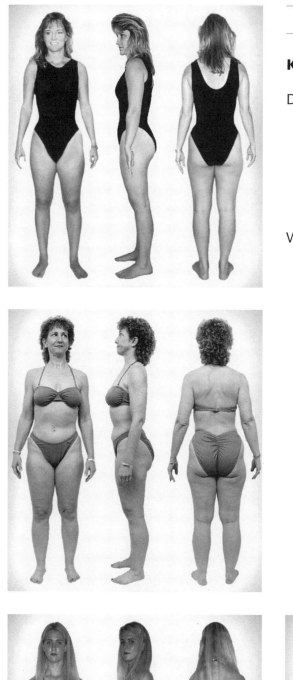

## Kidney Female

### Distinguishing Physical Features

- ▸ Long, oval face with V-shaped chin and high forehead
- ▸ Large, muscular thighs
- ▸ Buttocks rounded to prominent
- ▸ Lower back curvature average to swayed
- ▸ Height: generally petite to average

### Weight-Gain Pattern

- ▸ Initial gain in entire upper two-thirds of thighs, including upper inner thighs, which can extend to knees and inner knees
- ▸ Lower hips, buttocks
- ▸ Minimally, if at all, in abdomen
- ▸ Main weight gain in buttocks and thighs
- ▸ Prone to developing cellulite

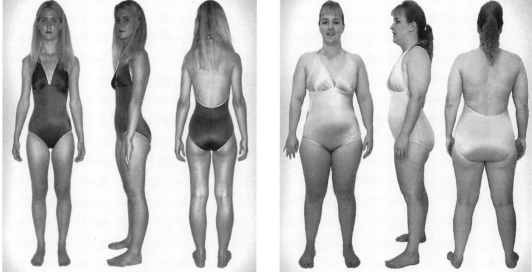

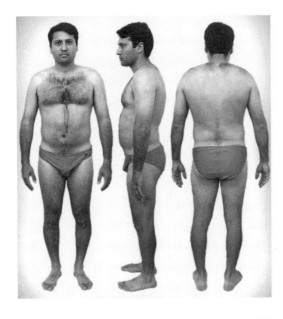

## LIVER MALE AND FEMALE

### Physical/Emotional

Personality Characteristics

- ▶ Exceptionally loyal and family oriented
- ▶ Good teachers
- ▶ Tend to put things together so they flow

### Liver Male

Distinguishing Physical Features

- ▶ Dominant, thick, straight torso
- ▶ Slender legs
- ▶ Relatively flat to rounded buttocks
- ▶ Height: average to very tall
- ▶ Solid, thick, stocky appearance
- ▶ Thick, heavy musculature

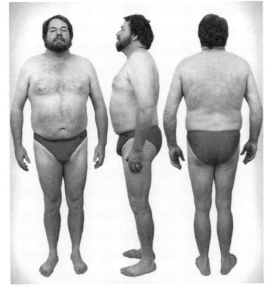

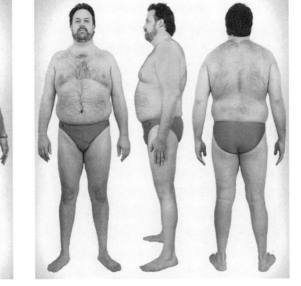

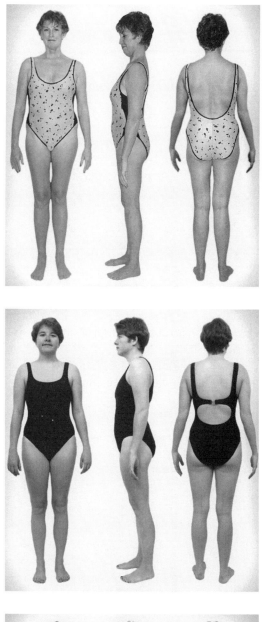

## Liver Female

### Distinguishing Physical Features

- ► Broad, thick torso with little weight gain in thighs
- ► Shoulders relatively even with or broader than hips
- ► Buttocks relatively flat to rounded
- ► Typically smaller lower body with narrow hips
- ► Dense, solid musculature with strong, sturdy appearance
- ► Height: petite to very tall

### Weight-Gain Pattern

- ► Initial gain in lower to entire abdomen
- ► Waist
- ► Upper, middle, and entire back
- ► Upper hips
- ► Upper inner thighs with slight gain in entire upper two-thirds of thighs

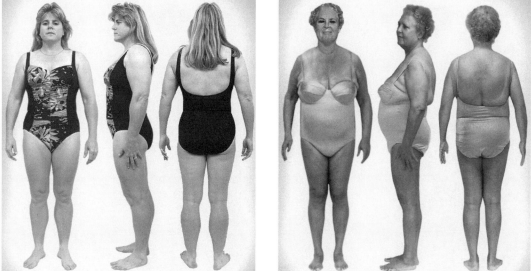

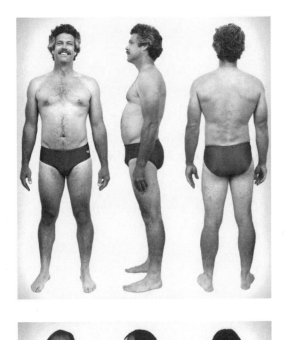

## LUNG MALE AND FEMALE

### Physical/Emotional

Personality Characteristics

- ▶ Mild-mannered
- ▶ Sensitive
- ▶ Strong nurturing qualities
- ▶ Physically creative and artistic, especially in music and dance
- ▶ Good with their hands
- ▶ Emotionally expressive
- ▶ Known for making the most of the moment

### Lung Male

Distinguishing Physical Features

- ▶ Torso appears relatively straight from front yet tapered and more dominant from back
- ▶ Shoulders moderately to markedly broader than hips
- ▶ Tendency to develop a rounded upper back, giving a stooped appearance
- ▶ Average musculature and torso
- ▶ Height: short to tall

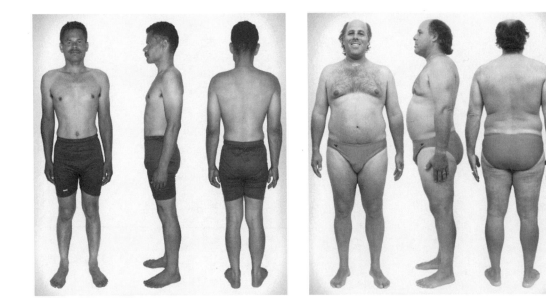

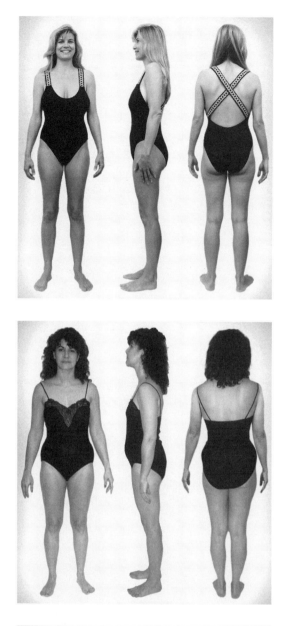

## Lung Female

### Distinguishing Physical Features

- ► High cheekbones with square or V-shaped jaw, often prominent chin; can be average oval or rectangular face
- ► Body may be a full size smaller above the waist than below
- ► Buttocks relatively flat to rounded
- ► Lower back curvature straight to average
- ► Height: petite to average

### Weight-Gain Pattern

- ► Initial gain in lower abdomen
- ► Waist
- ► Upper hips
- ► Slight to no weight gain in thighs

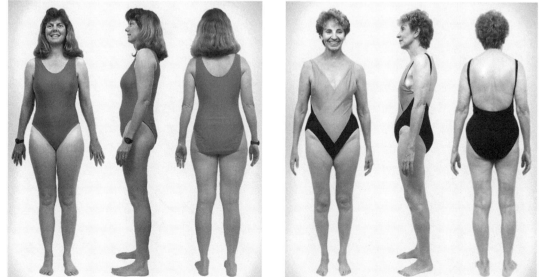

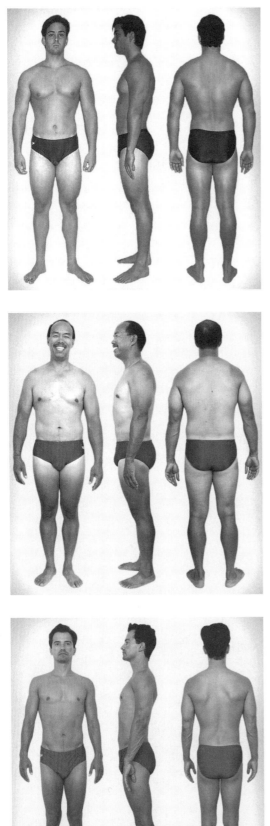

## LYMPH MALE AND FEMALE

### Physical/Mental

Personality Characteristics

- ► Playful, bright, and quick-witted
- ► Thrive on excitement; change, variety, and movement essential to happiness
- ► Physical or mental stimulation prevents stagnation
- ► Strong desire for physical exercise

### Lymph Male

Distinguishing Physical Features

- ► Typically athletic, muscular build
- ► Markedly broad shoulders
- ► Lower back curvature average to swayed
- ► Buttocks rounded to prominent
- ► Average, proportionate torso
- ► Well-defined musculature
- ► Height: average to tall

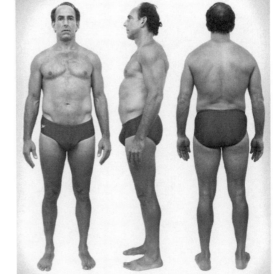

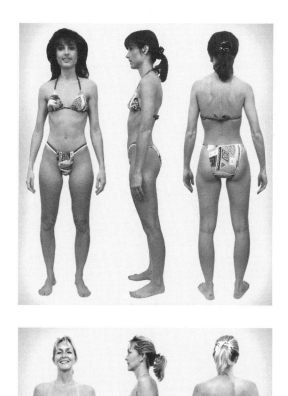

## Lymph Female

### Distinguishing Physical Features

- ▸ Athletic appearance, with broad to even shoulders
- ▸ Well-proportioned, attractive face and body
- ▸ Buttocks round to prominent
- ▸ Lower back curvature average to swayed
- ▸ Height: very petite to average
- ▸ Strong abdominal muscles and thighs
- ▸ Waist straight to defined

### Weight-Gain Pattern

- ▸ Initial gain in entire upper two-thirds of thighs including upper inner thighs
- ▸ Buttocks
- ▸ Possibly upper hips

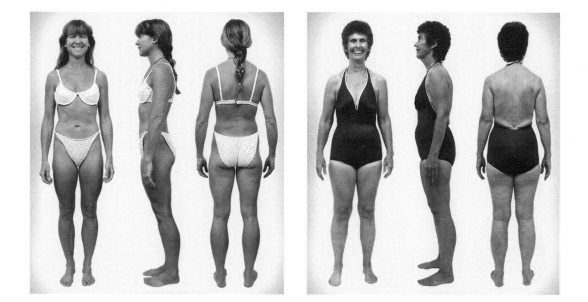

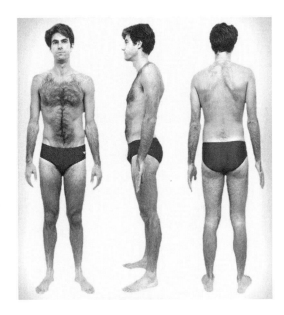

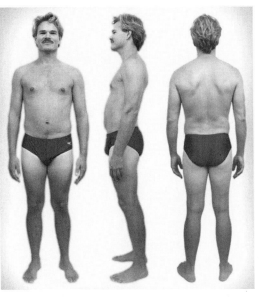

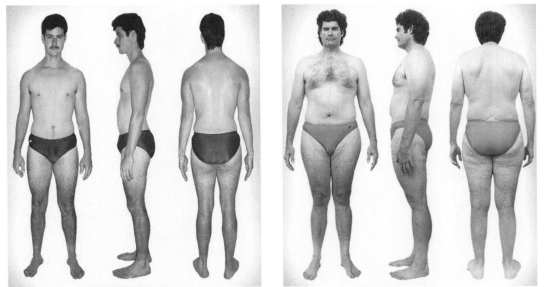

## MEDULLA MALE AND FEMALE

### Physical/Mental

Personality Characteristics

- ► Steady, stable, and persistent
- ► High sense of responsibility and loyalty
- ► Patient teachers
- ► Altruistic, kind, gentle, and helpful

### Medulla Male

Distinguishing Physical Features

- ► Typically low forehead, with heavy eyebrows
- ► Hair generally thick and full
- ► Height: average to tall
- ► Average, proportionate torso with average musculature
- ► May have difficulty gaining or maintaining weight

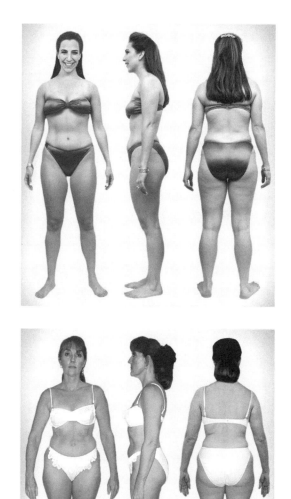

## Medulla Female

### Distinguishing Physical Features

- ▶ Typically low forehead (although can be high)
- ▶ Heavy eyebrows
- ▶ Buttocks relatively flat to rounded
- ▶ Height: average to tall
- ▶ Waist straight to defined
- ▶ Build muscle mass with regular exercise; require sustained exercise to lose weight

### Weight-Gain Pattern

- ▶ Initial gain in lower abdomen
- ▶ Entire upper two-thirds of thighs, including upper inner thighs
- ▶ Upper hips
- ▶ Waist
- ▶ Middle back

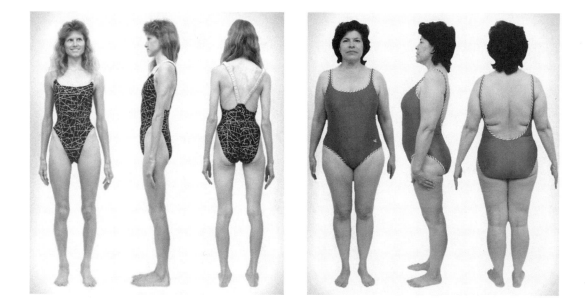

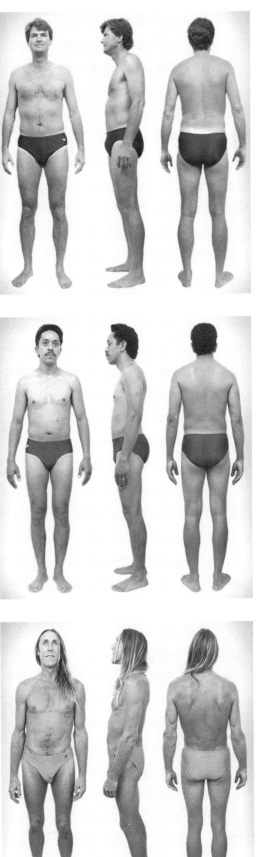

## NERVOUS SYSTEM MALE AND FEMALE

### Physical/Mental

Personality Characteristics

- ► High energy, with excellent stamina and determination
- ► Practical and efficient, with good common sense
- ► Known for accomplishing what they set out to do
- ► Quite verbal; natural communicators
- ► Enjoy introducing and connecting people

### Nervous System Male

Distinguishing Physical Features

- ► Long-limbed appearance, especially in arms
- ► Average, proportionate to long, slender torso
- ► Musculature average to well-defined
- ► Height: average to very tall
- ► Average to long oval or rectangular face
- ► May have difficulty gaining or maintaining weight

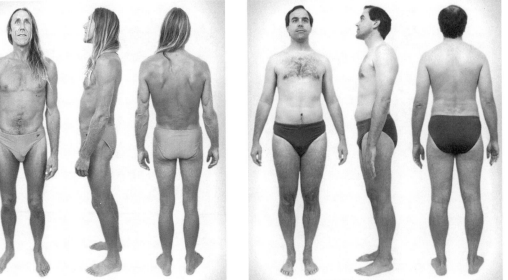

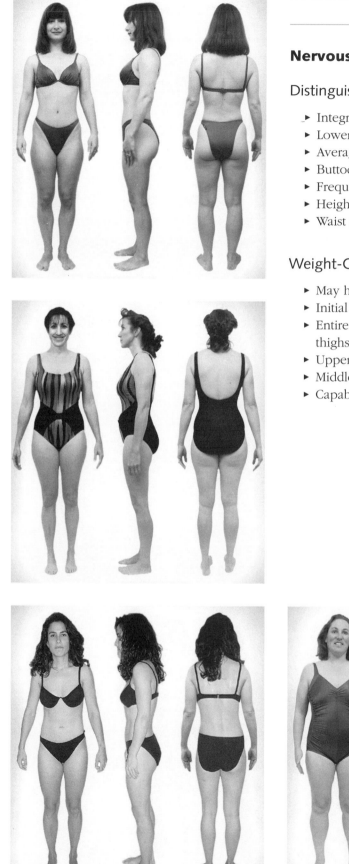

## Nervous System Female

### Distinguishing Physical Features

- ▶ Integrated, strong, solid body
- ▶ Lower back curvature average to swayed
- ▶ Average to large head, often high forehead
- ▶ Buttocks relatively flat to rounded
- ▶ Frequently have square or firm jaw
- ▶ Height: petite to very tall
- ▶ Waist straight to defined

### Weight-Gain Pattern

- ▶ May have difficulty gaining weight
- ▶ Initial gain either all over or in lower abdomen
- ▶ Entire upper two-thirds of thighs, including upper inner thighs
- ▶ Upper hips
- ▶ Middle back and waist
- ▶ Capable of putting on and losing large amounts of weight

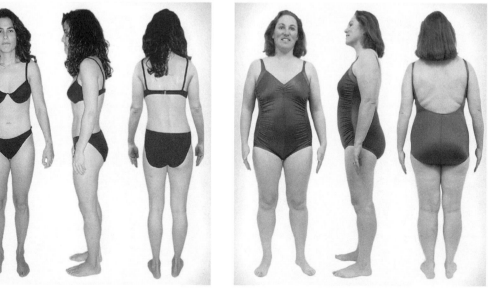

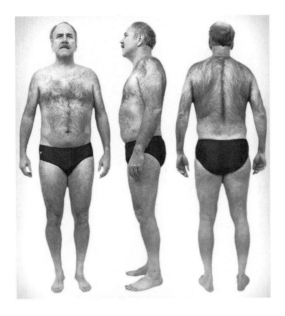

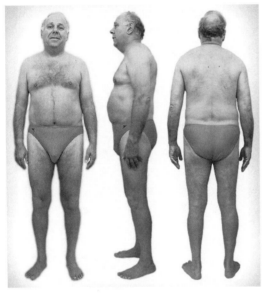

## PANCREAS MALE AND FEMALE

### Physical/Emotional

#### Personality Characteristics

- ► Known for bringing joy
- ► Particularly enjoy social activities centered around food
- ► Tendency toward "rut" eating—eating same foods for three to four days in a row

### Pancreas Male

#### Distinguishing Physical Features

- ► Thick, straight torso
- ► Solid, prominent abdominal paunch
- ► Height: generally average to very tall
- ► Hands can be small, or large with large bone structure
- ► Musculature average to soft layer
- ► Can easily put on large amounts of weight and have great difficulty losing and keeping it off

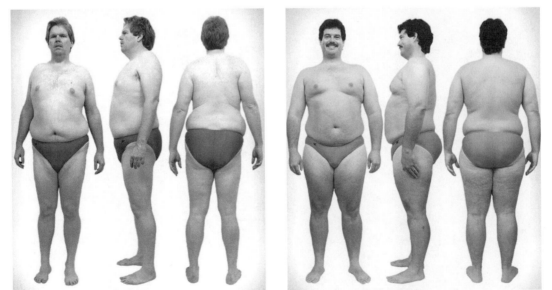

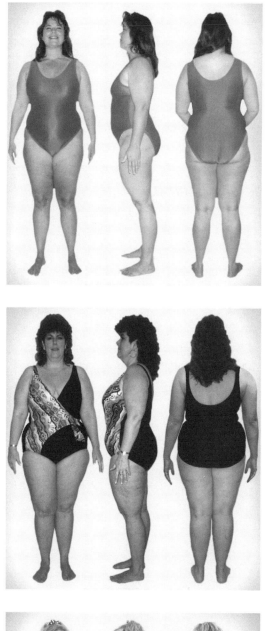

## Pancreas Female

### Distinguishing Physical Features

- ► Small hands and often small feet
- ► Little weight gain from knees to feet or elbows to hands
- ► Waist defined to well-defined
- ► Hair frequently thin or fine
- ► Height: generally petite to average
- ► Predominantly rounded in appearance, particularly noticeable from behind in upper hips and buttocks

### Weight-Gain Pattern

- ► Initial gain in lower abdomen
- ► Upper hips
- ► Upper inner thighs
- ► Inner knees
- ► Middle back
- ► Waist in firm rolls
- ► Excess fat initially firm, not flabby
- ► Can put on large amounts of weight and have difficulty losing and keeping it off

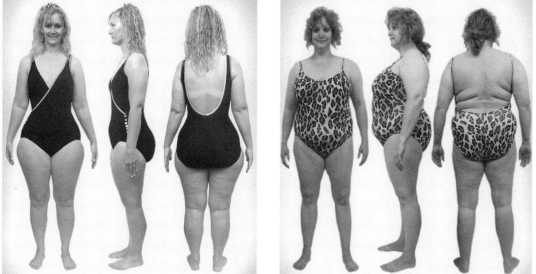

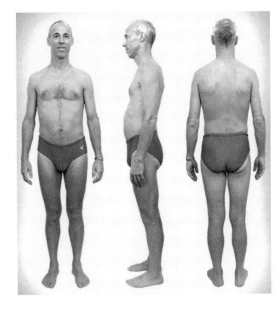

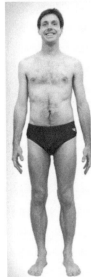

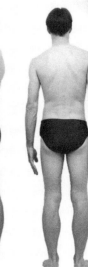

## PINEAL MALE AND FEMALE

### Spiritual/Mental

Personality Characteristics

► Prone to depression, mild to severe, when sunlight is unavailable
► Tend to be highly visual
► Need to know how and why things work, or are as they are
► Known for talking to collect or focus thoughts

### Pineal Male

Distinguishing Physical Features

► Small head in relationship to body
► Long, slender or average proportionate torso
► Average musculature
► Lower back curvature average to swayed
► Often have difficulty gaining or maintaining weight
► Height: ranges from short to very tall

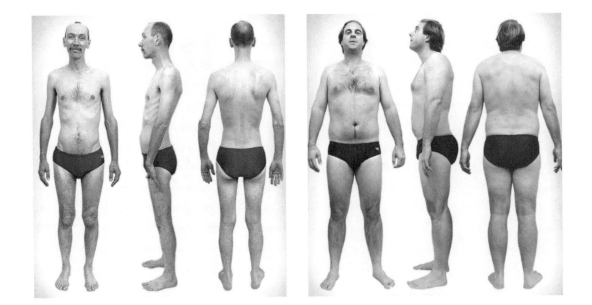

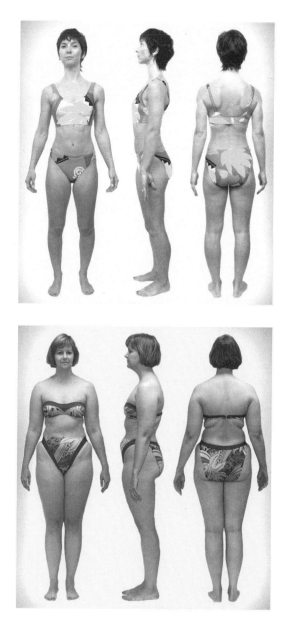

## Pineal Female

### Distinguishing Physical Features

- ▶ Small head in relationship to body
- ▶ Lower back curvature average to swayed
- ▶ Buttocks relatively flat to prominent
- ▶ Height: petite to tall
- ▶ Average to long oval or rectangular face with thin lips
- ▶ May be chronically underweight

### Weight-Gain Pattern

- ▶ Initial gain in lower abdomen
- ▶ Buttocks
- ▶ Waist
- ▶ Upper hips
- ▶ Entire upper two-thirds of thighs, including upper inner thighs

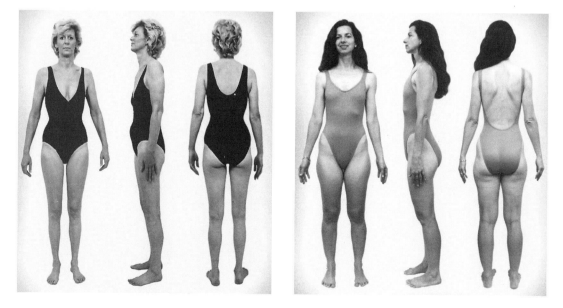

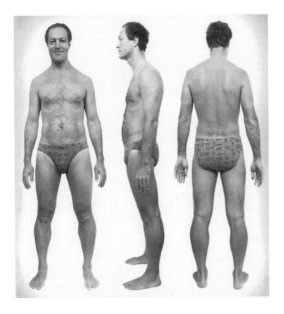

## PITUITARY MALE AND FEMALE

### Spiritual/Mental

Personality Characteristics

- ▸ Tend to make life fun; approach life with childlike openness and innocence
- ▸ Extremely responsible and capable
- ▸ Prefer mental to physical activity
- ▸ Stimulated by new ideas and concepts, which they use to bring happiness

### Pituitary Male

Distinguishing Physical Features

- ▸ Large head in proportion to rest of body, often with high, wide forehead
- ▸ Head usually rests forward of shoulders
- ▸ Average, proportionate torso with average musculature or soft layer
- ▸ Height: short to very tall

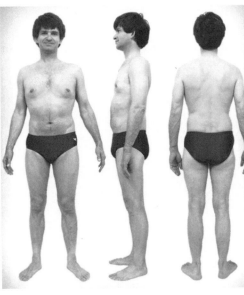

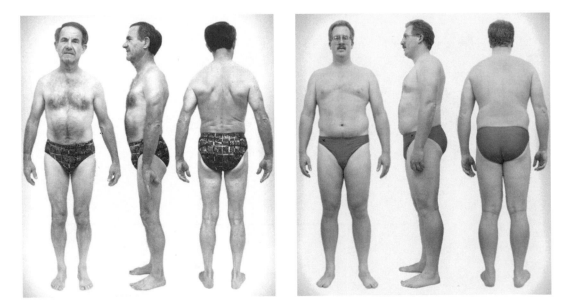

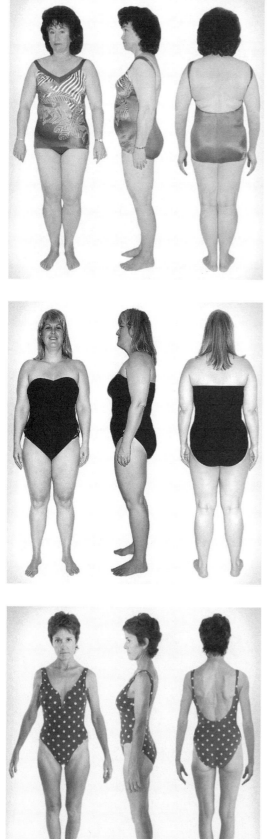

## Pituitary Female

### Distinguishing Physical Features

- ▶ Large head in proportion to rest of body
- ▶ Often high, wide forehead
- ▶ Head generally positioned in front of shoulders
- ▶ Soft, childlike, underdeveloped look
- ▶ Height: petite to tall

### Weight-Gain Pattern

- ▶ Initial gain evenly in soft rolls all over entire body, including hands and feet
- ▶ Waist and lower abdomen
- ▶ Upper hips
- ▶ Upper inner thighs or entire thighs
- ▶ Inner knees
- ▶ Alternative pattern: mostly in abdomen with little gain, if any, in the thighs

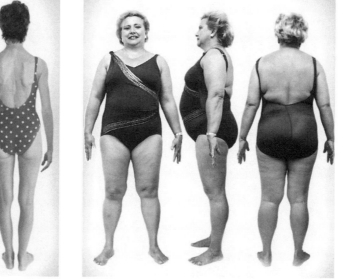

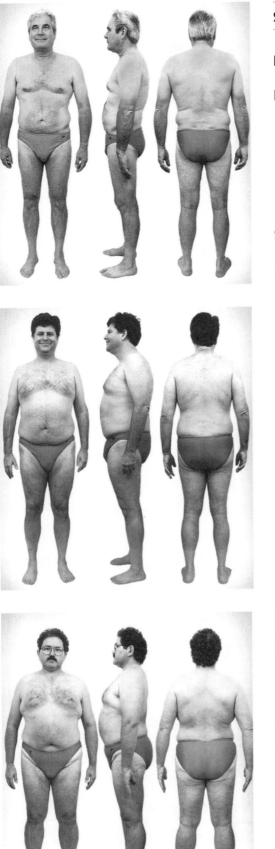

## SKIN MALE AND FEMALE

### Physical/Emotional

Personality Characteristics

- ► Communicate through touch
- ► Extremely sensitive to subtle energies and vibrations
- ► Highly visual
- ► Strong connection with the earth, nature, and animals
- ► Good sense of humor; like to play

### Skin Male

Distinguishing Physical Features

- ► Dominant, thick, straight torso, often with slender legs
- ► Soft layer of fat under skin covering muscle, minimizing muscle definition
- ► Square, flat upper back extending across the shoulders and shoulder blades
- ► Weight carried predominantly in torso in front of body
- ► Height: short to very tall

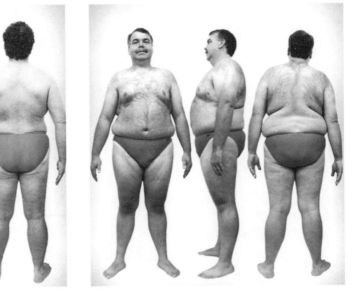

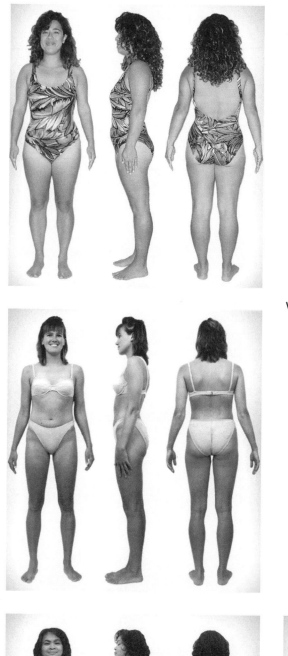

## Skin Female

### Distinguishing Physical Features

- ▶ Soft, gentle appearance
- ▶ Full face, which gets fuller with weight gain
- ▶ Square, flat upper back
- ▶ Straight to defined waist
- ▶ Rounded to prominent buttocks, generally firm and shapely (occasionally flat)
- ▶ Height: very petite (less than 5 feet) to tall
- ▶ Puffiness in hands and feet, so tendons in back of hands are not visible

### Weight-Gain Pattern

- ▶ Initial gain in lower abdomen
- ▶ Upper hips
- ▶ Waist
- ▶ Middle back
- ▶ Face
- ▶ Entire upper two-thirds of thighs, including upper inner thighs

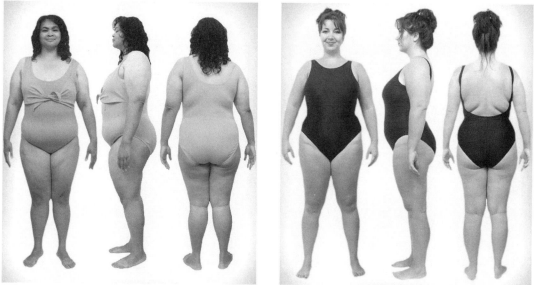

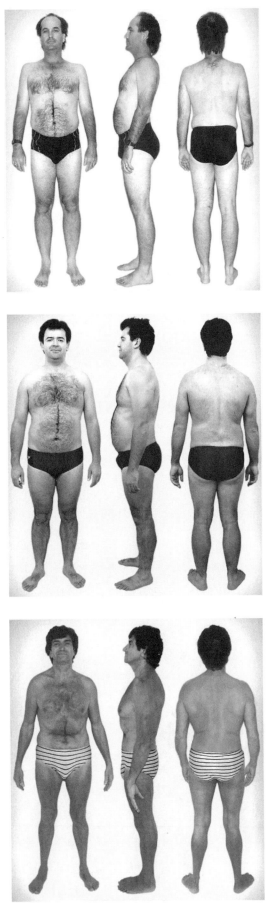

## SPLEEN MALE AND FEMALE

### Physical/Mental

Personality Characteristics

▶ Friendly, down-to-earth personality
▶ Can be intense, tenacious, determined, and strong-willed
▶ Known to make things happen by disseminating energy

### Spleen Male

Distinguishing Physical Features

▶ Striking or distinctive face
▶ Thick, straight torso
▶ Natural lower abdominal protrusion progressing to lower to entire abdominal paunch
▶ Average musculature that may be covered by soft layer of fat, making muscle definition moderate to difficult to attain
▶ Average to muscular thighs and calves

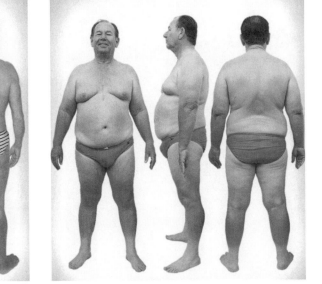

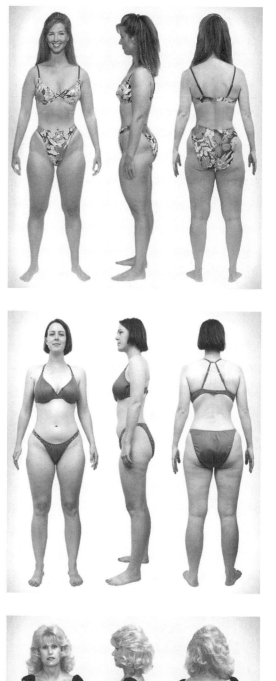

## Spleen Female

### Distinguishing Physical Features

- ▸ Buttocks rounded to prominent
- ▸ Lower back curvature straight to swayed
- ▸ Solid body with wide hips
- ▸ Height: petite to tall
- ▸ Hands small to average, often with short fingers
- ▸ Lower body often full size larger than upper body

### Weight-Gain Pattern

- ▸ Initial gain in lower abdomen
- ▸ Entire upper two-thirds of thighs, including upper inner thighs
- ▸ Buttocks
- ▸ Upper and lower hips
- ▸ Waist
- ▸ Middle back
- ▸ Often carry bulk of weight and cellulite in legs, which can appear chunky

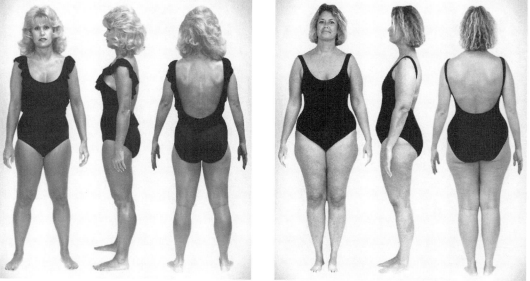

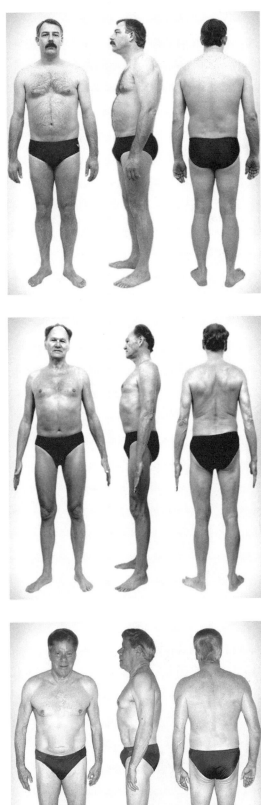

## STOMACH MALE AND FEMALE

### Physical/Mental

Personality Characteristics

- ▸ Passion and their intense mental focus enable them to accomplish their goals
- ▸ Exceptional ability to come in and take charge
- ▸ Give those they focus on the feeling of being embraced

### Stomach Male

Distinguishing Physical Features

- ▸ Dominant, thick, straight torso
- ▸ Slender legs
- ▸ Smaller lower body
- ▸ Average musculature
- ▸ Natural upper abdominal protrusion at breastbone that develops into upper to entire abdominal paunch or thick, heavy abdominal musculature
- ▸ Average to long oval head with thin to average lips
- ▸ Often have large or characteristic nose

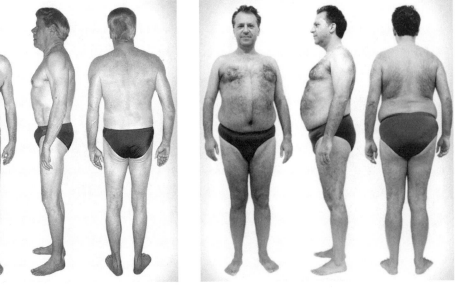

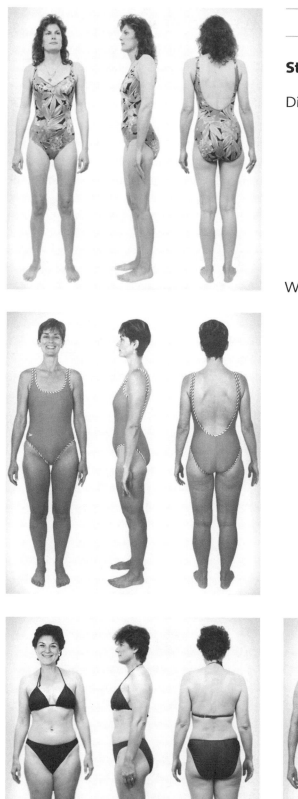

## Stomach Female

### Distinguishing Physical Features

- ▶ Average to large dominant striking head and face with prominent chin
- ▶ Characteristic head posture is lifting chin and tilting head backward
- ▶ Buttocks relatively flat to rounded
- ▶ Strong body with good stamina
- ▶ Waist straight to defined
- ▶ Height: petite to tall

### Weight-Gain Pattern

- ▶ Initial gain in lower abdomen
- ▶ Waist
- ▶ Upper hips
- ▶ Upper back under arms to middle back
- ▶ Entire upper two-thirds of thighs, including upper inner thighs
- ▶ Alternative pattern: upper to entire abdomen, upper hips, waist, and possibly breasts

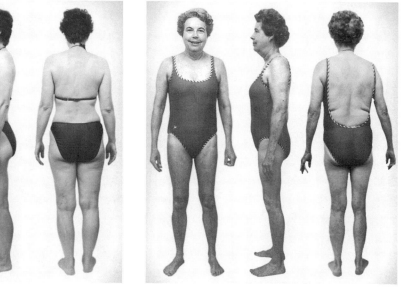

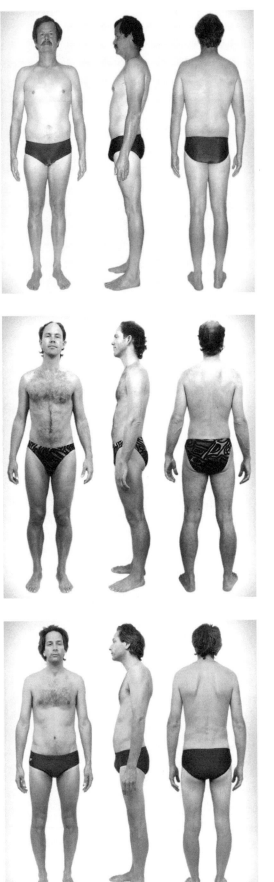

## THALAMUS MALE AND FEMALE

### Spiritual/Mental

Personality Characteristics

- ▸ Energy focus is predominantly in head
- ▸ Noted for collecting and evaluating information
- ▸ May have protruding ears as a child
- ▸ Music is essential, as it provides a direct link to their emotions

### Thalamus Male

Distinguishing Physical Features

- ▸ High, wide, and/or dominant forehead
- ▸ Long, slender oval or long to average rectangular face, often with small eyes
- ▸ Usually slender appearance, with long, proportionate, slender to average torso
- ▸ Continuous arching abdominal musculature with lower abdominal protrusion
- ▸ Lower back curvature average to swayed
- ▸ Height: average to very tall
- ▸ Buttocks relatively flat to rounded

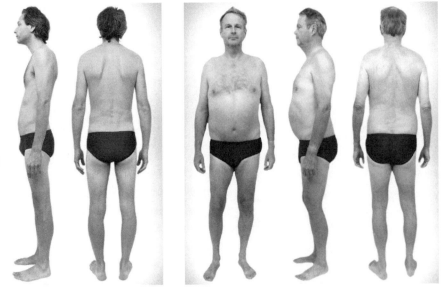

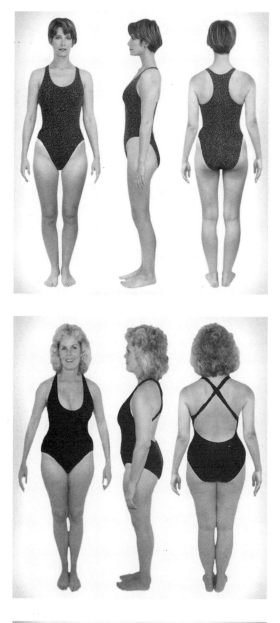

## Thalamus Female

### Distinguishing Physical Features

- ▶ High, wide, and/or dominant forehead
- ▶ Long, slender oval face or long to average rectangular face
- ▶ Continuous arching abdominal musculature with lower abdominal protrusion
- ▶ Typically slender, delicate appearance
- ▶ Lower back curvature average to swayed
- ▶ Buttocks relatively flat to rounded

### Weight-Gain Pattern

- ▶ Initial gain in lower abdomen
- ▶ Face
- ▶ Entire upper two-thirds of thighs, including upper inner thighs and upper hips
- ▶ May have difficulty gaining or maintaining weight

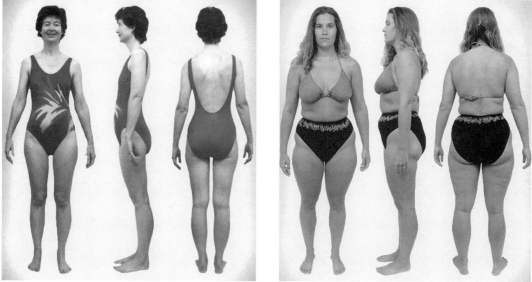

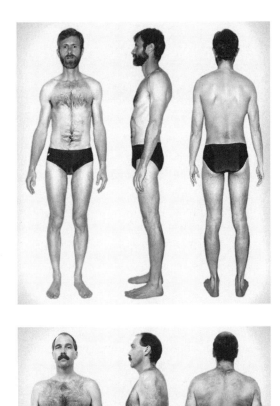

## THYMUS MALE AND FEMALE

### Physical/Mental

Personality Characteristics

▸ Strong sense of responsibility and loyalty
▸ Forceful presence
▸ Able to bring stability to their environment
▸ Well-meaning, take-charge demeanor (sometimes perceived as controlling)

### Thymus Male

Distinguishing Physical Features

▸ Tall to very tall, generally 5 feet 11 inches or taller
▸ Generally lanky
▸ Long, slender torso with long limbs
▸ Muscle definition in torso; moderate to easy to maintain

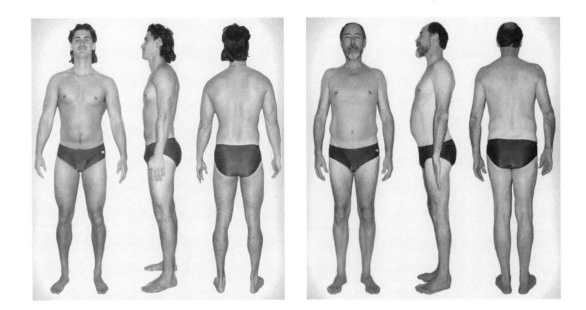

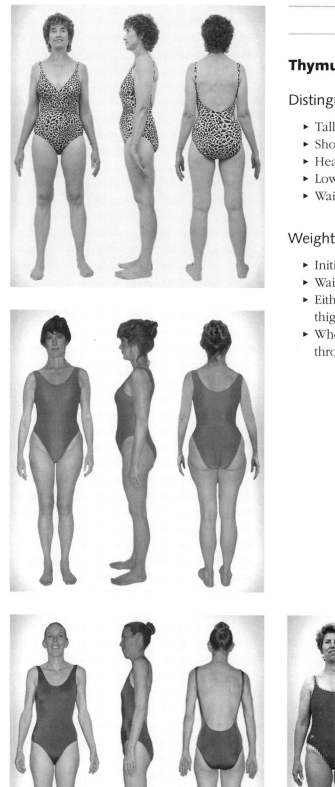

## Thymus Female

### Distinguishing Physical Features

- ▸ Tall to very tall with long-limbed appearance
- ▸ Shoulders relatively even with hips
- ▸ Head may appear small
- ▸ Lower back curvature straight to average
- ▸ Waist straight to defined

### Weight-Gain Pattern

- ▸ Initial gain in lower abdomen
- ▸ Waist and possibly upper hips
- ▸ Either entire upper two-thirds of thighs or only upper inner thighs
- ▸ When at ideal weight, generally have stable weight pattern throughout life

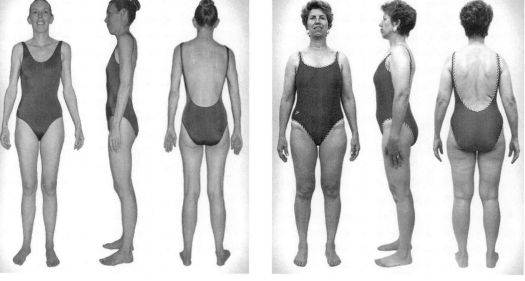

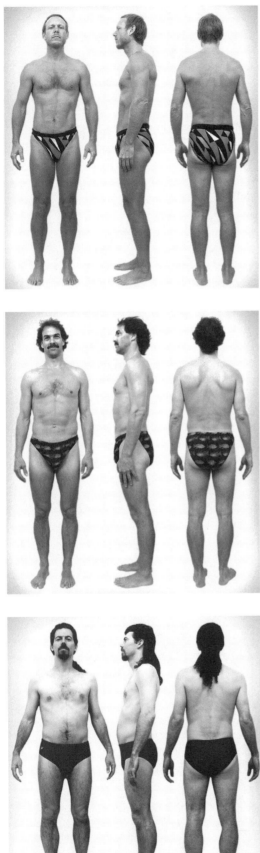

## THYROID MALE AND FEMALE

### Spiritual/Mental

Personality Characteristics

- ▸ Eyes reveal brightness and sensitivity
- ▸ Known for being able to see what needs to be done and getting it done
- ▸ Good at formulating and adjusting theories

### Thyroid Male

Distinguishing Physical Features

- ▸ Forehead high and full or slanted posteriorly
- ▸ Average, proportionate, or long, slender torso
- ▸ Musculature average to well-defined
- ▸ Often slight or slender build with small to average hands and narrow feet
- ▸ May have difficulty gaining or maintaining weight

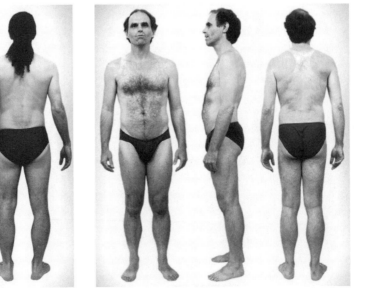

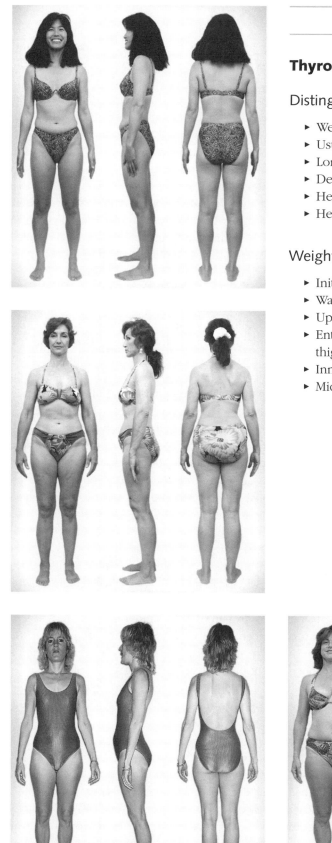

## Thyroid Female

### Distinguishing Physical Features

- ▸ Well-proportioned body, often delicate in appearance
- ▸ Usually delicate or slender hands
- ▸ Long, tapered fingers and narrow feet
- ▸ Defined to well-defined waist
- ▸ Height: petite to tall
- ▸ Healthy, abundant hair

### Weight-Gain Pattern

- ▸ Initial gain in lower abdomen
- ▸ Waist
- ▸ Upper hips
- ▸ Entire upper two-thirds of thighs, including upper inner thighs
- ▸ Inner knees
- ▸ Middle back

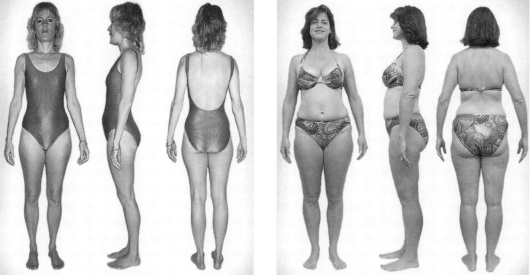

## STEP 3: Psychological Identity

This third step ties distinct psychological characteristics into the body type identification process. The following information about the essence and the aspects of your psyche will confirm the body type you have selected based on your physical characteristics.

### Identifying Your Essence

The *essence* embodies the basic nature of each body type. It ties the dominant gland to certain personality traits. The essence of each type is described below; read through the ones that pertain to the body types your physical characteristics and the photos point you toward for further confirmation of your body type.

### Adrenal Essence

Just as the adrenal glands are the strongest glands in the body, Adrenal body types are distinguished by their high energy, physical strength, and endurance. This dominant physical energy is reflected in their heavy, solid musculature, commanding presence, and physical comfort in the world. They are by nature outgoing, often charming and charismatic.

### Balanced Essence

The Balanced body type is not controlled by any single gland, organ, or system but is dependent upon everything working together synergistically. Balanced body types need balance in their world—balance between work and play, physical and spiritual expression, mental and emotional states, and personal and business relationships. Essentially playful and adventurous, they embody the synergy that brings about balance.

### Blood Essence

Just as the blood maintains harmony throughout the body by carrying oxygen and nutrients to all parts, Blood body types need to maintain harmony. Easygoing and personable, Blood types are social beings whose basic nature is warm, receptive, and nurturing. The slightest bit of disharmony, such as a minor misunderstanding, can have adverse effects on Blood types, physically as well as emotionally. They are noted for going to great lengths to maintain social and environmental harmony. Their strength lies in their ability to make others aware of the effect that disharmony has on people and on the earth.

### Brain Essence

Just as the brain is the information storage center of the body, Brain body types collect and store data. Brain types are noted for intensely gathering information in detail, as they like to have all possible knowledge on a subject before making a decision. Brain types know the value of doing everything right. This desire to do everything right leads them to be very precise in their speech and actions.

### Eye Essence

Just as our eyes link us to our outer world and environment and provide a window to our soul, Eye body types link their inner and outer worlds through implementing visions. They visualize what they want to manifest and then set out to make it happen.

### Gallbladder Essence

Just as the gallbladder can be depended upon to store bile manufactured by the liver (which is essential for the breakdown of fats) and release it as needed, the Gallbladder body type is dependable. Known for being helpful, loyal, and consistent, Gallbladder types create a steady, stable environment. They prefer to work behind the scenes, doing the jobs that are essential to keeping a home or business running. Their quiet, steady strength is often expressed in what appears to be a timid or shy nature. They are exceptionally reliable and loyal and feel most fulfilled when they are being useful.

### Gonadal Essence

Just as the gonads are a pleasure center in the body, the nature of Gonadal body types is to create pleasure and to be playful. However, Gonadal types are prone to being controlled by their emotions. Difficulty focusing or concentrating is typical when they are tired or stressed. To compensate, Gonadal types do no-brainer jobs like shopping, weeding the garden, or other routine tasks. Playtime or time to completely relax is essential, as it allows them to reconnect with their essence.

### Heart Essence

Just as the heartbeat regulates the flow of the blood throughout the body, Heart body types regulate the beat of their environment. Heart types can walk into a room and create either harmony or discord within a group. Their approach can be quite subtle, especially when they are in a new environment—first getting in step with what is going on, and then deciding whether to shift it. Being able to set the beat, they have the natural ability to influence the moods of those around them. Physically softer than most other types, they impress others as being sweet and lovable. Women are often round and heart-shaped, while men and boys are huggable like teddy bears.

## Hypothalamus Essence

Just as the hypothalamus gland is responsible for the involuntary functions necessary for life (regulating the heartbeat, body temperature, blood pressure, metabolism, and blood-sugar levels, as well as the pituitary gland, for example), Hypothalamus body types have an intense sense of responsibility for their behavior. They seem to be intuitively aware of the significance of their actions and have a need for accuracy in all they do. Consequently they approach life with a certain caution. They generally gather all the necessary tools, study the directions, and formulate a plan before starting a project.

## Intestinal Essence

Just as the intestines openly accept everything that comes in and then discern which nutrients to keep and which to release as waste, Intestinal body types are discerning. They approach life with an openness, taking everything in and then letting go of what isn't appropriate. This often leads to a thorough analysis of everything new and a prejudice ("to prejudge") against anything similar to something already analyzed in the past. While their initial response to life is emotional, they generally don't trust their emotions, so they gather as much information as possible to make a logical decision. New experiences are vital: if personal expansion doesn't occur mentally, emotionally, or spiritually, Intestinal types will expand physically.

## Kidney Essence

Just as the kidneys regulate body fluid levels and are responsive to arterial pressure, Kidney body types rise to the occasion when under pressure. They respond and function best when they are needed, particularly if under time or performance pressure. If sufficient outside pressure doesn't exist, they will create it, procrastinating until they get behind in their projects to the point of discomfort, which forces them to excel and move beyond their previous limits. Fearful by nature, their success in meeting challenges builds confidence and prepares them for their next experience, allowing them to move further than they had ever dreamed.

## Liver Essence

Just as the liver is in charge of converting nutritional substances into usable forms and filtering out what can't be used, Liver body types are noted for putting pieces together and fitting them into the flow of the day or project. Placing a high priority on family, loyalty, and stability, they excel at helping with whatever needs to be done. They create the desire that, when coupled with their tremendous physical strength, results in accomplishment. Teaching, often through leadership, is their way of ensuring that the knowledge gained by one generation can flow to the next.

## Lung Essence

Just as the lungs supply the oxygen needed for life, Lung body types give life to their world by expressing positive, supportive emotions. Nurturing and creative, their strength lies in being able to shift emotional energy; they can, for example, change hurt into creativity. This allows Lung types to express the energy of negative emotions in a safe, constructive, or positive manner. By respecting emotions and using them as an indicator rather than a response, Lung types can use their emotions to move into a greater richness and fullness of life, which is what enables them to excel at making the most of each moment.

## Lymph Essence

Just as the lymphatic system requires stimulation to move the waste away from the tissues, the Lymph body type needs continual stimulation in the form of movement and change. It's this constant movement that adds variety to life. Lymph types require a lot of variety through physical activity or mental stimulation to maintain mental clarity and a sense of vitality. Fun loving and playful, they are happiest when they feel excitement, and activity allows them to feel vibrant and alive. Consequently, stimulation, either mental or physical, is essential.

## Medulla Essence

Just as the medulla in the brain stem is responsible for controlling respiration and heart rate, functions that require steady perseverance, Medulla body types are known for their consistency and persistence. Undaunted by time or trends, Medulla types are unwavering in their activities and beliefs, staying with what they choose to be doing with unusual resolve. With an abundance of patience, Medulla types possess an intense sense of responsibility and remain loyal indefinitely, especially when they have identified with a group or cause. It's their high sense of responsibility that makes them patient teachers, and the appreciation of their students, patients, or clients makes it all worthwhile.

### Nervous System Essence

Just as the nervous system connects all parts of the body and keeps the brain informed of what is happening, Nervous System body types enjoy listening to others and connecting people according to their needs, desires, or interests. Practical and efficient, they are happiest when they are connecting people and ideas. Nervous System types tend to have an abundance of nervous energy and manifest it through a myriad of activities. For Nervous System types, listening to others is an adventure.

### Pancreas Essence

Just as the pancreas releases energy by breaking down carbohydrates or sugars, Pancreas body types release energy through their sense of joy. They love socializing, especially around food, and are usually the life of a party. Conscientious and reliable, Pancreas types can be quite dynamic when their energy is channeled into a particular area. They are the ones who continually release the energy that keeps an organization running. With their genuine concern for people and their ability to use laughter to burst out of the most uncomfortable situations, they are known for bringing joy to their environment.

### Pineal Essence

Just as the pineal gland is sensitive to light and regulates the sleep cycle, Pineal body types listen to their intuition. The pineal gland is derived from a third eye that begins to develop early in the embryo and later degenerates. Similarly, our intuition is present early in life but is too often later suppressed. Pineal types tend to retain their intuition longer and more strongly than most types. Generally sensitive on all levels, they must learn to listen to their intuition accurately and balance it with their mental acuity. Being highly susceptible to a barrage of internal information, they use talking as a way of focusing and as a means of sorting out what is most appropriate.

### Pituitary Essence

Just as the pituitary gland controls hormones necessary for a child's growth, Pituitary body types manifest the childhood quality of making life fun. They approach life with a childlike openness and wide-eyed innocence that makes them fun to be around. As the master gland in charge of directing the entire body, the pituitary gland has to be extremely responsible. Likewise, Pituitary types are naturally capable, responsible people. Lighthearted and creative, they are stimulated by new ideas and concepts, which they use to bring happiness.

### Skin Essence

Just as the skin communicates between the inner and outside worlds, Skin body types communicate by using feelings to receive information. While they are generally very open to others and their environment, when stressed they retreat by detaching, disassociating, or essentially closing down and turning their focus inward. Strongly attached to and affected by their environment, Skin types have a strong connection with the earth, nature, and animals, which allows them to recharge naturally. Highly visual, they generally see, remember, and learn through pictures. Many are extremely sensitive, easily picking up on subtle energies and vibrations, including sounds and voice inflections.

### Spleen Essence

Just as the spleen acupuncture point draws energy into the body to be disseminated through the blood as needed, Spleen body types disseminate energy. They have a strong ability to organize and delegate, making sure projects get done, many of which often involve food and social or group interaction. Noted for their tenacity, Spleen types stay with a subject until they get the results they want. They are most comfortable when they can solve a problem in a logical step-by-step fashion and are noted for providing the sustaining energy needed to get a job done right.

### Stomach Essence

Just as the stomach focuses all its attention on the food it's digesting, Stomach body types focus on what's in front of them, which allows them to ignite their passion and truly live in the present moment. It's their focus, passion, and physical stamina that enable them to accomplish their goals. When dealing with a problem, they often talk it out, either alone or with someone else, chewing the data until they have sufficiently digested it. They make their best decisions after they have thoroughly processed the material. Their passion brings vitality to everything they undertake, which is especially apparent when expressed through music and dance.

## Thalamus Essence

Just as the thalamus collects information and files it for storage in the cerebral cortex or brain, Thalamus body types collect and evaluate information. They like to be effective and tend to be perfectionists. Just as they readily take in information, they are just as willing to let it go as new data becomes available, making them open-minded and willing to change.

## Thymus Essence

Just as the thymus gland eliminates unknown protein—generally bacteria and viruses—to keep the body's internal environment safe, Thymus body types stabilize their environment. They are protective of their own and go to great lengths to keep their environment constant, generally resisting change of any kind. Judging everything as good or bad, right or wrong, makes maintaining a constantly stable environment easier. Because being safe is generally associated with known situations, they have a deep-seated fear of change. Their innate desire to protect and keep life constant gives rise to a sense of loyalty and responsibility that towers above that of most other body types.

## Thyroid Essence

Just as the thyroid gland regulates the metabolism, ensuring the adequate release of energy into the body, Thyroid body types are known for getting things done. Extremely responsible, they go to great lengths to fulfill their obligations, often at their own expense. Thyroid types thrive on doing things that are worthwhile and are often idealistic, wanting to make a contribution to their world. With an affinity for both the theoretical and the practical, Thyroid types are constantly formulating theories, then testing and refining them based on their practical application. Bridging the gap between the head and the body, or the mind and the emotions, Thyroid types are able to see both sides of an issue, distill it, and communicate its essence.

## Identifying Your Aspects

Each of the 25 body types is dominated by one or more of four traits, or aspects: mental, emotional, physical, and spiritual. Identifying your two strongest aspects will take you a long way in accurately determining your type.

The first step is to identify your two dominant or connected aspects. These are the aspects you identify with most. They are the ones that reflect your basic nature. Through personal development, you may have strengthened other areas, but your challenge is to identify the dominant aspects you were born with, your natural way of relating to the world. For example, some people think about what they should do, while others rely on their gut feelings for guidance. We all have a stronger connection with either our mind (the mental aspect) or our feelings (the emotional aspect), which makes one of our dominant aspects either mental or emotional. The same applies to the physical and spiritual aspects; you relate more easily to either your body (the physical aspect) or your intuition (the spiritual aspect).

| SPIRITUAL<br>Intuition | MENTAL<br>Recognition &<br>Understanding |
|---|---|
| EMOTIONAL<br>Feelings | PHYSICAL<br>Body Awareness |

Following are some of the qualities associated with each aspect. Look at each list of words and select, based on your first impression, the list where you relate to the most words. If you are not sure, answer the questions that follow and choose the set of statements that is most true of you. (Answer according to what you know to be true and not from what someone else has told you!) Select your basic nature, not what you are currently working on or what you have trained yourself to do to be successful in the world.

### Mental versus Emotional

| MENTAL | EMOTIONAL |
|---|---|
| Think | Feel |
| Rely on mind | Rely on feelings |
| Logic | Gut feeling |
| Focused | Let it be |
| To the point | Expansive |
| Linear | Random |
| Peace | Warm fuzzies |
| Ambition | Commitment |
| Passion | Belief |
| Drive | Action |

What aspect do you ultimately rely on most heavily, mental or emotional? This is often your first impulse or your strongest influence. When faced with a difficult situation, do you rely most heavily on your ability to think it through logically (mental), or do you connect with your feelings, relying most heavily on your gut sense of how to handle the situation (emotional)?

### Mental

- I generally think first, feel later.
- At home, I respond best to reasonable requests.
- I tend to approach my feelings and those of others from a detached, analytical, point of view.
- I prefer conversations to be logical, orderly, and unemotional.

### Emotional

- My initial response to a situation is a feeling; then I think about it.
- At home, I respond best to direct requests.
- I tend to become immersed in feelings, both mine and others'.
- I prefer conversations that deal emotionally with issues.

## Physical versus Spiritual

Are you more mental or emotional, or an emotional personality who doesn't display feelings?

| PHYSICAL | SPIRITUAL |
| --- | --- |
| Sturdy | Fragile |
| Tangible | Invisible |
| Ground | Air |
| Solid | Delicate |
| Step-by-step | Random Access |
| Factual | Intuitive |
| Scientific | Magical |
| Precise | Conceptual |
| Literal | Ethereal |
| Solid | Delicate |
| Sensory | Sensitive |
| Manifestation | Idea |

Do you relate or identify more with your body or your spirit? Are you a spirit with a body or a body with a spirit? If you identify most with your body, your reality is closely associated with your physical body, strength, or physical presence. If you identify most with your spirit, your reality is closely associated with sensitivity, intuition, and an inner knowing.

### Physical

- I prefer life to be orderly and straightforward.
- I prefer to hear a new idea several times before I try it.
- I go from the details to the big picture.
- I am a body with a spirit.

### Spirit.ual

- I prefer life to occur with a natural ebb and flow.
- I enjoy trying new ideas or concepts immediately.
- I go from the big picture to the details.
- I am a spirit with a body.

## Aspects and Body Types

Select the two aspects that best describe you and verify them by reading the body type sets below. Select the types that match your body type in Chapter 2.

- PHYSICAL/MENTAL BODY TYPES: Adrenal, Lymph, Medulla, Nervous System, Spleen, Stomach, Thymus

To physical/mental personalities the tangible world is reality. They need to see it, touch it, and understand how it works for it to be real. Physically strong and mentally focused, they can achieve whatever they set out to do.

- SPIRITUAL/MENTAL BODY TYPES: Balanced, Brain, Eye, Hypothalamus, Pineal, Pituitary, Thalamus, Thyroid

To spiritual/mental body types, ideas, ideals, and concepts are reality. Figuring out how to synthesize bits of information and insights to express in physical form for the good of humankind is their strength, making them primarily more task oriented than socially oriented.

- PHYSICAL/EMOTIONAL BODY TYPES: Blood, Gallbladder, Gonadal, Kidney, Liver, Lung, Pancreas, Skin

Emotions and physically expressing feelings are reality for physical/emotional personalities, so family and social relationships are their highest priority.

- SPIRITUAL/EMOTIONAL BODY TYPES: Heart, Intestinal

Extremely sensitive from both the spiritual and the emotional aspects, spiritual/emotional personalities generally learn to focus on physical and mental aspects early in life to survive. Their power lies in using their strengths.

## STEP 4: Confirmation

After identifying your unique physical characteristics, matching them to the photos of various body types, and considering the essence and aspects of your personality and of each body type, you have probably zeroed in on the body type that fits you. But if you're still not 100 percent sure or if you want to double-check your choice, take a close look at the psychological profile that is given for each body type in Part 2 of this book. Here you'll find information about charac-

teristic traits and motivations, along with descriptions of each type's potentially best and worst behavior.

## Ready, Set, Go!

All the work involved in body typing is in this chapter. Once you take the time to find the type that best fits you, you have everything you need to begin the Body Type Diet, which will bring you optimum health and weight control. The following chapter gives information about implementing the Body Type Diet that is vital to successfully using this program. Be sure to read it carefully and then move to Part 2, where you'll find all the details about your particular body type.

# CHAPTER 3

# Implementing the Body Type Diet

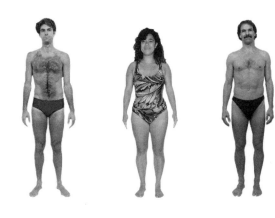

Now that you know your body type, you can begin to implement your personalized Body Type Diet. Although you are a unique individual, there are some aspects of your body type and diet that can be generalized to all in your body type category. But if you find that something in the suggested diet just doesn't feel right or is difficult for you to maintain, listen to your body. Apply what works for you and substitute in areas that don't. It will take a little experimenting, but it won't be long before you learn to understand the messages your body sends you about the strengths and weaknesses of the foods you fuel it with.

When you look up your particular body type in the following chapters, you'll see a section in each called Dietary Profile. This information includes diet tips and guidelines that specifically support the needs of your unique body type. This chapter explains how best to apply the guidelines of dietary emphasis, how to use the food lists to find your ideal weight and optimum health, how to schedule your meals, and how to convert the sample menus into a blueprint for life.

## How to Read the Dietary Emphasis Section of Your Profile

The Dietary Emphasis section in each body type profile gives you general dieting tips as well as specific information regarding your intake of fats, proteins, dense proteins, and amino acids. It suggests how to adjust your diet to support your health when you are physically or emotionally weak. And it outlines weight-loss and weight-gain tactics. The following guidelines will help you get the most out of the Dietary Emphasis information.

### Calories, Proteins, Fats, and Dense Proteins

Body types vary in the percentage of proteins, fats, and dense proteins they require for support, for weight loss, and for weight gain. You'll see that each of these percentages is listed as a suggested range. Your requirement for fat, for example, might read "from 10 to 30 percent of your calories." This range gives you some flexibility and freedom in choosing the foods that are best for you. You do not have to worry about getting an exact amount—these are only estimates. Ideally, if you are in good health, you should try to stay in the middle or lower end of the range. But if you are rebuilding your body, try to stay in the higher end of the range. You may also want to start in the higher end of the range if you've been sick or have low energy. In any case, don't let these numbers make you crazy. They are general guidelines, not absolute law.

Your body does require certain amounts of calories, proteins, fats, and dense proteins every day, but the requirements listed in your body type chapter are guidelines to the big picture. In other words, if you have a day when you eat dense protein that is high in fat and this raises your fat percentage above the suggested average, don't worry—the next day, just eat more fish, which is still high in protein but lower in fat. You should try to make your menus balance out to meet your fat and protein requirements over several days; don't make yourself nuts worrying about the percentages of fat and protein at every meal.

Use the charts below as guidelines to the most common breakdowns for fat, protein, and dense protein. But remember that your body is not as exact as a black-and-white chart. If you crave fish one day, eat fish, even if it increases your dense protein count above the suggested percentage. Listen to your body's needs, and make an effort to balance your intake in the long run.

From the Total Percentage of Fat Grams and Calories per Day chart you can see, for example, that if the recommended intake of fat for your body type is

25 percent of an 1,800-calorie day, you should try to eat 50 grams of fat at 450 calories. See the chart titled Food Calories, Protein, and Fat Examples (page 78) for an overview of foods that fit this profile.

From the Total Percentage of Protein Grams and Calories per Day chart you can see that if the recommended intake of protein for your body type is 30 percent of an 1,800-calorie day, you should try to eat 135 grams of protein at 540 calories. See the Food Calories, Protein, and Fat Examples chart for an overview of foods that fit this profile.

The Food Calories, Protein, and Fat Examples chart will help you apply the percentages of fat and protein given in your body type dietary profile. For example, if it is recommended that 20 to 30 percent of your calories are to come from fat, you can use the Total Percentage of Fat Grams and Calories Per Day chart to see that on an 1,800-calorie diet you can eat 40 to 60 grams of fat per day (using 360 to 540 of your total daily calories). Food Calories, Protein, and Fat Examples gives you examples of the kinds of foods that fit those requirements.

## Watch Your Supply of Amino Acids

When you're going through a lot of changes in your life or a period of personal growth, the amino acids threo-

### TOTAL PERCENTAGE OF FAT GRAMS AND CALORIES PER DAY

| Total Calories per Day | 20% Grams | 20% Calories | 25% Grams | 25% Calories | 30% Grams | 30% Calories | 35% Grams | 35% Calories | 40% Grams | 40% Calories |
|---|---|---|---|---|---|---|---|---|---|---|
| 1,000 | 22 | 200 | 27 | 250 | 33 | 300 | 38 | 350 | 44 | 400 |
| 1,500 | 33 | 300 | 41 | 375 | 50 | 400 | 58 | 525 | 66 | 600 |
| 1,800 | 40 | 360 | 50 | 450 | 60 | 540 | 70 | 630 | 80 | 720 |
| 2,000 | 44 | 400 | 56 | 500 | 67 | 600 | 77 | 700 | 88 | 800 |
| 2,200 | 49 | 440 | 60 | 550 | 73 | 660 | 85 | 770 | 98 | 880 |

### TOTAL PERCENTAGE OF PROTEIN GRAMS AND CALORIES PER DAY

| Total Calories per Day | 20% Grams | 20% Calories | 25% Grams | 25% Calories | 30% Grams | 30% Calories | 35% Grams | 35% Calories | 40% Grams | 40% Calories |
|---|---|---|---|---|---|---|---|---|---|---|
| 1,000 | 50 | 200 | 62 | 250 | 75 | 300 | 87 | 350 | 100 | 400 |
| 1,500 | 75 | 300 | 93 | 375 | 112 | 450 | 131 | 525 | 150 | 600 |
| 1,800 | 90 | 360 | 112 | 450 | 135 | 540 | 157 | 630 | 180 | 720 |
| 2,000 | 100 | 400 | 125 | 500 | 150 | 600 | 175 | 700 | 200 | 800 |
| 2,200 | 110 | 440 | 137 | 550 | 165 | 660 | 192 | 770 | 220 | 880 |

## FOOD CALORIES, PROTEIN, AND FAT EXAMPLES

| FATS | Fat Grams | Protein Grams | Cal. | PROTEIN | Fat Grams | Protein Grams | Cal. |
|---|---|---|---|---|---|---|---|
| 1 oz. almonds dry roasted, toasted | 14.4 | 5.8 | 166 | 6 oz. T-bone steak | 36 | 42 | 507 |
| 1 med. avocado | 14.9 | 4 | 324 | 6 oz. Porterhouse steak | 36 | 42 | 519 |
| 1 oz. Brazil nuts | 18.8 | 4.1 | 186 | 6 oz. roasted tenderloin | 47 | 40 | 600 |
| 1 oz. Brie cheese | 7.9 | 5.9 | 94 | 6 oz. round tip | 30 | 44 | 467 |
| 1 tsp. butter | 3.8 | 0.1 | 34 | 6 oz. top sirloin | 29 | 47 | 458 |
| 1 oz. cashews dry roasted or salted | 13.2 | 4.4 | 163 | 6 oz. roasted chicken dark meat, no skin | 17 | 47 | 348 |
| 1 oz. cheddar cheese | 9.4 | 7.1 | 114 | 6 oz. roasted chicken breast meat, no skin | 6 | 53 | 281 |
| 1 oz. coconut dried, unsweetened | 19.6 | 1.5 | 194 | 6 oz. roasted turkey dark meat, no skin | 12 | 49 | 318 |
| 1 oz. cottage cheese | 1.3 | 3.5 | 29 | 6 oz. roasted turkey white meat, no skin | 6 | 51 | 267 |
| 1 oz. cream cheese | 9.9 | 2.1 | 99 | 6 oz. pork chops lean, broiled | 18 | 54 | 393 |
| 1 oz. feta | 6 | 4 | 75 | 6 oz. lamb chops lean, broiled | 17 | 51 | 358 |
| 1 oz. kefir | 1 | 1.2 | 33 | 6 oz. leg of lamb roasted | 13 | 48 | 326 |
| 1 oz. mozzarella part skim milk | 4.5 | 6.9 | 72 | | | | |
| 1 tbs. olive oil | 14 | 0 | 120 | 6 oz. fresh tuna | 11 | 51 | 314 |
| 1 tbs. sesame oil | 14.2 | 0 | 126 | 6 oz. canned tuna packed in water | 1 | 50 | 222 |
| 1 tbs. peanut butter | 7 | 4 | 90 | 6 oz. fresh rainbow trout | 7 | 45 | 257 |
| 1 oz. pecans | 20 | 2 | 190 | | | | |
| 1 oz. pumpkin seeds roasted | 12 | 9.4 | 148 | 6 oz. halibut | 5 | 45 | 238 |
| 1 oz. ricotta part skim milk | 2.2 | 3.2 | 39 | 6 oz. haddock | 2 | 41 | 190 |
| 1 oz. sesame seeds | 14.1 | 5 | 162 | 6 oz. salmon | 13 | 47 | 315 |
| 1 oz. sunflower seeds | 14.1 | 6.5 | 162 | 6 oz. sole, flounder | 3 | 41 | 200 |
| 1 oz. Swiss cheese | 7 | 8 | 100 | 6 oz. shrimp | 2 | 36 | 168 |
| 1 oz. tahini (sesame butter) | 14.5 | 5.1 | 169 | 2 oz. (1) beef frankfurter | 17 | 7 | 181 |
| 8 oz. yogurt plain, low-fat | 3.5 | 11.9 | 144 | 1 egg, large | 5 | 6.3 | 75 |

Source: Corinne T. Netzer, *The Corinne Netzer Encyclopedia of Food Values,* (New York: Dell Books, 1992.)

nine, isoleucine, and cystine can become depleted. This puts your body in a highly stressed state. The Dietary Emphasis section tells you which foods are the best sources of these amino acids for your body type.

## Consider Special Dietary Needs

The Dietary Profile section for your body type also supplies guidelines to follow if your diet goal is to rebuild your body, lose weight, or gain weight.

## Sensitive Types

If you are in poor or moderate health, have a sensitive digestive system, or are going through a lot of stress and don't have a lot of energy to spend digesting your food, you can use the information listed for sensitive individuals to take the stress off your body so it can rebuild. These will help you increase the fat and dense protein your body requires to support your overall health and provide your body with the nutrients necessary to attain balance.

## Weight Loss and Weight Gain

Once your body is strong and balanced it can begin the job of shedding excess weight or adding weight, depending on your body's needs. Guidelines headed For Weight Loss and For Weight Gain will help you adjust the amount of fat, protein, and dense protein you take in each day to support your efforts to control your weight.

Because gaining weight is the first symptom of an imbalance in the body, the initial step to losing weight is to rebalance your body. The healthy and sensitive diets are designed to accomplish this goal. But there are a couple of pitfalls I'd like to caution you about. Occasionally, as individuals begin eating the foods they have deprived themselves of (sometimes for years), they experience weight gain. It is not uncommon to experience an increase in appetite for a short period before the system stabilizes. Also, some types have a strong tendency to go overboard on certain foods, especially if they have been deprived of them. If the foods happen to be high in fat or in calories, weight gain can result, particularly if the diet is not adjusted accordingly. Another common problem is quantity of food. The amount you eat is left to your discretion as it will vary according to your activities and diet earlier in the day or week. Naturally, if you have been eating large meals, you may be ready for less food. However, if your food consumption has been low, your body may be needing more fuel.

If you use the Body Type Diet to lose weight, be prepared for a surprise. Weight loss on this diet may cause you to drop a clothing size or two while you actually gain weight. This happens because the body is rebuilding itself. On a poor diet, when adequate nutrients are not available, muscle is cannibalized and often replaced with fat stores. On the Body Type Diet, this muscle is rebuilt and fat is eliminated. Because muscle weighs more than fat, body size may decrease (most often recognized when clothes begin to feel looser), while body weight actually increases. So don't let the scale fool you—initially look for changes in your body size, not your body weight. Typically, two weeks on the Body Type Diet are sufficient to provide the nutrients that may have been missing to adequately support complementary systems so the body can rebuild. Then the actual dieting can begin.

## How to Use Your Personalized Food List

In each of the body type sections you will find an extensive list of foods that support the needs of that particular body type. The lists are designed to be as complete as possible, so don't let unfamiliar foods scare you. You don't have to eat something just because it's listed. However, because no one food contains all the vitamins, minerals, and amino acids, and every food contains some of them, variety is essential. By adding the nutrients from different foods to your diet, you provide your body with more complete nutrition than you would with a diet of limited food selections.

The lists are divided into three categories: Ultra-Support Foods, Basic Support Foods, and Stressful Foods.

▶ ULTRA-SUPPORT FOODS: Ultra-Support Foods are those that best support your particular body type and that should be eaten most often, which means they can be included in three to seven meals per week. When you are hungry and can't think of anything that you especially want to eat, look at your Ultra-Support list for ideas. Just make sure you also get variety by including Basic Support Foods rather than relying exclusively on the same foods over and over.

▶ BASIC SUPPORT FOODS: Basic Support Foods offer variety in your diet. These are the foods you might eat one to two times a week. Keep in mind that the suggested frequency refers to individual foods, not to entire groups. For example, it's not grains that you need only once or twice a week—it's specific types of grains.

---

### SUBSTITUTE

You can often substitute the following:

- Instead of mayonnaise, use creamy Italian or avocado dressing.
- Instead of margarine, use butter.
- Instead of bread, eat rice, pasta, potatoes, or tortillas.
- Instead of diet soda, drink water with lemon or peppermint, or herbal teas.
- Instead of coffee, drink strong herbal teas.
- Instead of cow's milk, drink rice, oat, or nut milk.

You might eat semolina pasta twice a week, corn once as corn tortillas and once again as corn bread, and rye once as rye crackers and later as rye bread. This way you have a variety of grains.

▶ STRESSFUL FOODS: Stressful Foods are those that you should eat no more than once a month. While these foods aren't the best for you, it won't hurt to eat them once in a while, and eating them eliminates the feeling of deprivation so common on other weight-loss diets (especially if something you love happens to be on a forbidden list). It's the Stressful Foods you eat 80 percent of the time that cause you problems!

What happens if you eat Stressful Foods frequently? They tax your body by taking away more energy than they provide, usually through excessively stimulating your dominant gland or overloading your digestive system. You may not experience an immediate stomachache or headache after eating a Stressful Food, but you can get a delayed reaction, ranging from mild to severe, that could include queasiness, upset stomach, mouth sores, lethargy, fatigue, constipation, diarrhea, dry or burning lips, dry skin, immune system weakness, nervousness, hyperactivity, or a craving for sweets. Symptoms may also be vague or hard to associate with a given food. Weight gain is often the result of eating too many Stressful Foods because the body often stores what it can't easily assimilate.

As you look over these food lists, remember that although you belong to a particular body type group, you are also a unique individual within this group. You may find foods in the Ultra-Support and Basic Support categories that do not appeal to you at all. Don't feel as though you must eat each of these foods. It may be that your individual body simply does not like them. If, for example, you are unable to eat dairy and cheese, don't discard the entire menu and diet plan. Just substitute food from another category that will supply the necessary protein. (You may find an increased tolerance for dairy and cheese after rebuilding your body!)

Note that some foods on your food lists are *italicized*. These are the foods that can be difficult for your particular body type to assimilate. You don't have to avoid every one of them, only the ones that are difficult for you. If you have food sensitivities, these are the foods that are most likely to cause trouble. As you get stronger you may find you can reintroduce these foods into your diet.

## Why Scheduling Meals Is Important

The Scheduling Meals section will help you to create an eating schedule that gives your body the right foods at the right time of day. Some types, like the Pituitary, Kidney, Medulla, and Pineal (and sometimes the Pancreas), for example, do not assimilate dense protein well in the evenings. For others, the time of day that fruit is eaten affects the way the body is able to maintain even blood-sugar levels. Different body types need different foods at different times of the day.

For each meal, as well as for snacks, you will be told what time of day it is best eaten, whether the meal should be heavy, moderate, or light, and what food groups should be included. These food groups are listed according to their emphasis. (You obviously would not include every food group with every meal.) The mealtimes listed are the ideal for your body type. Do the best you can to accommodate your lifestyle. If you work nights, for example, the times given may not work for you. Use this information to find the eating plan that fits your schedule best.

## Guidelines for Using Your Sample Menu

Each of the 25 body type diets includes an individualized Sample One-Week Menu. This menu gives you a week's worth of meal ideas you can use as a blueprint. This sample menu is designed to show you how to implement the Body Type Diet for a lifetime.

**1. Pay attention to your body.** Often the foods have been selected for the way they work together. Wrong combinations of foods can cause symptoms ranging from mild indigestion, a heavy or sluggish feeling, nausea, bloating, fatigue, irritability, and weight gain to stomachaches and allergic reactions. *Note that some foods listed on the menus are in parentheses. These foods are not necessary to the food combination and can be eliminated without upsetting the supportive balance. Eating compatible combinations gives you a point of reference.*

**2. Feel free to substitute.** You should not use these menus exactly as they are written week after week. You can switch foods and meals and mix and match from one day to another. You can eat Monday's meals on Thursday; you can eat Saturday's breakfast on Tuesday. If you don't like a particular meal, substitute other foods from the alternative menus.

**3. Rotate your foods.** It's important to add as much variety to your diet as possible. Your body gets different nutrients from different foods, so when you substitute, be careful that you continue to choose a wide variety of foods.

Remember, these menus are intended to give you an idea of how you can schedule foods that support your body type. To begin, you can rearrange days or substitute from the list of alternative menus provided. Soon you will be creating your own menus.

### Cleanse

In the suggested menu plan, you will notice a one-day cleanse. Giving your body a chance to rest and cleanse is important in maintaining health and eliminating excess weight. The suggested cleanse is gentle and can be done one day a week or one day every two weeks, especially when your digestive system feels overloaded. We know it is important to include whole raw foods in our diet. Here are some simple suggestions that are easy to incorporate.

Eat the white part of the watermelon rind and chew the seeds along with the sweet part.

Raw almonds and pumpkin, sunflower, and sesame seeds are easiest to digest when soaked for 24 hours. Use your drinking water for soaking and give the water to your plants when you pour it off. Keep the soaked almonds and seeds in the refrigerator for up to two days after soaking. They make wonderful snacks especially with vegetables and fruit.

### Cooking

While microwave cooking is convenient, it is a cause of excess weight gain and immune system stress. Research shows that the molecular changes in food caused by microwave radiation make the food unrecognizable to the body and therefore toxic, resulting in an immune system overload. Additional information can be found in the 1989 "Microwave News" report by the University of Vienna, first published in the *Lancet,* which stated that milk heated in a microwave oven forms neurotoxic compounds (substances that have a toxic effect on nerve tissues) because of molecular changes in some of the amino acids. Researchers at the Stanford University School of Medicine reported in the April 1992 issue of the *Journal of Pediatrics* that microwaving breast milk to warm it destroyed 98 percent of its immunoglobulin-A antibodies. These antibodies are necessary for the passive immunity breast milk gives the infant, as well as 96 percent of its liposome activity, which inhibits bacterial growth. Alternative cooking methods include steaming, using a fifth burner, and convection or toaster ovens.

### What If Members of the Same Family Have Different Body Types?

If different members of your family have different body types, you may wonder how you can prepare meals that support each one's needs. The easiest way is to prepare a healthy meal that avoids foods from the Stressful Foods list of each family member. You'll also want to plan ahead so that everyone's scheduling needs can be met. If Mom is a Pituitary type who needs protein in the morning but not for dinner, for example, and Dad is a Stomach type who needs protein for dinner, Mom can still fix the usual dinner and eat the vegetables, saving her protein for breakfast the next morning.

### Will You Get Fast or Slow Results?

Your level of health and your past dietary habits have an effect on how fast you can implement a new diet. If you presently enjoy good health and if you find that this diet includes the foods you are already most accustomed to eating, your body will easily adjust to the Body Type Diet. You will probably find that the Body Type Diet validates what you know to be true and fills in the gaps. It may be as simple as avoiding fruit for breakfast or making sure you have your heaviest meal at lunch. Simply shifting the recommended foods into the pattern that supports your body type may have an immediate, gratifying effect on your energy, stamina, and weight.

On the other hand, sudden changes in what you eat, even when you go from a poor diet to a healthy one, can produce negative effects in your system. For example, a system used to highly refined junk food learns to need its fats and sugars, which are easily metabolized for quick energy. These are stimulants that keep the system going (although destroying health at the same time). If healthy foods like whole grains, dense protein, and raw vegetables can't immediately be assimilated by your unbalanced system, suddenly dropping all processed and junk foods can leave you devoid of energy. This alone might encourage you to abandon the new diet and go back to unhealthy eating, which at least will supply the energy necessary to function.

To avoid this kind of discouragement, make drastic dietary changes slowly. You might change only your breakfast meal for a week, then begin to choose your lunch foods from your Ultra-Support Foods list as well. Broth soups are easy to digest and a good place to start. Wean yourself slowly from diet sodas. Finally, after a few weeks, change your dinner and snack habits. After a month you should be weaned off your unhealthful foods and find yourself enjoying the good health and vitality of the full Body Type Diet.

## Tips for Vegetarians

If you are a vegetarian, you will find that your ability to maintain optimum health on the Body Type Diet depends on your body type's need for dense protein. If the daily percentage required (as stated in your body type section) begins at zero, you can easily adjust the foods on the sample menu to fit your vegetarian needs. This applies to the following body types: Adrenal, Brain, Gallbladder, Gonadal, Hypothalamus, Intestinal, Kidney, Lung, Lymph, Medulla, Pancreas, Pituitary, and Skin.

However, if your body type needs a higher percentage of dense protein for good health, you are faced with a decision. You can decide for the sake of your overall health to *gradually* introduce dense protein like fish and eggs into your diet to support your particular body type. Or, if you choose to stay away from animal products, you can still use the information in your body type section to help you be the healthiest vegetarian you can be. You will find a variety of the vegetable protein sources that are most compatible with your body's needs. If your protein levels are particularly low, you may wish to include additional concen-

trated protein sources. Use your Ultra-Support Foods list to create meals that emphasize the vegetables, legumes, nuts, seeds, grains, and fruits most beneficial to your body type. You can also use the information in these chapters to learn which vegetarian foods and beverages stress your body and should be avoided.

## Benefits of Maintaining Your Body Type Diet

The Body Type Diet is neither a fad nor an instant cure. It is about making permanent, long-term change. This lifetime eating program is based on sound dietary practices and what is individually right for each body type.

To get the greatest value out of your specific eating program, you'll need to change your eating patterns to the ways that truly support your body. In this process you will become more aware of when changes are necessary. Once you experience what it's like to feel really healthy, you will also know when your body is out of balance as well as how to regain that balance.

Here's how some of my patients began to incorporate this program into their lives.

"I looked at the diet, familiarized myself with what was ideal for me, and then compared it to what I was currently doing. I incorporated the parts that were easy for me, adding a single item I was attracted to, and put the diet away until I was ready for more."

"I changed a pattern of eating sweets, like ice cream, cookies, candy, or pastries, from anytime during the day to only when my body could easily handle them. Now I save the sweets for later and, if I still want them, eat them as an evening or bedtime snack."

"I shifted the time of day that I ate my largest meal from dinner to lunchtime. It dramatically changed my energy level."

"I looked at the diet and realized that I really liked most of the right foods but had been avoiding them because of the different health tips that worked for my friends. I was excited to have them back in my diet. I just needed to rearrange when I ate them and eliminate a few Stressful Foods. After three or four days my sugar cravings left entirely and the amount of increased energy and stamina was simply amazing. Although I was overweight, my main priority was increasing energy and vitality, and even though my focus was not on weight loss, I lost 7 pounds in six weeks. The weight loss is probably attributed to finally feeling satisfied after eating meals. I no longer spent my evenings 'grazing' for something to eat that satisfied me."

"I started keeping a diary of what I ate and how I felt after each meal. I read my diary while I'm riding my stationary bicycle. This motivates me to stay with my diet and keeps me from sliding back into my old habits. When I first started following my diet a year ago, I felt great. Then I felt I was invincible and could eat anything. It worked for a while, but then I gradually started slipping back into my old habits. My headaches returned, my energy was down, and I became irritable and short-tempered. I went back on my diet and felt dramatically better. That's when I realized I needed to keep a diary to keep reminding me that I can feel great and what it takes to do it."

# PART 2

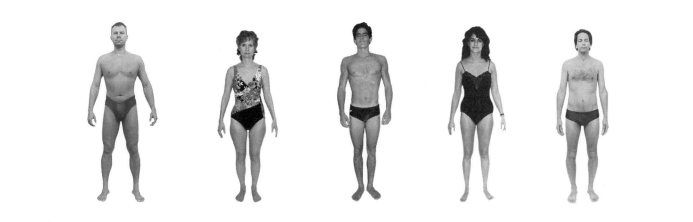

# The 25 Body Types:
# Profiles and Diets

# Adrenal

*The Adrenal body type is symbolized by a lightning bolt. Forceful and dynamic, Adrenal types are characterized by high energy, physical strength, and endurance. Charming and charismatic, they readily make their presence known.*

FAMOUS PEOPLE: Oprah Winfrey, Whoopi Goldberg, Arnold Schwarzenegger, Bruce Willis

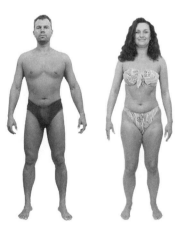

**ADRENAL**
**Location and Function**

The adrenal gland is either of a pair of organs situated on top of each kidney in the lower back at the level of the lower ribs. The adrenal glands are the strongest glands in the body; they produce hormones (including adrenaline) that are secreted under stress to prepare for the "fight or flight" response.

## Psychological Profile

### Characteristic Traits

Adrenal types thrive on excitement and obvious success. They possess a quick, powerful energy and approach life with a see-and-touch attitude. They are dynamic leaders who can easily control and lead a crowd. Highly competitive, they often gravitate toward sales and contact sports.

With inquiring, investigative minds, Adrenal types like to examine things from alternative perspectives. They are good at surveying the facts and are geared to practical, down-to-earth solutions. Predominantly visually oriented, they readily examine and see solutions to physical problems. Easily bored, they prefer to move on to something else once a task becomes routine. Mentally quick and alert, they don't like to stay with a task too long, making them appear to have a relatively short attention span. They prefer to see what needs to be done, delegate the tasks, then oversee the work.

Independent minded and prone to act, Adrenal types like to be in total control of a task or situation so that they alone can determine the outcome. With their quick, strong initiating energy, they are the first to dive into a project, even when not really sure how to do it.

### Motivation

Adrenal types tend to be unaware of their emotions and may not know that something is bothering them until their feelings have become strongly aroused. When the internal pressure builds up to a certain point, they are likely to undergo a sudden emotional discharge that may include bursts of anger or tears or outbreaks of excitement. Verbally uninhibited, Adrenal types think nothing of asking questions or making comments that would embarrass other types. Likewise, when stressed they readily blow off steam. The angry outburst ends as suddenly as it began and without any lingering hard feelings. Once Adrenal types are able to express their feelings and get rid of the bottled-up energy, they're prepared to forgive just about anything and to resume the relationship as though nothing had happened.

A basic fear of rejection causes Adrenal types to have difficulty saying no for fear of being left out. They tend to be "people pleasers" who strive to make a good impression. Consequently, they often commit to an activity and fail to follow through. As they gain more emotional maturity, their fear of rejection becomes less of a motivation.

Recognition and approval from others is often closely linked to self-esteem. Being externally directed, Adrenal types need career success and validation from outside themselves for a sense of well-being. Self-worth can hinge on doing well in their chosen line of work, and women Adrenal types often experience a need to prove themselves in "a man's world." Especially sensitive to rejection, Adrenal types are strongly motivated to make a good impression, making them extremely concerned about their image and how well they're accepted by others.

## "At Worst"

When under stress, Adrenal types experience an adrenaline rush that disturbs their ability to channel their energy productively. They may get scattered, hyperactive, or depressed. When their energy is high and their excess energy is not dissipated through exercise, they experience mood swings and emotional volatility. Sensitive to rejection, they defend themselves through verbal attacks or blaming when they don't get the approval they are seeking and their self-esteem is threatened.

The tendency to overeat to soothe their emotions can easily culminate in an addiction to food, alcohol, or drugs. Thriving on excitement and immediate success, Adrenal types can also easily become addicted to thrill-seeking and adrenaline rushes. Feeling physically indestructible, they often go through a period of living on the wild side and push their bodies to the limit.

With their inherent strength, Adrenal types can easily become overpowering, controlling, tactless, and pushy. They may become physically aggressive, particularly when their fear of rejection has been numbed through drugs or alcohol. Verbally, they are often too forceful at the expense of the feelings and opinions of others. They can become overly analytical and critical, demanding that things be done their way, refusing advice or assistance from others. When the going gets rough, when they hit a snag, or when their success is not readily assured, Adrenal types tend to lose patience with themselves, others, or with a task. This often results in lack of follow-through on the project at hand. The tendency is to try to quickly power through the problem, and if that doesn't work, to delegate or ignore it.

Basic Adrenal type philosophies are "Nothing succeeds like success" and "To be successful, you have to look successful." Their nature is to emphasize the physical expression and appearance of success. They use money to impress, often insisting on picking up the check even when they can't afford it. Their attitude is one of "Here today and gone tomorrow." High rolling and gambling, their easy-come-easy-go philosophy and living only for the moment result in money problems; there never seems to be enough to sustain all their wants and impulses.

## "At Best"

Adrenal types are at their best when they redefine success by placing value on their intuition, internal validation, and the spirit. Success is then measured by their personal growth and emotional maturity and the development of their connection with a source of inner guidance.

Once Adrenal types have developed their intuition through their spiritual connection, life really works for them. They are then able to get off the emotional roller coaster and focus their attention, so that productivity increases and social situations are more harmonious. Life takes on new meaning, with a richness, joy, and excitement unattainable through thrill-seeking and adrenaline rushes.

Validated from within, no longer dependent upon others' responses and reactions to them, Adrenal types become balanced and can live with harmony and self-esteem. Their spiritual connection provides the peace that creates a stable inner environment. This emotional maturity comes through self-knowledge and insight.

Learning to flow with life rather than force or try to control it allows Adrenal types to channel their high energy effectively. Once they let go of their need to be in charge, they step into the universal flow, which allows them to experience abundance and prosperity in the physical world.

## Dietary Profile

### Main Focus

- ► Maintain a low-fat, low-protein diet.
- ► Eat raw vegetables, salads, fruit, dairy (yogurt, cottage cheese, and cheese).
- ► A vegetarian diet is ideal unless stressed; then increase protein, particularly chicken and fish. Include soups and cooked vegetables.
- ► Have a light breakfast.
- ► Have a moderate to heavy lunch and dinner.

## Dietary Emphasis

- From 20 to 25 percent of your calories are to come from fat.
- Best fat sources: almonds and dairy (yogurt, cottage cheese, cheese). If intolerant of dairy, include chicken, turkey, and fish.
- From 10 to 30 percent of your calories are to come from protein.
- From 0 to 30 percent of your calories are to come from dense protein.
- Best sources of the three amino acids threonine, isoleucine, and cystine: sesame seeds, cottage cheese, and light or white fish.
- Caloric intake: 1,500 to 1,800 calories a day for women and 1,700 to 2,000 calories a day for men. If you are engaging in intense exercise (competition type) or heavy labor, increase calories.
- Drink a minimum of 64 ounces of water a day. Drink water before and after meals, not with meals.
- Drinking mineral water and/or parsley tea can help reduce appetite and cleanse the body.
- Occasional desserts are best as an evening snack.
- When healthy, eat more raw vegetables than cooked (sensitive require more cooked); whole grains; fruit (up to 40 percent of diet); protein, mainly from poultry or fish; and dairy.

## For Weight Loss

- Fat and dense protein: 20 to 30 percent of daily calories.
- If fats drop below 20 percent of calories, weight loss will be hindered.
- Protein: 20 to 40 percent of caloric intake.
- Dense protein: 20 to 30 percent, particularly fish, turkey, and chicken to rebuild the adrenals. Dense protein is necessary when there is excess weight gain (over 20 pounds), fatigue, and/or a general feeling of being stressed.
- Reduce food quantity, especially carbohydrates (including breads, rice, pasta, and potatoes).
- May, if tolerated, use appetite suppressants.
- Best not to snack, but may include midafternoon and evening snacks.
- May include grains for lunch, or breakfast and dinner, but not for lunch and dinner.
- Exercise at least 40 minutes daily.
- Eat raw fruits and vegetables, salads, protein, and soups.

## For Weight Gain

- Protein: 20 to 30 percent of daily calories.
- Increase food quantity.

## Healthy Foods List

There is no need to sacrifice delicious and filling foods to maintain a healthy Adrenal body type. The following lists will help you focus on foods that support your health, and avoid foods that can stress your system.

*You'll notice that some foods are printed in italics; these foods take more energy to assimilate and could be ones you will want to avoid when you are in a sensitive state due to any physical or emotional stresses.*

Be sure to read Chapter 3, "Implementing the Body Type Diet," for lots of important information about how to use these many foods to gain their full benefit.

## Ultra-Support Foods

Foods to include in 3 to 7 meals a week. Refers to each food in the entire category but does not require eating foods from each category.

**Dense Protein:** chicken, chicken broth, chicken livers, Cornish game hen, turkey; anchovy, bass, bonita, catfish, cod, haddock, halibut, herring, mackerel, mahimahi, perch, roughy, sardines in tomato sauce, shark, red snapper, swordfish, tuna; calamari (squid)

**Dairy:** *milk* (whole, 2%, raw, goat's), sour cream, yogurt (regular, low fat, nonfat, plain, or flavored), *butter*

**Cheese:** cream, feta, Monterey Jack, Muenster, Parmesan, ricotta, Romano, Swiss

**Nuts and Seeds:** almonds (raw, roasted), almond butter, hazelnuts, macadamias (raw, roasted), macadamia butter; sesame seeds (raw, roasted), sesame seed butter

**Legumes:** beans (lima, pinto)

**Grains:** amaranth, buckwheat, *corn,* corn grits, *corn tortillas,* hominy, millet, quinoa, rice (*white or brown basmati, short grain brown,* Japanese, white, wild), rice cakes, brown rice bread, Chinese rice noodles, cream of rice

**Vegetables:** asparagus, avocados, bamboo shoots, green beans, bok choy, broccoli, cabbage (green, napa, red), carrots, cauliflower, celery, cilantro, corn, garlic, greens (beet, collard, mustard, turnip), kale, kohlrabi, romaine lettuce, okra, black olives, parsley, parsnips, peas, snow pea pods, bell peppers (green, red, yellow), potatoes (red, russet, *White Rose,* Yukon Gold), pumpkin, radish, sprouts (alfalfa, mung bean, radish), squash (acorn, banana, butternut, spaghetti, yellow [summer]), Swiss chard, *tomatoes* (*canned, hothouse, vine-ripened*), turnips

**Fruits:** apricots, bananas, berries (blueberries, strawberries), cherries, *dates, grapes* (*black, green,* red), *lemons, limes, oranges,* peaches, pears

**Sweeteners:** stevia

**Condiments:** ginger, Vege-Sal

**Salad Dressings:** *creamy Italian*

## Basic Support Foods

Foods to include in 1 to 2 meals a week.

**Dense Protein:** beef broth, buffalo, calf's liver, lamb, *pork, ham, bacon, sausage,* veal, venison, organ meats (heart, brain); duck; flounder, salmon, sardines, sole, trout; abalone, clams, eel, lobster, mussels, octopus, oysters; eggs

**Dairy:** *nonfat milk,* half-and-half, sweet cream, buttermilk, kefir, *frozen yogurt,* ice cream (Alta Dena, Ben & Jerry's, Breyers, Dreyer's, Häagen-Dazs, Swensen's, Baskin 31 Robbins)

**Cheese:** American, blue, Brie, Camembert, cheddar, Colby, low-fat cottage, Edam, goat, Gouda, Limburger, mozzarella

**Nuts and Seeds:** Brazils, coconut, hazelnuts, peanuts (raw, roasted), peanut butter, pecans, pine nuts (raw, roasted), walnuts (black, English), water chestnuts; seeds (raw or roasted caraway, pumpkin, *sunflower*), *sunflower seed butter*

**Legumes:** beans (adzuki, black, garbanzo, Great Northern, kidney, lima, red, soy), lentils, black-eyed peas, split peas; hummus; miso, *soy milk, tofu*

**Grains:** barley, couscous, oats, popcorn, long grain brown rice, rice bran, unsalted rice cakes, *rye,* triticale, *whole wheat,* wheat bran, wheat germ, refined wheat flour, *flour tortillas,* breads (corn, corn/rye, French, garlic, Italian, *multigrain,* oat, rye, *sevengrain,* sourdough, sprouted grain, white, *whole wheat*), plain bagels, croissants, English muffins, Ry-Krisp, *pasta* (plain, artichoke, vegetable), udon noodles, cream of rye, *cream of wheat*

**Vegetables:** artichokes, *arugula,* yellow wax beans, beets, broccoflower, brussels sprouts, eggplant, jicama, leeks, lettuce (butter, endive, *iceberg, red leaf*), mushrooms, green olives, onions (chives, brown, green, red, Vidalia, white, yellow), chili peppers, pimientos, daikon radishes, rutabaga, sauerkraut, seaweed (arame, dulse, kelp, nori, wakame), shallots, spinach, sprouts (clover, *sunflower*), sweet potatoes, *watercress, yams,* zucchini

**Vegetable Juices:** *carrot, carrot/celery,* celery, parsley, spinach, *tomato,* V-8

**Fruits:** *apples* (*Golden or Red Delicious, Granny Smith, Jonathan, McIntosh, Pippin, Rome Beauty*), berries (*blackberries, boysenberries,* cranberries, gooseberries, *raspberries*), figs (*fresh, dried*), grapefruit (*white, red*), guavas, kiwi, kumquats, loquats, mangoes, melons (*cantaloupe, casaba, Crenshaw, honeydew, watermelon*), nectarines, papayas, persimmons, plums (*black, purple, red*), pineapples, pomegranates, prunes, raisins, rhubarb, tangelos, tangerines

**Fruit Juices:** *apple, apple cider, apple/apricot, apricot,* black cherry, cherry, cranapple, cranberry, *grape* (*purple,* red, *white*), *grapefruit, guava, lemon, orange, papaya, pear, pineapple, pineapple/coconut, prune, tangerine*

**Vegetable Oils:** all-blend, *almond,* avocado, coconut, *corn, peanut, flaxseed, olive, safflower, sesame, soy, sunflower*

**Sweeteners:** *fructose, honey, molasses,* sorghum, *sugar* (*brown, date, raw, refined cane*), syrup (barley malt, brown rice, *corn, maple*), *succonant*

**Condiments:** *catsup, mustard, mayonnaise, horse-radish, barbecue sauce, pesto sauce, soy sauce,* salsa, tahini, *margarine,* vinegar, sea salt
**Salad Dressings:** *blue cheese, French,* ranch, *creamy avocado, Thousand Island,* vinegar and oil, lemon juice and oil
**Desserts:** *custard, tapioca, chocolate, desserts containing chocolate, sherbet (orange, raspberry)*
**Chips:** *bean, corn (blue, white, yellow), potato*
**Beverages:** *coffee,* tea (*black,* green, herbal, Japanese, Chinese oolong); mineral water, sparkling water; lemonade; *beer, barley, champagne, gin,* liqueurs, *malt liquor, regular sodas, root beer, sake, scotch,* sherry, *vodka, whiskey;* wine (*red, white*)

## Stressful Foods

Have no more than once a month.

**Dense Protein:** *beef, beef liver; crab, scallops, shrimp*
**Dairy:** *most ice creams*
**Nuts and Seeds:** *cashews (raw, roasted), cashew butter, pistachios*
**Grains:** *crackers (oat, saltines, wheat)*
**Vegetables:** *cucumbers*
**Vegetable Oils:** *canola*
**Sweeteners:** *aspartame, Equal, NutraSweet, saccharin, Sweet'n Low*
**Condiments:** *salt, MSG*
**Beverages:** *diet sodas*

## Scheduling Meals

### Healthy

When healthy, eating a large breakfast results in the desire to eat all day long. Schedule your meals as follows:

*Breakfast:* 6–8 A.M. Light, with fruit, dairy, vegetables, and/or grain.
*Lunch:* 12–2 P.M. Moderate but may be heavy if dinner is moderate, with vegetables, grain, legumes, nuts, seeds, dairy, protein, and/or fruit.
*Dinner:* 7–9 P.M. Heavy, or moderate if lunch was heavy, with grain, vegetables, protein, dairy, legumes, nuts, seeds, and/or fruit.

### Snacks (optional)
*Midmorning:* vegetables, fruit, grain, dairy

*Midafternoon:* vegetables, fruit, grain, dairy, protein, nuts
*Evening:* fruit, vegetables, grain, protein, dairy, nuts, sweets

### Sensitive or Exhausted Adrenals

*Breakfast:* moderate-to-heavy, with protein and vegetables.
*Lunch:* moderate, with soups, salads, vegetables, grain, dairy, and/or legumes.
*Dinner:* moderate-to-heavy, with protein, dairy, nuts, seeds, legumes, vegetables, fruit, and/or grain.

## Sample One-Week Menu

DAY 1
*Breakfast:* celery and cream cheese
*Lunch:* calamari, rice, and broccoli
*Dinner:* lamb, hummus, lettuce or celery, and/or cilantro
*Snack:* grapes

DAY 2
*Breakfast:* banana
*Lunch:* steamed cauliflower, broccoli, carrots, and onions w/melted mozzarella cheese
*Dinner:* red snapper and a salad of romaine lettuce, tomato, onion, and alfalfa sprouts w/vinegar and oil
*Snack:* apple and cheese

DAY 3
*Breakfast:* cottage cheese w/pineapple
*Lunch:* sushi and miso soup
*Snack:* jicama w/rice vinegar
*Dinner:* chicken and a salad of butter lettuce, mushrooms, onions, tomato, and bell pepper w/creamy Italian dressing
*Snack:* vanilla yogurt

DAY 4
*Breakfast:* carrot/celery juice (or parsley/spinach) or apple
*Lunch:* cheese ravioli w/spaghetti sauce and a salad of iceberg lettuce, radishes, sprouts, and zucchini w/olive oil and red wine vinegar
*Snack:* rice cakes or corn tortillas and beans w/salsa
*Dinner:* swordfish, asparagus, and a salad of tomato, red leaf lettuce, onions, jicama, and parsley w/lemon and oil dressing
*Snack:* California roll/ginger/wasabi w/soy sauce

DAY 5: CLEANSE

*Breakfast:* watermelon or fruit all day; or raw/steamed vegetables all day; or juice

*Lunch:* salad of endive lettuce, green beans, bok choy, and garlic w/lemon juice dressing; or juice of carrot/celery (parsley/spinach)

*Dinner:* soaked raw almonds, pumpkin, and/or sunflower seeds

DAY 6

*Breakfast:* banana smoothie—bananas, milk, and almonds

*Lunch:* salad of romaine lettuce, tomato, onion, cheese, broccoli, and avocado w/ranch or Italian dressing

*Snack:* almonds (raw or roasted, unsalted)

*Dinner:* bass and a salad of spinach, peas, beets, red or green onions, and radishes w/Italian dressing

*Snack:* fruit yogurt

DAY 7

*Breakfast:* cheese

*Lunch:* chicken, potato, snow peas, and carrots

*Snack:* pear

*Dinner:* salad of tuna, avocado, romaine lettuce, red cabbage, green onions, and beets w/blue cheese dressing

*Snack:* strawberries

## Alternative Menus

*(Foods in parentheses may be omitted)*

### Breakfast

Fruit, such as strawberries, peaches, pears, cherries, or red grapes

Chicken, cheese and salad, or avocado

Orange roughy and asparagus

Plain yogurt w/protein powder and almonds

Salmon and green beans or peas

Chicken Caesar salad

Carrot juice

### Lunch or Dinner

Turkey and a salad of romaine lettuce, tomato, onion or scallion, and broccoli (cheese and/or avocado) w/Italian dressing or vinegar and oil

Salad of fresh tuna and tomato (pickles)

Greek salad—celery, tomato, black olives, and feta cheese

Romaine lettuce salad and cheese

Wild rice, mushrooms, and broccoli

Stir-fried vegetables and rice

Black beans w/garlic and Parmesan cheese

Vegetable soup or stew

Spaghetti w/meatless tomato sauce, Parmesan cheese, or garlic pesto sauce

Chicken soup

Chicken fajita and salad

# Balanced

*The Balanced body type is symbolized by the yin-yang sign. Dependent upon everything working together synergistically, Balanced body types need balance between work and play as well as all other aspects of life. Essentially playful and adventurous, they embody the synergy that brings about balance.*

FAMOUS PEOPLE: Fred Astaire, Gwyneth Paltrow, Tina Turner, Neil Diamond

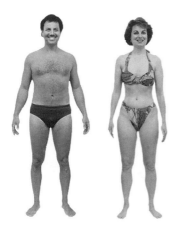

**BALANCED**
**Location and Function**

No one gland or organ is dominant in the Balanced body type. All glands, organs, and systems must work together harmoniously for optimal functioning.

## Psychological Profile

### Characteristic Traits

Sensitive by nature, Balanced types have a fragile equilibrium and will go to great lengths to maintain their delicate balance. On the outside they are often light, playful, personable, and entertaining, while on the inside they are reserved, reluctant to share their true feelings. They are generally quite social, and people are readily attracted to them but rarely allowed to get very close emotionally until they've proven they can be trusted.

Balanced body types have a strong sense of adventure and like to travel or move frequently, giving them the opportunity to meet new people and try new things. They love performing or being the center of attention and, since they are typically in their glory when interacting with people, will often be the life of the party. They mix well with others and can be quite good at making favorable impressions. They are basically easygoing, forgiving, optimistic, and open-minded individuals, with a positive attitude toward life.

A sense of adventure creates an aliveness and a love of life that are often expressed as new ideas, concepts, and designs. Imaginative and creative, with a strong attraction to the arts, Balanced types have a need for order and structure that allows them to be extremely precise in their music, dance, or creative expression. Sensitive and artistic, they are also practical, logical, and technically adept. Their acute sight, hearing, and touch are balanced with a natural rhythm and timing, which they often use to discover their inner sense of stability and balance.

### Motivation

Balanced types have a heightened need for security and stability. This need causes them to go to great lengths to control their environment. They need to work in situations that ensure maximum predictability and harmony. They often find it difficult to delegate tasks or supervise others and feel that it's faster and more effective to do a job personally. Consequently they prefer to work alone, taking full responsibility for the outcome and offering their personal guarantee that the job will be done right. By working alone they also avoid the unpleasant task of criticizing or correcting coworkers.

Despite the care they take in projecting a positive image, Balanced types are also known to undermine their own efforts. For example, because they place such a high value on honesty, their truthfulness can override diplomacy and result in tactless comments. They have a tendency to speak without self-censorship. They have difficulty keeping secrets and don't like others to be secretive, often becoming very impatient when others withhold information.

Being intuitively aware of the dangers relationships pose, and taking commitments seriously, they are cautious about making them. Consequently, as a protective mechanism, they may have a fear of intimacy, which compels them to distance themselves from others and limit close friends to a select few. They need to develop relationships slowly and to know others well before they are willing to reveal their innermost thoughts and feelings.

## "At Worst"

Balanced types can become extremely impatient both with themselves and others when things go wrong and when their need for order and balance isn't satisfied. Unless they've developed considerable self-control, they may display anger or even rage and then regret it later. They can overreact with rigidity and intolerance or retreat from problems through compulsive/addictive behavior in the form of an activity, a relationship, or substance abuse.

If Balanced types haven't developed an inner sense of stability, they typically look to others to provide it. Since relationships can never fulfill what can only come from within, expecting to gain stability from relationships makes them prone to disillusionment, or to settle for relationships that are detrimental to their personal growth and inner peace.

Motivated by a need for acceptance by others, Balanced types often suppress or even deny their feelings, causing them to appear distant, detached, or preoccupied. Their fear of rejection can cause them to keep their feelings hidden to avoid upsetting themselves or others. These suppressed emotions generally surface as physical complaints, like headaches or digestive problems. Balanced types use play and adventurous activities to release stored-up emotional energy. When out of balance, they can get so caught up in their play and fantasies that they lose sight of reality.

## "At Best"

Balanced types are persistent, goal-oriented self-starters who like to be in control of their work, gladly accepting responsibility for the completion of a task. They are good at getting to the heart of a matter, focusing more on the big picture or the main objective than on technicalities. While they are not primarily detail oriented, they'll make sure the details are correct before finally releasing a project. Conscientious and competent, they can be depended upon to fulfill their promises and are often found working late into the night to finish a project.

Balanced types get rid of pent-up stress and revitalize themselves through play, engaging in adventurous activities and daring pursuits that capture their imagination and challenge their problem-solving abilities. They find the balance between work and play by pursuing their passion and making work and play synonymous. Balancing work with play helps them find the harmony they need for a sense of well-being. This in turn helps them maintain an optimistic, open-minded, positive attitude toward life that enables them to bounce back from adversity.

Balanced types at their best are self-contained and at peace within themselves. Having developed an inner sense of harmony and balance, they have an easygoing, forgiving, and humorous nature that brings lightness and balance into the lives of those they touch.

## Dietary Profile

### Main Focus

- ► Balance is essential in all aspects of life.
- ► Get adequate protein and fat, especially at lunch.
- ► For breakfast, emphasize carbohydrate with moderate fat.
- ► For lunch, emphasize protein and fat.
- ► For dinner, emphasize vegetables.
- ► Rotation and variety of foods is essential.

### RECOMMENDED EXERCISE

The initial benefit of exercise for the Balanced body type is emotional. It gets energy moving, lifts spirits, adds variety to daily activities, and activates the physical body by getting the lymphatics moving. Sunlight is beneficial, and being around water is often important. Variety is essential. Exercise may include Pilates, dancing, walking, hiking, bicycling, swimming, rebounding, weight lifting, baseball, or tennis.

## Dietary Emphasis

- From 20 to 35 percent of your calories are to come from fats.
- Best fat sources: dense protein (chicken, turkey, eggs, fish, and beef) and butter.
- From 25 to 40 percent of your calories are to come from protein.
- From 10 to 30 percent of your calories are to come from dense protein.
- Best sources of the three amino acids threonine, isoleucine, and cystine: tuna, sunflower seeds, and ricotta cheese.
- Caloric intake: 1,500 to 1,800 calories a day for women and 1,700 to 2,000 calories a day for men. If you are engaging in intense exercise (competition type) or heavy labor, increase calories.
- Drink a minimum of 64 ounces of water a day. Drink water before and after meals, not with meals.
- Balance raw and cooked vegetables.
- Restrict fruit to breakfast and midmorning and evening snacks.
- Balance choices from all food groups.
- May include snacks.
- Occasional desserts are best as an evening snack.
- When rebuilding body, increase protein. Breakfast may be heavy with protein.

## For Weight Loss

- Protein: 25 to 35 percent of daily calories.
- Avoid caffeine, sugar, and stimulants (including mahuang and alcohol).
- Eat a light dinner, consuming most of calories at breakfast and lunch.
- Eliminate starches at dinner, especially breads and grains with wheat.
- Reduce dairy, dried fruit, and honey.
- Emphasize protein and vegetables.

---

### RECOMMENDED CUISINE

Balanced body types need protein, grain combinations, and foods that are moderately seasoned. Best cuisine bets are Chinese, Thai, Japanese (including sushi), Moroccan, Mexican, French, and Italian.

---

## For Weight Gain

- Fat: 25 to 40 percent of daily calories.
- Dense protein: 20 to 35 percent of daily calories.

## Healthy Foods List

There is no need to sacrifice delicious and filling foods to maintain a healthy Balanced body type. The following lists will help you focus on foods that support your health and avoid foods that can stress your system.

*You'll notice that some foods are printed in italics; these foods take more energy to assimilate and could be ones you will want to avoid when you are in a sensitive state due to any physical or emotional stresses.*

Be sure to read Chapter 3, "Implementing the Body Type Diet," for lots of important information about how to use these many foods to gain their full benefit.

### Ultra-Support Foods

Foods to include in 3 to 7 meals a week, listed by category.

**Dense Protein:** chicken (white), *Cornish game hen,* turkey (white); anchovy, tuna; octopus

**Dairy:** milk (whole, raw), nonfat plain yogurt, butter

**Cheese:** cheddar, cream, feta, mozzarella, Muenster, Parmesan, ricotta, Swiss

**Nuts and Seeds:** almonds (raw, roasted), almond butter, coconut, water chestnuts; sunflower seeds (raw, roasted), sunflower seed butter, pumpkin seeds (roasted)

**Grains:** oats, oatmeal, rice (brown or white basmati, *long or short grain brown,* Japanese), breads (corn, oat, *seven-grain*), *bagels,* pasta, vegetable pasta, cream of rice

**Vegetables:** avocados, green beans, carrots, eggplant, jicama, bell peppers (green, red, yellow), mung bean sprouts, sweet potatoes, yams

**Fruits:** cantaloupes, cherries, dates, Mission figs (soaked), nectarines, Fuyu persimmons, pineapples, pomegranates

**Sweeteners:** stevia

**Beverages:** coffee with cream (morning), decaf coffee (morning or evening), café au lait, espresso

## Basic Support Foods

Foods to include in 1 to 2 meals a week.

**Dense Protein:** beef, *beef broth, beef liver,* veal, *buffalo,* pork, organ meats (heart, brain); *chicken* (dark, broth, livers), turkey (dark); bonita, catfish, cod, flounder, haddock, halibut, herring, mackerel, mahimahi, perch, orange roughy, salmon, sardines, shark, red snapper, sole, swordfish, trout with cornmeal; abalone, *calamari* (squid), crab, clams, eel, *lobster,* mussels, oysters, *scallops, shrimp;* eggs

**Dairy:** nonfat or low-fat milk, half-and-half, sweet cream, sour cream, buttermilk, kefir, regular or low-fat yogurt (plain, black cherry, raspberry, boysenberry, lemon, strawberry, cinnamon apple, apricot, pineapple/coconut), *frozen yogurt,* ice cream (Ben & Jerry's, Breyers, Dreyer's)

**Cheese:** American, blue, Brie, Camembert, Colby, cottage, Edam, goat, Gouda, kefir, Limburger, Monterey Jack, low-fat mozzarella, Romano

**Nuts and Seeds:** Brazils, raw cashews, *hazelnuts, macadamias (raw, roasted), macadamia butter, peanuts (raw, roasted), pecans, pine nuts (raw, roasted),* pistachios, *walnuts (black, English);* caraway seeds (raw, roasted), *pumpkin seeds (raw), sesame seeds (raw, roasted)*

**Legumes:** *beans (adzuki, black, garbanzo, Great Northern,* kidney, *lima,* pinto, *red, soy),* lentils, *black-eyed peas, split peas;* hummus; miso, soy milk, tofu

**Grains:** *amaranth, buckwheat,* corn, corn grits, corn tortillas, couscous, hominy grits, popcorn, *quinoa,* wild rice, rice bran, rice cakes, rye, triticale, refined white flour, whole wheat, wheat bran, wheat germ, flour tortillas, breads (corn, corn/rye, French, *garlic,* Italian, multigrain, *rice,* rye, *sourdough,* sprouted grain, *white),* croissants, English muffins, crackers (oat, rye, saltines), udon noodles, Chinese rice noodles, cream of rye, cream of wheat

**Vegetables:** *artichokes, arugula, asparagus, bamboo shoots, yellow wax beans, beets, bok choy, broccoflower, broccoli, brussels sprouts,* raw cabbage (green, napa, red), *cauliflower,* celery, *cilantro, corn,* cucumber, garlic, *greens (beet, collard, mustard, turnip),* kale, *kohlrabi,* leeks, *lettuce (Boston,* butter, *endive,* iceberg, red leaf, romaine), *mushrooms, okra, olives (green, ripe),* cooked onions (chives, brown, green, red, Vidalia, white, yellow), parsley, parsnips, *green peas, snow pea pods,* chili peppers, pimientos, potatoes (purple, red, russet, White Rose, Yukon Gold), pumpkin, radish, daikon radish, rutabaga, sauerkraut, seaweed (arame, dulse, kelp, nori, wakame), shallots, spinach, sprouts (alfalfa, clover, radish, sunflower), squash (acorn, banana, butternut, spaghetti, yellow [summer], zucchini), Swiss chard, cooked or *raw tomatoes* (canned, hothouse, vine-ripened), turnips, watercress

**Vegetable Juices:** carrot, *carrot/celery,* carrot/celery/parsley, *celery,* parsley, spinach, tomato, V-8; *green juice*

**Fruits:** apples (Golden or Red Delicious, Granny Smith, Jonathan, McIntosh, Pippin, Rome Beauty), apricots, bananas, berries (blackberries, blueberries, boysenberries, cranberries, gooseberries, raspberries), figs (fresh, dried), guavas, kiwi, kumquats, lemons, limes, loquats, mangoes, melons (casaba, Crenshaw, honeydew, watermelon), papayas, peaches, pears, Hachiya persimmons, *prunes,* raisins, rhubarb, tangelos, tangerines

**Fruit Juices:** apple, apple cider, apple/apricot, apricot, black cherry, cherry, cranapple, cranberry, grapefruit, guava, lemon, orange/mango, papaya, pear, pineapple, pineapple/coconut, *prune,* tangerine, watermelon

**Vegetable Oils:** all-blend, almond, avocado, coconut, corn, flaxseed, olive, safflower, sesame, soy, sunflower

**Sweeteners:** *fructose, honey, molasses, sorghum, sugar (brown, date, raw, refined cane), syrup (barley malt, brown rice, corn, maple), succonant*

**Condiments:** *catsup, mustard, horseradish, barbecue sauce, pesto sauce, soy sauce,* salsa, tahini, vinegar, salt, sea salt, Vege-Sal

**Salad Dressings:** *blue cheese, French, ranch, creamy Italian, creamy avocado, Thousand Island,* vinegar and oil, lemon juice and oil

**Desserts:** *custards, tapioca, puddings, pies, cakes, sherbet (orange, raspberry)*

**Chips:** *bean, corn (blue, white, yellow), potato*

**Beverages:** coffee, tea (*black,* green, herbal, Japanese, Chinese oolong); mineral water, sparkling water; *wine (white, red); root beer, diet soda, regular soda*

## Stressful Foods

Have no more than once a month.

**Dense Protein:** *lamb, ham, bacon, sausage, venison; duck; sea bass*

**Dairy:** *milk (2%, goat's), nonfat yogurt (mandarin orange, strawberry/banana), regular or low-fat yogurt (vanilla), most ice creams*

**Nuts and Seeds:** *roasted cashews, cashew butter, peanut butter, sesame seed butter*

**Grains:** *barley, millet, polished rice, wheat crackers, whole wheat breads*

**Vegetables:** *cooked cabbage, raw onions*

**Vegetable Juices:** *beet*

**Fruits:** *grapefruit (red, white), grapes (black, green, red), oranges, plums (black, purple, red), strawberries*

**Fruit Juices:** *grape (purple, red, white), orange/grapefruit/tangerine*

**Vegetable Oils:** *canola, peanut*

**Sweeteners:** *saccharin, aspartame, Equal, NutraSweet, Sweet'n Low*

**Condiments:** *mayonnaise, margarine*

**Desserts:** *chocolate, desserts containing chocolate*

**Beverages:** *sake, beer, barley malt liquor, champagne, gin, scotch, vodka, whiskey, margaritas, regular Pepsi, diet Pepsi, diet Coke*

## Scheduling Meals

Balanced body types should avoid heavy meals. If sensitive, avoid fruit with lunch or dinner. Schedule your meals as follows:

*Breakfast:* 7–8 A.M. light to moderate, with grain and/or fruit, vegetables, dairy, nuts, and/or seeds. Emphasize carbohydrates, with moderate fats.

*Lunch:* 12–2 P.M. moderate, with protein, grain, vegetables, and/or dairy. Emphasize protein. Avoid fruit.

*Dinner:* 7–9 P.M. moderate, with grain, vegetables, legumes, protein, and/or dairy. Emphasize grain and vegetables. Avoid fruit.

### Snacks (optional)

*Midmorning:* grain, vegetables, fruit

*Midafternoon:* protein, vegetables, grain, nuts

*Evening* (10 P.M.–2 A.M.): vegetables, fruit, seeds, grain, sweets

## Sample One-Week Menu

DAY 1

*Breakfast:* omelette w/cheese, spinach, mushrooms, and onions

*Lunch:* roasted chicken breast and baby green salad

*Dinner:* turkey, pasta, and kale

*Snack:* mixed nuts (peanuts, almonds, walnuts, pecans, and cashews)

DAY 2

*Breakfast:* sweet potato or yam w/butter

*Lunch:* pot roast, potatoes, onions, garlic, carrots, and celery

*Dinner:* fish and cabbage

DAY 3

*Breakfast:* egg foo yung w/grated carrots, zucchini, and bean sprouts

*Lunch:* ahi tuna steak, asparagus, and basmati rice

*Dinner:* tri color salad—beet, watercress, carrots—and sunflower sesame rissoles

DAY 4

*Breakfast:* eggs, broccoli, and onions

*Lunch:* roasted chicken (white), mashed potatoes, spinach and tomato salad with creamy Italian dressing

*Dinner:* spaghetti and meatballs

DAY 5: CLEANSE

*Breakfast:* juice of lemon in water; baked potato and/or steamed broccoli

*Lunch:* soaked raw almonds

*Snack:* raw broccoflower and cauliflower and/or steamed brussels sprouts; and/or juice of celery, carrot, carrot/celery, carrot/celery/parsley, parsley, greens

*Dinner:* steamed asparagus

*Snack:* carrots or carrot juice

*Bedtime:* juice of lemon in water

DAY 6

*Breakfast:* blueberry muffin and apple

*Lunch:* fillet of salmon, polenta, and a salad of jicama, cucumber, and tomato

*Dinner:* tuna, avocado, and a salad of romaine lettuce, tomato, red bell pepper, carrots, and sprouts w/balsamic vinegar

DAY 7

*Breakfast:* oatmeal w/butter, banana, and raspberries

*Lunch:* Cornish game hen, green beans, and sweet potato or yam w/butter

*Dinner:* lentil soup and potato

## Alternative Menus

*(Foods in parentheses are optional.)*

### Breakfast

Eggs fried in butter, with rice and avocado (Braggs Liquid Aminos)

Scrambled tofu and Kashi

Croissant and smoked salmon

Granola w/fruit and nuts and milk

Grape-Nuts w/banana and soy milk

Puffed wheat w/banana, berries, and soy milk

Bagel w/smoked salmon (capers, cream cheese, and tomato)

### Lunch

Tuna fillet, broccoli, carrots, and red potatoes w/butter

Meat loaf, mashed potatoes w/gravy, and mixed vegetables such as carrots and peas

Jicama, cabbage, and fish

Potatoes and bread w/butter

Salad of chicken, romaine lettuce, tomatoes, alfalfa sprouts, and avocado w/vinaigrette dressing

Porterhouse steak, baked potato w/butter, and asparagus

Roasted chicken breast on salad of baby greens, peas, and tomatoes w/poppy seed dressing, and corn bread w/butter

Omelette w/ground turkey, spinach, black olives, mushrooms, and shredded Monterey Jack cheese

### Lunch or Dinner

Lobster, asparagus, and brown rice w/mushrooms

Turkey, mashed potatoes, and asparagus

### Dinner

Vegetable soup

Baked potato and green beans

Chicken salad

Caesar salad w/chicken breast

Vegetable burrito (beans)

Chicken stir-fry and rice

Chicken livers, parsleyed potatoes, and pickled beet salad

Lentil soup w/chicken and corn bread

Split pea soup, meat loaf, and cauliflower

# Blood

*The Blood body type is symbolized by a drop of blood. Blood maintains harmony by carrying oxygen and nutrients and by removing wastes. Greatly affected by emotional and environmental stress, this body type will go to great lengths to maintain harmony.*

FAMOUS PEOPLE: Jack Nicholson, Phylicia Rashad, Tiger Woods, Roma Downey

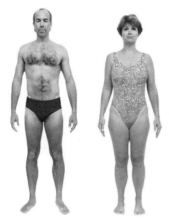

## BLOOD
### Location and Function

Blood is located throughout the body, circulating through the heart, arteries, capillaries, and veins. Blood essentially serves as a transport mechanism. It consists of plasma, red blood cells (which specifically carry oxygen and nutrients to cells throughout the body), white blood cells (designed to fight infection), and platelets.

## Psychological Profile

### Characteristic Traits

Easygoing and personable, Blood body types are social beings whose basic nature is warm, receptive, and nurturing. Sensitive and considerate, they have a genuine concern for others, particularly those who aren't able to speak out on their own behalf. They are intensely drawn to the young, the old or disabled, animals, and to nature.

With their strong desire to experience life, Blood body types are generally open-minded and willing to try new things, including the unorthodox. Internally driven to find a meaning in life, they often study a subject in depth and become so immersed in it that other things get ignored or forgotten. They may even concentrate so much on individual details that they temporarily lose sight of the whole. However, being practical and flexible, once they have experienced it, they let go of what isn't right for them and keep what works.

While Blood body types are supported by social interaction and contact, they are highly task oriented, self-motivated, and responsible. When they commit to a project, they make it their main focus, getting it done well with utmost efficiency. They can even be so meticulous as to border on the obsessive/compulsive. In their efforts to understand something, they do much analyzing and processing of events and situations.

### Motivation

Harmony is of utmost importance to Blood body types, and they will do almost anything to achieve and maintain it. All too often they compromise long-term harmony for short-term peace, choosing to suppress their feelings rather than confront conflict. When they do find the courage to speak up, if things are not resolved, they will deny the existence of the problem in order to maintain the appearance of calm. Unfortunately, unresolved conflict eventually undermines their inner tranquillity and sense of well-being, preventing them from experiencing true harmony. Suppressing unresolved conflict causes stress and tension to be turned inward and causes physical problems (more so than with any of the other types).

When unable to deal with a situation or process feelings, the tendency of Blood body types is to deny them or to stop expressing them, denying parts of themselves. Unfortunately, these blocked emotions—

especially those stemming from anger or confrontation—back up in the veins and arteries of the body, particularly around the heart, and eventually result in coronary heart disease.

Respect is a motivating factor for Blood body types—respect for themselves and respect for others as well as respect from others. Self-respect can be a challenge for Blood body types, as they are often torn between being true to themselves and giving others what they want in order to maintain harmony. Often raised in a family where they were not allowed to express anger, many learned that they needed to repress parts of themselves to get their needs met.

Valuing outside appearances, Bloods may try to please by overcommitting physically, financially, or emotionally. They need social approval, and the world's perception of them is extremely important, so making a favorable impression on others is essential. Consequently their outward presentation is generally cordial and obliging—even when their true feelings are less so. Harmony is not only essential in their emotional world but in their physical world as well. Having things in their life clear, ordered, and balanced provides them with a sense of security and well-being.

## "At Worst"

Highly emotional, Blood body types may react without knowing why, experiencing feelings but being unable to grasp their basis mentally. Unable to verbalize logically, they often express their feelings through tears. Crying is a way of dissipating or shutting off feelings. Frequently there is underlying anger, hurt, or sadness. When fear sets in they can become paranoid, anxious, compulsive, overly emotional, unreasonable, irritable, critical, and short-tempered.

Blood body types often refuse to take personal responsibility for their feelings. They may react in a childlike fashion by letting their feelings be easily hurt and then turning the hurt into inappropriate anger. They can get into an "I don't care" or "Whatever you do is not enough" attitude.

Blood body types have a tendency to "stuff" their emotions (later to be expressed through the body) and lose confidence in themselves. Unwilling to stand up in the world, they can become codependent in relationships, living off someone else and stifling their own identity. A common defense is drinking, as alcohol numbs the emotions and creates isolation.

Having a plan gives Blood body types a sense of mental security. This can cause them to be obsessive about details, such as time schedules, with no flexibility. They want to know the rules and what to expect. They may start out being very accommodating and in complete agreement with the plan for the day or trip, but if things don't go the way they planned, particularly when things take longer than expected, they can become irritable, nitpicky, demanding, impatient, paranoid, emotional, and unreasonable.

## "At Best"

At their best, Blood body types recognize that true harmony can only exist when there is complete inner harmony. By discovering what is true for them, they can know, honor, and respect themselves and achieve the spiritual harmony they need. True integration occurs when they are able to move their energy from the emotional to the spiritual to the mental and express it physically. Being in harmony provides a sense of security that allows them to experience genuine happiness and freedom.

Positive and easygoing, Blood body types maintain harmony by spreading optimism and encouragement throughout their sphere of influence. With their ability to "read" others and their good sense of humor, it's easy for them to make others feel at ease. Having superior social skills, they're one of the most companionable of all the body types. More than socially adaptive, they contribute to the cohesiveness of the group while also tending to the needs of individual members. Sensitive to others' feelings and genuinely interested in helping others, they are at their best when they can express their well-developed humanitarian impulses.

When Blood body types learn to confront their anger by getting in touch with their feelings, they are able to communicate in a calm, loving fashion. Once they are able to let go of their anger, the universe supports

### RECOMMENDED EXERCISE

The most significant benefit of exercise for Blood body types is emotional. Exercise provides a means of clearing the mind and releasing emotional stress. Moderate exercise is beneficial in losing or maintaining weight as well as improving vascular integrity. Heavy exercise is often contraindicated. Ideal activities include swimming, rebounding, walking, bicycling, and dancing.

them. By "letting go and letting God," by trusting their own inner knowledge, and by being true to themselves, they are able to be the true peacemakers on earth.

## Dietary Profile

### Main Focus

- Have protein, principally at lunch.
- Eat vegetables and grains, particularly at dinner.
- May include fruit for breakfast but not with lunch or dinner.
- Clear emotional stress.

### Dietary Emphasis

- From 20 to 30 percent of your calories are to come from fats.
- Best fat sources: avocados, chicken, fish, cheese, and pumpkin seeds.
- From 20 to 35 percent of your calories are to come from protein, primarily at lunch.
- From 5 to 35 percent of your calories are to come from dense protein (includes fish).
- Best sources of the three amino acids threonine, isoleucine, and cystine: chicken, sesame and sunflower seeds.
- Caloric intake: 1,500 to 1,800 calories a day for women and 1,700 to 2,000 calories a day for men. If you are engaging in intense exercise (competition type) or heavy labor, increase calories.
- Drink a minimum of 64 ounces of water a day. Drink water before and after meals, not with meals.
- To rebuild body, focus on protein, particularly chicken and fish with vegetables.
- Occasional desserts are best as an evening snack.
- Avoid eating potato or squash with dense protein.
- Broth soups are easy to digest; use low sodium.
- Consume a minimum of 4 ounces of dense protein 3 times a week.
- Generally, Blood body types experience fatigue when not consuming enough protein.
- The following foods support the body only when eaten in these combinations:
    Eggs and Swiss cheese
    Beef and eggs
    Beef and rice
    Ham and tomato
    The above combinations should be consumed no more than once a week. Other foods may be added to these combinations.

### RECOMMENDED CUISINE

Blood body types benefit from pasta dishes, including fish and pasta combinations. Enjoy Italian, Mexican, Chinese, soup, and salad.

- Turkey w/celery, mustard, or bacon may be consumed up to 5 times a week.

### For Weight Loss

- Eliminate all dairy (except butter), including cheese, yogurt, and milk.
- If fats from ideal sources fall below 15 percent of calories, weight loss will be hindered.
- Reduce breads.
- Avoid vegetable oils.
- Avoid mayonnaise; may use creamy Italian dressing as a substitute.

### For Weight Gain

- Include dairy.
- Increase quantity of food.

## Healthy Foods List

There is no need to sacrifice delicious and filling foods to maintain a healthy Blood body type. The following lists will help you focus on foods that support your health, and avoid foods that can stress your system.

*You'll notice that some foods are printed in italics; these foods take more energy to assimilate and could be ones you avoid when you are in a sensitive state due to any physical or emotional stresses.*

Be sure to read Chapter 3, "Implementing the Body Type Diet," for lots of important information about how to use these many foods to gain their full benefit.

### Ultra-Support Foods

Foods to include in 3 to 7 meals a week, listed by category.

**Dense Protein:** buffalo, *lamb;* chicken, chicken broth, chicken livers, Cornish game hen, turkey; *anchovy,* bass, bonita, catfish, cod, flounder, haddock, halibut, herring, mackerel, mahimahi, perch, red snapper, roughy, salmon, sardines, shark, swordfish, trout; clams, eel, *mussels,* octopus

**Dairy:** *goat milk,* sweet cream, sour cream, kefir

**Cheese:** Camembert, cream, goat, Parmesan, Romano

**Nuts and Seeds:** almonds (raw, roasted), coconut, macadamias (raw, roasted), peanuts (raw, dry-roasted), pine nuts (raw, roasted), pistachios; pumpkin seeds (raw, roasted)

**Grains:** popcorn, rice (white or brown basmati)

**Vegetables:** avocados, celery, eggplant, garlic, parsley, spinach

**Fruits:** melons (cantaloupe, watermelon), raisins

**Condiments:** *tahini*

**Sweeteners:** stevia

**Beverages:** black tea

## Basic Support Foods

Foods to include in 1 to 2 meals a week.

**Dense Protein:** beef liver, beef broth, bacon, pork, ham, sausage, veal, *venison,* organ meats (heart, brain); duck; sole, tuna; abalone, calamari (squid), crab, lobster, oysters, scallops, *shrimp; eggs*

**Dairy:** *buttermilk, plain or flavored yogurt,* frozen yogurt, ice cream (Ben & Jerry's, Breyers, Dreyer's), butter

**Cheese:** American, blue, Brie, *Colby,* cottage, Edam, *feta,* Gouda, kefir, Limburger, Monterey Jack, *mozzarella,* Muenster, ricotta, Swiss

**Nuts and Seeds:** *almond butter,* Brazils, cashews (raw, roasted), *cashew butter, hazelnuts, macadamia butter,* peanuts (roasted, salted), *peanut butter, pecans,* walnuts (black, English), *water chestnuts;* raw or roasted seeds (caraway, sesame, sunflower), sesame seed butter, sunflower seed butter

**Legumes:** beans (adzuki, black, garbanzo, Great Northern, kidney, lima, navy, pinto, red, soy), lentils, black-eyed peas, split peas; hummus; miso, soy milk, tofu

**Grains:** amaranth, barley, buckwheat, *corn, corn grits, corn tortillas,* couscous, *hominy grits,* millet, oats, quinoa, rice (long or short grain brown, Japanese, wild), rice bran, rice cakes, rye, triticale, whole wheat, wheat bran, wheat germ, refined wheat flour, flour tortillas, breads (*corn, corn/rye, French, garlic, Italian, multigrain, oat, rice, rye, seven-grain, sourdough, sprouted grain, white,* whole wheat), *bagels, croissants, English muffins, crackers* (oat, rye, saltines, wheat), pasta, Chinese rice noodles, udon noodles, cream of rice, cream of rye, cream of wheat

**Vegetables:** artichokes, asparagus, bamboo shoots, beans (green, yellow wax), beets, bok choy, *broccoflower,* broccoli, brussels sprouts, cabbage (green, napa, red), carrots, cauliflower, cilantro, corn, cucumbers, greens (beet, collard, mustard, turnip), *hominy,* jicama, kale, kohlrabi, leeks, lettuce (Boston, butter, endive, *iceberg,* red leaf, romaine), mushrooms, okra, olives (green, ripe), onions (chives, brown, green, red, Vidalia, white), parsnips, peas, snow pea pods, bell peppers (green, red, yellow), chili peppers, pimientos, potatoes (purple, red, russet, White Rose, Yukon Gold), pumpkin, *radishes,* daikon radishes, rutabaga, seaweed (arame, dulse, kelp, nori, wakame), sauerkraut, shallots, sprouts (alfalfa, clover, mung bean, radish, sunflower), squash (acorn, banana, butternut, spaghetti, yellow [summer], zucchini), sweet potatoes, *Swiss chard,* tomatoes (canned, vine-ripened), turnips, watercress, yams

**Vegetable Juices:** carrot, carrot/celery, celery, tomato, V-8

**Fruits:** apples (Golden or Red Delicious, Granny Smith, Jonathan, Pippin, McIntosh, Rome Beauty), apricots, *bananas,* berries (blackberries, blueberries, boysenberries, cranberries, gooseberries, raspberries), cherries, dates, figs (fresh, dried), grapes (black, green, red), grapefruit (red, white), guavas, kiwi, kumquats, lemons, *limes,* loquats, mangoes, *nectarines, oranges,* papayas, peaches, pears, *persimmons,* pineapples, pomegranates, plums (black, purple, red), *prunes,* rhubarb, tangelos, *tangerines*

**Fruit Juices:** *apple,* apple cider, apple/apricot, apricot, black cherry, red cherry, cranapple, cranberry, grape (purple, red, white), *grapefruit,* guava, lemon, orange, papaya, pear, pineapple, pineapple/coconut, prune, *tangerine,* watermelon

**Vegetable Oils:** all-blend, *almond,* avocado, coconut, *corn, peanut, flaxseed, sesame, sunflower*

**Sweeteners:** *fructose,* molasses, *sorghum, sugar* (*brown, raw*), syrup (barley malt, brown rice, corn), *succonant*

**Condiments:** *catsup, mustard, horseradish,* green chilies, *barbecue sauce, pesto sauce, soy sauce,* salsa, *margarine,* vinegar, ginger, lemon pepper, salt, sea salt, Vege-sal, *MSG*

**Salad Dressings:** *blue cheese, French, ranch, creamy Italian, creamy avocado, Thousand Island,* vinegar and oil, lemon juice and oil

**Desserts:** *custards, tapioca, puddings, pies, cakes, chocolate, desserts containing chocolate, sherbet (orange, raspberry)*

**Chips:** *bean, blue corn, potato*

**Beverages:** decaf coffee, Swiss mocha; tea (green, herbal [mint, raspberry], Japanese, Chinese oolong); plain or flavored mineral water; *white wine (chardonnay or zinfandel), champagne;* tonic water w/lime

## Stressful Foods

Have no more than once a month.

**Dense Protein:** *beef*

**Dairy:** *milk (whole, 2%, low fat, nonfat, raw), half-and-half, most ice creams*

**Cheese:** *cheddar*

**Nuts and Seeds:** *trail mix*

**Grains:** *polished rice*

**Vegetables:** *arugula, hothouse tomatoes*

**Vegetable Juices:** *parsley, spinach*

**Fruits:** *melons (casaba, Crenshaw, honeydew), strawberries*

**Vegetable Oils:** *canola, olive, safflower, soy*

**Sweeteners:** *honey, sugar (date, refined cane), maple syrup, saccharin, aspartame, Equal, NutraSweet, Sweet'n Low*

**Condiments:** *mayonnaise*

**Chips:** *corn (white, yellow)*

**Beverages:** *regular coffee; carbonated sparkling water; red wine, sherry, sake, liqueurs, beer, barley malt liquor, gin, scotch, vodka, whiskey,* margaritas; *sodas (diet, regular)*

**Other:** *salty and fried foods*

## Scheduling Meals

### Healthy

Schedule your meals as follows:

*Breakfast:* 7–9 A.M. Light to moderate, with vegetables, protein, dairy, grain, and/or fruit.

*Lunch:* 12–2 P.M. Moderate to heavy, with protein, nuts, seeds, grain, and/or vegetables. Avoid fruit.

*Dinner:* 6–9 P.M. Moderate, with protein, nuts, seeds, dairy, grain, legumes, and/or vegetables. Emphasize carbohydrates. Avoid fruit.

### Snacks (optional)

*Midmorning:* fruit, vegetables, grain, nuts, and seeds

*Afternoon or anytime:* dairy, nuts, seeds, grains, legumes, vegetables

*Evening* (10 P.M.–2 A.M.): dairy, nuts, seeds, grain, vegetables, fruit, sweets, desserts

### Sensitive

Limit lunch and dinner to protein and/or grain.

*Breakfast:* Light to moderate, with vegetables, protein, dairy, grain, and/or fruit.

*Lunch:* Moderate to heavy, with protein and/or grain.

*Dinner:* Light to moderate, with protein and/or grain.

## Sample One-Week Menu

DAY 1
*Breakfast:* cantaloupe
*Lunch:* chicken breast, green beans, and onion
*Dinner:* orange roughy, mushrooms, and pasta

DAY 2
*Breakfast:* bagel and cream cheese, orange juice, and herbal tea such as lemon/ginger
*Lunch:* shrimp or seafood rice bowl
*Dinner:* pasta primavera and a salad of romaine lettuce, carrots, and red onion w/balsamic vinegar and grape seed oil

DAY 3
*Breakfast:* dates and cream cheese
*Lunch:* roasted turkey w/garlic and a salad of celery and cucumber slices
*Dinner:* baked potato, mushrooms, and steamed zucchini

DAY 4
*Breakfast:* oatmeal w/sunflower seeds
*Lunch:* sesame chicken (rice)
*Dinner:* salmon ravioli and a spinach salad

DAY 5: CLEANSE
*Breakfast:* cantaloupe or papaya
*Lunch:* raw bell pepper or spinach (w/avocados);

steamed artichoke, asparagus, broccoli, and zucchini and/or carrot/celery (spinach) juice

*Dinner:* soaked raw almonds and/or pumpkin seeds w/steamed artichoke or asparagus and/or raw bell pepper and/or carrot/celery/spinach juice

## DAY 6

*Breakfast:* baked potato w/salsa or chives

*Lunch:* kabobs of lamb, onions, and bell peppers w/tahini dressing

*Dinner:* angel-hair pasta w/Thai spices and vegetables, such as broccoli, red peppers, onions, and/or mushrooms

## DAY 7

*Breakfast:* sesame bagel and avocado

*Lunch:* roast beef, Yorkshire pudding, broccoli, and cauliflower

*Dinner:* vegetable rice soup or minestrone soup

## Alternative Menus

*(Foods in parentheses may be omitted.)*

### Breakfast

Papaya

Watermelon

Carrot/celery (beet) juice

Oatmeal w/raisins

Oat bran muffin (herbal tea, such as spice, mint, orange, or peppermint)

Eggs, Swiss cheese, and ham

Egg and Swiss cheese omelette

Beef, eggs, and fruit or toast

Omelette w/mushrooms, Swiss cheese, and onions (green chilies and salsa, shrimp or crab)

### Lunch

Calamari, rice, and broccoli

Chicken and rice w/peas

Steamed clams and a spinach and avocado salad

Spinach quiche and ham (cheese)

Chicken and a salad of lettuce, avocado, and celery w/creamy Italian dressing

Open taco w/black beans, rice, and lettuce

*Carne asada* (beef) burrito and rice

Turkey, mustard, and lettuce on sourdough bread

Fish and pasta

Clam linguini

Tuna on tomato or green salad

Chicken, mushrooms, and broccoli (rice)

Chef salad w/turkey, celery, and bell peppers

### Dinner

Tuna or swordfish and green beans w/slivered almonds

Sautéed chicken and basmati rice w/garlic, onions, carrots, and pumpkin seeds

Couscous and steamed vegetables

Chicken, boiled red potatoes, peas, and carrots

Red potatoes w/parsley, tomatoes, and zucchini (onions)

Baked potato w/plain yogurt and a green salad of red leaf lettuce, avocados, celery, and clover sprouts w/lemon juice and canola oil dressing

Rice bowl of short grain white rice, teriyaki chicken, broccoli, carrots, bok choy, and celery w/soy sauce

Mahimahi, steamed rice, carrots, and zucchini

Chicken, pasta, and eggplant or a spinach salad

Lamb chops, wild rice, and broccoli

Rice and broccoli (spinach)

Turkey, basmati and/or wild rice, and celery (spinach salad)

# Brain

*The Brain body type is symbolized by a computer. Meticulously collecting and storing data for ready access, Brain body types like to have all the information before making a decision. With a strong desire to do everything right, they are extremely precise in their speech and actions.*

FAMOUS PEOPLE: Jerry Seinfeld, Meryl Streep, Andre Agassi, Uma Thurman

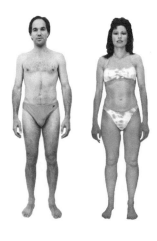

## BRAIN
### Location and Function

The brain is nervous tissue within the skull or cranium. It includes the cerebrum, cerebellum, and pons. It controls and directs the activities of the mind and body.

## Psychological Profile
### Characteristic Traits

Mentally oriented, Brain body types are most comfortable when they have all the information available before they make a decision. Inclined to precision, they apply themselves conscientiously to whatever they undertake. Typically self-directed and independent, they can be quite diligent and persevering in carrying out projects. Brain types tend to think in ways less conventional and more creative than most other types and are quite analytical. They enjoy investigating a variety of topics and do so with resourcefulness and a lively curiosity. Sensitive and intuitive as well, Brain types are comfortable dealing with abstract and conceptual realities. Their personal identity is often associated with their career, and academic recognition often provides the desired type of status in society.

Brains usually have a strong drive to find the meaning of life and specifically their personal direction. Their reason for being here may take the form of needing to feel they are needed, being involved in a worthwhile project, doing something that offers a mental challenge, or feeling their skills are well utilized in their job or career.

It is extremely important for Brain types to do things right. They are not comfortable unless they can function at the highest possible level. Consequently, before accepting any new theory or development, they want to make sure it is scientifically proven, with sufficient reasons, explanations, and facts to support it.

### Motivation

Brains are overly concerned with the possibility of making mistakes or appearing stupid. Consequently they are thorough, meticulous, hardworking, and completely honest, with a great desire for accuracy. Brain types may belabor their points, assuming that otherwise people won't listen or won't understand them or that they'll be perceived as naive or even stupid. By being verbose, they can seem cold and hard, without warmth. While their intention is not to be antagonistic, their mode of delivery often comes across as such. In reality they are generally nice people who have a genuine concern for others and are usually very sweet and endearing.

Soft-spoken and not wanting to make waves, Brain types prefer to avoid conflict, which tends to upset their rather delicate equilibrium. Basically sensitive and often somewhat shy or timid, they usually acquiesce with the ideas of those around them. They may even withhold certain negative or disturbing communications because of their desire to please others or win approval. Their apprehension about the possibility of doing something wrong can sometimes cause them to be passive or indecisive. While they prefer to handle life in a harmonious manner, they can be quite tenacious when it comes to getting what they want.

Generally self-contained, with active minds, they are perfectly content to stay at home or in their ivory tower research centers. To feel safe, they gather as much information as they can. They have a tendency to spend too much time thinking about concepts and not enough time applying them, which results in a thwarting of their basic need to produce tangible results.

## "At Worst"

Brain types can become extremely rigid, locked into their own belief structures, with a bias against anything new or different and with a "Prove it to me" attitude. They may intellectualize too much, needing to know every detail about something before making a decision, which others can find extremely annoying. Their excessive mental activity may cause them to get lost in details and lose sight of the whole picture. They can easily get sidetracked by distractions or withdraw into their own world.

Brain types can become mentally defiant to the extent that the mental realm becomes an arena for challenge or opposition. An example is insisting that everything have scientific, documentable proof. They tend to reject anything that doesn't fit into their reality, rather than accept or allow other realities to coexist. Their initial attitude toward anything that is not their idea is negative, pessimistic, and cynical. They use the mental arena to compensate for their basic underlying insecurities.

Easily stressed by mental or emotional upsets, once exhausted they go "brain-dead" and are unable to make the simplest decision. Their fear of being wrong and appearing stupid or doing something wrong immobilizes them. Wary of taking risks, they shy away from new adventures and experiences. They can easily stay too long in the ordinary and wind up feeling dissatisfied. Unless they have outside support and encouragement, their fear of failure makes it difficult for them to make needed changes.

It's easy for Brain types to get spaced out and lose touch with practical reality. Their perceived lack of self-worth leads to perfectionism and compulsive aloofness. Depression is common, as is playing the role of the victim, and constantly asking why. With low self-esteem, it's easy for them to get caught in a feeling of hopelessness and become addicted to food, alcohol, drugs, or codependent relationships. Their feelings of insecurity and self-doubt can keep them distanced from the physical and social worlds, causing them to miss out on opportunities that would give them their sense of direction.

## "At Best"

Intuitive, sensitive, and empathic, Brain types can be very effective in working with people. Because they typically use language with precision, they can be outstanding communicators and frequently excel in the teaching and counseling fields. In addition to being good at transmitting knowledge, they are also able to guide others in finding self-knowledge. With their innate patience, perseverance, and tenacity, Brain types can effectively apply themselves and resolve the most intricate problems.

Gifted with the ability to tune in to the needs of those around them, Brain types are able to use this sensitivity and understanding to guide others in productive ways. They have good minds and can be very focused, able to take the information they receive and articulate it carefully and precisely. Insightful and inventive, they're often able to explain things so that they make sense to others, helping them see what had previously been cloudy or confusing. They are a lot of fun, supportive of others, and willing to be out in front.

Intuitive and practical, Brain types can take the information they receive and distill it into a tangible form. They are likely to excel in academics and pursuits that appeal to their inquiring nature. They are

---

### RECOMMENDED EXERCISE

Exercise is physically beneficial for Brain body types. It's essential to move to get energy from the head distributed throughout the body. Dance, aerobics, tennis, walking, biking, and moderate weight training are good basics. It's important for Brain types to connect their feelings to their intellect, so exercise needs to be fun or nurturing, such as getting up early and going for a meditative walk.

often found among distinguished researchers and scientists. Though especially good at abstract analysis, they can also be quite imaginative and artistic. Recognizing the power that the mind has in controlling their lives, they maintain a positive attitude. Once Brain types are clear about who they are and what they want, they have the direction they need to be successful, both professionally and socially.

## Dietary Profile

### Main Focus

- Make lunch the largest meal.
- Smaller meals are supportive and may include snacks.
- Have no protein before 11 A.M.
- Tofu is an excellent protein source.
- Eat grains and fruit for breakfast (not fruit alone).

### Dietary Emphasis

- From 20 to 30 percent of your calories are to come from fats.
- Best fat sources: pistachios, pecans, sunflower seeds, olive oil, eggs, chicken, turkey, and dairy (including yogurt and cottage cheese).
- From 25 to 35 percent of your calories are to come from protein.
- From 0 to 25 percent of your calories are to come from dense protein.
- Best sources of the three amino acids threonine, isoleucine, and cystine: turkey, clams, and beef.
- Caloric intake: 1,500 to 1,800 calories a day for women and 1,700 to 2,000 calories a day for men. If you are engaging in intense exercise (competition type) or heavy labor, increase calories.
- Drink a minimum of 64 ounces of water per day. Drink water before and after meals, not with meals.
- Parsley assists kidneys.
- Use soy sauce in place of salt.
- Occasional desserts are best as an evening snack.

### For Weight Loss

- Limit dense protein and bread.
- Ideal meal schedule is 10 A.M. for breakfast, 2 P.M. for lunch, and between 6 and 7 P.M. for dinner.
- Problem of weight loss is largely mental. You need to get a mind-set about being thin.

### RECOMMENDED CUISINE

Thai, soup and salad bars, Japanese, Italian, Greek, Mexican. Rarely: fast foods, French.

### For Weight Gain

- Increase food quantity.

### Sensitive

- May add vegetables or yogurt to fruit and grain for breakfast.
- Eliminate dense protein, nuts, seeds, and/or dairy at dinner.

## Healthy Foods List

There is no need to sacrifice delicious and filling foods to maintain a healthy Brain body type. The following lists will help you focus on foods that support your health and avoid foods that can stress your system.

*You'll notice that some foods are printed in italics; these foods take more energy to assimilate and could be ones you will want to avoid when you are in a sensitive state due to any physical or emotional stresses.*

Be sure to read Chapter 3, "Implementing the Body Type Diet," for lots of important information about how to use these many foods to gain their full benefit.

### Ultra-Support Foods

Foods to include in 3 to 7 meals a week, listed by category.

**Dense Protein:** beef broth, beef liver; chicken broth, chemical-free turkey; anchovy, bass, bonita, catfish, cod, flounder, haddock, halibut, herring, mackerel, mahimahi, perch, orange roughy, salmon, sardines, shark, red snapper, sole, swordfish, trout; calamari (squid), clams, eel, lobster, mussels, octopus, oysters, scallops

**Dairy:** half-and-half, butter

**Cheese:** kefir, Limburger

**Legumes:** beans (adzuki, garbanzo, lima, pinto, red, soy), lentils, hummus, tofu

**Grains:** popcorn, brown or white basmati rice, English muffins, pasta
**Vegetables:** brussels sprouts, carrots, celery, red leaf lettuce, parsley, zucchini
**Fruits:** cooked apples, bananas, grapes (black, green, red), grapefruit (red, white), guavas, red plums, raspberries
**Fruit Juices:** apple/apricot, grape (purple, red, white)
**Sweeteners:** stevia
**Condiments:** soy sauce
**Beverages:** tea (mint, peppermint, Tension Tamer)

## Basic Support Foods

Foods to include in 1 to 2 meals a week.

**Dense Protein:** buffalo, *pork, bacon, ham, sausage, lamb,* veal, venison, organ meats (heart, brain); chemical-free chicken, chicken livers, Cornish game hen, duck; tuna (fresh or canned); abalone, crab, shrimp; eggs
**Dairy:** milk (*whole,* 2%, nonfat, *raw, goat's*), sweet cream, sour cream, kefir; yogurt (regular, low fat, nonfat, plain, or flavored), frozen yogurt with nuts, ice cream (Ben & Jerry's, Dreyer's)
**Cheese:** American, blue, Brie, Camembert, cheddar, *Colby,* cottage, cream, Edam, feta, goat, Gouda, *Monterey Jack, mozzarella,* Muenster, Parmesan, ricotta, Romano, Swiss
**Nuts and Seeds:** almonds (raw, roasted), almond butter, Brazils, cashews (raw, roasted), cashew butter, coconut, hazelnuts, macadamias (raw, roasted), macadamia butter, peanuts (raw, roasted), peanut butter, pecans, pine nuts (raw, roasted), pistachios, walnuts (black, English), water chestnuts; raw or roasted seeds (caraway, pumpkin, sesame, sunflower), sesame seed butter, sunflower seed butter
**Legumes:** beans (black, Great Northern, kidney), black-eyed peas, split peas; miso, soy milk
**Grains:** amaranth, barley, buckwheat, corn, corn grits, corn tortillas, couscous, hominy, millet, oats, quinoa, rice (long or short grain brown, Japanese, wild), rice bran, rice cakes, rye, triticale, refined wheat flour, whole wheat, wheat bran, wheat germ, flour tortillas, breads (corn, corn/rye, French, garlic, Italian, multigrain, oat, rice, rye, sourdough, sprouted grain, white, whole wheat), bagels, croissants, crackers (oat, rye, saltines, wheat), udon noodles, Chinese rice noodles, whole wheat noodles, cream of rice, cream of rye, cream of wheat

**Vegetables:** artichoke, arugula, *asparagus,* avocados, bamboo shoots, beans (green, yellow wax), beets, bok choy, broccoflower, broccoli, cabbage (green, napa, red), cauliflower, cilantro, corn, cucumbers, eggplant, garlic, greens (beet, collard, mustard, turnip), jicama, kale, kohlrabi, leeks, lettuce (Boston, butter, endive, iceberg, romaine), mushrooms, okra, olives (green, ripe), onions (chives, brown, green, red, Vidalia, white, yellow), parsnips, peas, snow pea pods, bell peppers (green, red, yellow), chili peppers, pimientos, *potatoes (all varieties),* pumpkin, radish, daikon radish, rutabaga, sauerkraut, seaweed (arame, dulse, kelp, nori, wakame), shallots, spinach, sprouts (alfalfa, clover, mung bean, radish, sunflower, wheat), squash (acorn, banana, butternut, yellow [summer], spaghetti), sweet potatoes, Swiss chard, tomatoes (canned, *hothouse, vine-ripened*), turnips, watercress, yams
**Vegetable Juices:** carrot, carrot/celery, celery, parsley, spinach, tomato, V-8
**Fruits:** *raw apples (all varieties),* apricots, berries (blackberries, blueberries, boysenberries, cranberries, gooseberries, strawberries), dates, figs (fresh, dried), kiwi, kumquats, lemons, limes, loquats, mangos, melons (cantaloupe, casaba, Crenshaw, honeydew, watermelon), nectarines, oranges, papayas, peaches, pears, persimmons, *pineapples,* plums (black, purple), pomegranates, prunes, raisins, rhubarb, tangelos, tangerines
**Fruit Juices:** apple, apple cider, apricot, black cherry, red cherry, cranapple, *cranberry,* grapefruit, guava, lemon, orange, papaya, pear, pineapple, pineapple/coconut, prune, tangerine, watermelon
**Vegetable Oils:** all-blend, *almond,* avocado, coconut, *corn,* olive, *peanut, flaxseed, safflower, sesame, soy,* sunflower
**Sweeteners:** *fructose, molasses, sorghum, sugar (brown, date, raw, refined cane),* syrup (barley malt, brown rice, *corn,* maple), *succonant*
**Condiments:** *horseradish, pesto sauce,* tahini, vinegar, sea salt, Vege-Sal
**Salad Dressings:** *blue cheese, French, ranch, creamy Italian, creamy avocado, Thousand Island,* vinegar and oil, lemon juice and oil
**Desserts:** *custards, tapioca, puddings, pies, cakes, sherbet (orange, raspberry)*
**Chips:** *bean,* corn (*blue,* white, yellow), *potato*
**Beverages:** *coffee;* tea (*black,* green, herbal, Japanese, Chinese oolong); mineral water, sparkling water; *wine (red, white), sake, beer, barley malt liquor,*

*sherry, liqueurs,* champagne, *gin, scotch, vodka, whiskey;* root beer, regular sodas, diet sodas

## Stressful Foods

Have no more than once a month.

**Dense Protein:** *beef; chemical-fed chicken, turkey*
**Dairy:** *buttermilk, frozen yogurt, most ice creams*
**Grains:** *polished rice*
**Fruits:** *cherries*
**Vegetable Oils:** *canola*
**Sweeteners:** *honey, saccharin, aspartame, Equal, NutraSweet, Sweet'n Low*
**Condiments:** *catsup, mustard, mayonnaise, salsa, barbecue sauce, margarine, salt*
**Desserts:** *chocolate, desserts containing chocolate*

## Scheduling Meals

### Healthy

Schedule your meals as follows:

*Breakfast:* 10 A.M. Light to moderate, with grain and fruit (not fruit alone). Protein after 11 A.M.
*Lunch:* 2 P.M. Moderate to heavy, with protein, nuts, seeds, dairy, legumes, grain, and/or vegetables.
*Dinner:* 6–7 P.M. Light to moderate, with protein, nuts, seeds, dairy, legumes, grain, vegetables, and/or fruit.

### Snacks (optional)

*Midmorning* (12 P.M.): fruits, vegetables
*Midafternoon:* grain, nuts, seeds, dairy, fruit, vegetables
*Evening:* dairy, nuts, seeds, grain, vegetables, fruit, sweets

### Sensitive

Adjust your intake as follows:

*Breakfast:* Light to moderate, with grain and fruit, vegetables, or yogurt and fruit. Avoid dense protein.
*Lunch:* Moderate to heavy, with protein, nuts, seeds, dairy, legumes, grain, and/or vegetables. Avoid fruit.
*Dinner:* Light to moderate, with grain, legumes, vegetables, and/or fruit.

## Sample One-Week Menu

Snacks are optional.

DAY 1
*Breakfast:* rice cereal cooked w/apple, cinnamon, and butter
*Lunch:* salmon teriyaki over red leaf lettuce, steamed zucchini
*Snack:* sunflower seeds
*Dinner:* braised tofu w/soy sauce baked in the oven w/chopped parsnips, brussels sprouts, and onions and a little olive oil or butter
*Snack:* celery w/cream cheese and olive chutney

DAY 2
*Breakfast:* yellow corn grits w/butter and bananas
*Lunch:* roasted (chemical-free) turkey and baked butternut squash w/cashews
*Dinner:* vegetable soup or clam chowder
*Snack:* yogurt w/pecans

DAY 3
*Breakfast:* shredded wheat w/grape juice
*Lunch:* halibut w/lemon garlic sauce, steamed artichoke w/lemon garlic sauce, and a Caesar salad
*Dinner:* carrots and celery w/hummus dip

DAY 4
*Breakfast:* buckwheat pancakes (made w/orange juice) and berries
*Lunch:* scallops sautéed in olive oil, baby squash, zucchini, onion, and mung bean sprouts
*Dinner:* spinach salad w/tofu
*Snack:* apple and cheese

DAY 5: CLEANSE
*Breakfast:* watermelon including seeds and white part of rind or raw carrots
*Snack:* watermelon
*Lunch:* raw bell pepper, celery, cucumbers, jicama and/or steamed asparagus, cauliflower, and/or juice, carrot/celery (parsley, spinach, tomato)
*Snack:* raw bell peppers (green, red, yellow), radishes, and/or steamed greenbeans and/or green or carrot/celery (parsley, spinach, tomato) juices
*Dinner:* watermelon or raw bell peppers, cucumbers, carrots, and/or steamed broccoli, cauliflower, onion
*Snack:* watermelon

DAY 6

*Breakfast:* whole wheat English muffin and baked apple w/cinnamon or apple butter

*Lunch:* salad of tuna and raw spinach, parsley, tofu, alfalfa, sunflower or wheat sprouts, raw carrots, broccoli, and kelp powder

*Snack:* pistachios

*Dinner:* lentils, rice, fresh tomatoes

DAY 7

*Breakfast:* granola w/apple juice

*Lunch:* turkey tenders (chemical free) sautéed w/butter, shiitake mushrooms, and Marsala wine, served over basmati rice

*Snack:* grapes

*Dinner:* vegetarian or beef chili

## Alternative Menus

*(Foods in parentheses are optional.)*

### Breakfast

Oatmeal and bananas

Oatmeal, apple, and pecans

Cream of wheat and cooked apples

Shredded wheat and rice milk (raisins and/or banana)

Waffles w/strawberries

Toasted English muffin w/strawberry jelly

Bagel and jam or banana

Plain yogurt w/strawberries, blueberries, orange, apple, or prunes

Baked White Rose or Yukon Gold potato w/butter

Spaghetti squash w/butter

### Lunch

Chemical-free turkey, rice, and broccoli

Chemical-free chicken, pinto beans, rice, and avocado

Cheddar cheese, corn or flour tortilla, and spinach salad w/olive oil and vinegar (radishes)

Brussels sprouts, tofu, and rice

Soybeans, broccoli, and cauliflower (plain yogurt)

Adzuki beans and corn or flour tortilla

Chicken vegetable soup—chicken, chicken broth, Swiss chard, carrots, celery, zucchini, and corn

### Lunch or Dinner

Chemical-free turkey, broccoli, cauliflower, zucchini, and carrots

Turkey loaf, corn, mashed or baked potato, and vegetable juice

Fish, rice, and corn on the cob

Lentils, rice, and yams (green beans or zucchini or carrots or brussels sprouts or salad)

Duck, yams, peas, zucchini, and broccoli

Chemical-free chicken, Spanish rice, pinto beans, and vegetable juice

Rice and eggs

Tofu, lettuce, cucumber, and carrots

Tofu, manicotti or lasagna, and zucchini

Hot and sour soup and stir-fried vegetables w/tofu, soy sauce, and rice

### Dinner

Lentils and steamed broccoli, cauliflower, and carrots

Rice, summer squash, and peas

Beans, rice, and brussels sprouts

Steamed carrots, onions, and lima beans

Brussels sprouts, tofu, and rice

# Eye

*The Eye body type is symbolized by an eye. Just as our eyes link us to our outer world, Eye body types link the world by implementing their visions. Witty and creative, they have the ability to see the good in even the bleakest situations.*

FAMOUS PEOPLE: Calista Flockhart, Patrick Stewart, Jessica Tandy, Will Smith

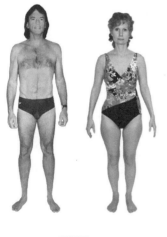

**EYE**
**Location and Function**

The eye is found in the bony orbits of the face. Its function is as an organ of vision (sight).

## Psychological Profile

### Characteristic Traits

As the main function of the eyes is to see, Eye body types are distinguished by their acute vision, both inner and outer. They access their inner vision through daydreaming or visualization, while externally they tend to see things that others don't notice. Besides discerning visual details, they pick up on subtle differences in voice and body language and even intuitive information. Often visionaries, they have a unique ability to see the big picture and the myriad of options available on a project they are involved in, or anything else that catches their eye.

While the basic nature of Eye types tends to be quiet, gentle, and controlled, underneath there's a witty, rebellious side just waiting to surface. Eye types have their own particular sense of humor, which is often described as being dry and a bit on the "far side." They can see the good in even the bleakest situations.

Eye types are intuitive, yet practical. Their ability to see is closely linked to an ability to bring their visions into practical reality. They are exceptionally adept with their hands and often find that their creativity comes through doing what they see needs to be done. Known for making things work, Eye types are also proficient in the realms of analysis and the abstract. The common thread of expertise between the practical and the theoretical is an eye for details and the ability to see how they connect to create a whole system. Eye types are both conscientious about the components and able to perceive the big picture.

### Motivation

Eye body types need personal experiences to integrate what they see into the physical world around them. Because they see the larger picture and are constantly looking for ways to make life better, they want to see their visions implemented. This leads them to wanting to do things differently or in their own way. It's their rebellious side that stimulates growth and motivates them to move out of their previous restrictions. Refusing to follow directions is a form of quiet rebellion that leads them to discover new ways of doing things. The question "Is there a better way?" evokes their creativity.

Being self-motivated and determined, Eye types often channel their creative energy through work. Applying themselves to a task for many hours at a time is quite normal for them, and they can show great perseverance in completing endeavors that are elaborate or complex. True to type, Eye types know that their projects are completed when they look right. While they derive satisfaction from seeing the fruits of their labor visually, to feel validated they need occasional reassurance. Because they can see all the little imperfections, a pat on the back helps them to focus on what is right and what they have already accomplished.

As a particularly sensitive type, Eye types often have problems dealing with elements of harshness in the world. In particular, issues of personal insecurity can cause difficulties relating to other people. Not knowing how to deal effectively with their negative emotions or feelings of vulnerability, Eye types internalize their emotions. This in turn leads to physical problems or illness. They may also feel empty and frustrated due to an inability to connect deeply and establish intimacy.

## "At Worst"

When stumped or overly stressed (generally from physical ailments, fatigue, or blocked emotions), Eye types become overwhelmed, sit in a daze, and wait to be rescued. Mentally exhausted, they are unable to see a way out of their dilemma. The problem looks too big, so working toward a solution seems hopeless, and they'll fall into a depression. Then they wait to be taken by the hand and led through a step-by-step solution, expecting constant approval and reassurance along the way.

Seeing multiple options, Eye types can get stuck in indecisiveness. Lacking confidence in their ability to pick the best course or to carry it out, they are reluctant to make a commitment to any single alternative. They may hold themselves back for lack of the courage of their convictions, or they may see what needs to be changed but feel the situation is hopeless. As a result, they often postpone taking action or making a decision for as long as possible, waiting to be pushed into it by something or someone else.

When they are unable to express what they see, their visual energy can turn inward, causing them to be short-sighted or stuck in limited viewpoints, seeing only one side of things rather than the whole picture. Then their tendency is to withdraw. Because this pattern is present during childhood, it can manifest itself physically through the need for glasses early on when children close down their sight to minimize seeing what they don't want to see. Closing down can cause

Eye types to retreat into the mental world, becoming too serious, rigid, and skeptical. If they get stuck in worry, they may escape into work, with an overemphasis on production as a means of gaining personal recognition, making them even more emotionally unavailable in their relationships.

## "At Best"

Able to see the big picture and all the available options, Eye types are also able to reach their goals effectively. They can sort through a profusion of details and figure out a variety of problems, and their ability to see more than one way of solving a problem can enable them to make decisions quickly and act upon them. Eye types are resourceful, flexible, and adaptable. Meticulous, persevering, logical, and strong on common sense, they are not afraid of hard work and are willing to do whatever it takes to accomplish what they set out to do.

Inner-directed, Eye types work well independently and often prefer to do so. Being intuitive as well as practical and efficient, they are able to see what needs changing, make the changes, and bring the project into being. They tend to be quite efficient and are able to get to the heart of the matter. They are manually adept and are usually able to figure out how to repair, fix, or build almost anything.

Sensitive and compassionate, Eye types are fair-minded, giving, and responsive to others. They're gifted in their ability to speak, to empower, and to demonstrate. When they trust in their intuitive guidance, they can be comfortable in the public eye, going where they need to go and doing what they are guided to do. The emotional fire to fulfill their desires

### RECOMMENDED EXERCISE

A minimum of 1 hour of exercise every other day is essential for Eye body types. This amount benefits all levels of health; it is particularly helpful in aiding digestion, maintaining mental clarity, and reducing stress. When stress is high, increase exercise to 4 to 6 times a week and include activities such as stomping and karate kicking to discharge anger held in the lower body. Other good exercise activities are free-style dancing, Callanetics, yoga, treadmill, water sports, skiing, in-line skating, walking, skipping, jumping rope, and biking.

comes through their passion about what they believe in. For Eye types, there is nothing more exhilarating than making a difference in the world, and particularly in the lives of those they encounter.

## Dietary Profile

### Main Focus

- Eat meals high in fat and with adequate dense protein.
- Variety and rotation of foods are essential.
- Trust your body and how it feels.
- Smaller meals with snacks are often helpful.
- Eat as many different foods as possible.

### Dietary Emphasis

- From 25 to 40 percent of your calories are to come from fats.
- Best fat sources: dense protein, butter, olive oil, avocado, nuts, and seeds.
- From 10 to 40 percent of your calories are to come from protein.
- From 10 to 40 percent of calories are to come from dense protein.
- Best sources of the three amino acids threonine, isoleucine, and cystine: clams, shrimp, lobster, and beef.
- Caloric intake: 1,500 to 1,800 calories a day for women and 1,700 to 2,000 calories a day for men. If you are engaging in intense exercise (competition type) or heavy labor, increase calories.
- Drink a minimum of 64 ounces of water a day. Drink water before and after meals, not with meals.
- Occasional desserts are best as an evening snack.
- Emphasize shellfish and foods high in vitamin A, including carrots, kelp, sweet potatoes, spinach, and yams.

### For Weight Loss

- Protein: 20 to 40 percent of daily calories.
- Dense protein: 20 to 35 percent of daily calories (includes fish).
- Avoid caffeine.
- Limit sugar, including fruit, fruit juice, fructose, and refined carbohydrates, to 2 times a week.
- Avoid all varieties of bread, especially whole wheat. If you must eat bread, sourdough is the best choice, but no more than 2 times a week.

### RECOMMENDED CUISINE

Seafood, Chinese, Japanese, Thai, Mexican, Italian, Greek, Indian (curry dishes), and standard American fare, both home-style cooking and highly seasoned, spicy foods. Focus on fish or meat and vegetables, chicken or meat and rice.

- Snacking is OK for weight loss; choose protein or dense protein as snacks, including cheese, nuts, and seeds.
- Minimize milk, yogurt, and ice cream.
- Reduce grains to 1 or 2 times a day.
- Potatoes may be included 5 to 7 times a week; choose different varieties.
- Have a heavy breakfast 4 to 5 times a week. Emphasize a large portion of dense protein with a variety of other foods.

### For Weight Gain

- Protein: 30 to 45 percent of daily calories.
- Dense protein: 30 to 40 percent of daily calories.
- Increase food quantities.
- Resolve any deep-seated emotional stress.

## Healthy Foods List

There is no need to sacrifice delicious and filling foods to maintain a healthy Eye body type. The following lists will help you focus on foods that support your health, and avoid foods that can stress your system.

*You'll notice that some foods are printed in italics; these foods take more energy to assimilate and could be ones you will want to avoid when you are in a sensitive state due to any physical or emotional stresses.*

Be sure to read Chapter 3, "Implementing the Body Type Diet," for lots of important information about how to use these many foods to gain their full benefit.

### Ultra-Support Foods

Foods to include in 3 to 7 meals a week, listed by category.

**Dense Protein:** beef, beef broth, beef liver, buffalo, lamb; chicken, chicken broth, chicken livers, Cornish game hen, turkey; anchovy, sea bass, cod, flounder, haddock, herring, mackerel, mahimahi, orange roughy, perch, smoked salmon, sardines, shark, red snapper, swordfish, trout; calamari (squid), eel, clams, lobster, mussels, octopus, oysters, scallops; eggs

**Dairy:** butter

**Cheese:** American, Brie, cheddar, Colby, cream, feta, Monterey Jack, mozzarella, Muenster, Parmesan, ricotta, Romano, Swiss

**Nuts and Seeds:** cashews (raw, roasted), cashew butter, hazelnuts, macadamias (raw, roasted), macadamia butter, pine nuts (raw, roasted), pistachios, water chestnuts; sesame seeds (raw, roasted), sesame seed butter

**Grains:** amaranth, buckwheat, rice (brown or white basmati, long or short grain brown, Japanese, wild), rice bran, rice cakes, refined wheat flour, white bread, yeastless wild rice spelt bread, Kavli crispbread, croissants, cream of rice, cream of rye

**Vegetables:** artichokes, avocados, bamboo shoots, beans (green, yellow wax), beets, bok choy, brussels sprouts, carrots, corn, greens (beet, collard, mustard, turnip), *eggplant,* jicama, kale, kohlrabi, leeks, mushrooms, okra, olives (green, ripe), onions (chives, green, red, Vidalia, white), parsley, peas, snow pea pods, pumpkin, rutabaga, scallions, seaweed (arame, dulse, kelp, nori, wakame), spinach, sprouts (alfalfa, clover, mung bean, radish, sunflower), acorn squash, sweet potatoes, Swiss chard, watercress, yams

**Fruits:** apples (Red or Golden Delicious, Granny Smith, Jonathan), berries (gooseberries, strawberries), grapes (black, green, red), guavas, kiwi, limes, mangoes, nectarines, papayas, pears, pineapples, pomegranates, prunes, tangelos, tangerines

**Fruit Juices:** black cherry, grapefruit, papaya

**Vegetable Oils:** *flaxseed,* sesame

**Sweeteners:** *honey, maple syrup,* stevia

**Condiments:** pickled ginger, sweet pickles, hot mustard, *barbecue sauce,* Braggs Liquid Aminos

**Beverages:** Japanese tea; barley malt liquor; ginger ale, *root beer*

## Basic Support Foods

Foods to include in 1 to 2 meals a week.

**Dense Protein:** pork, ham, bacon, sausage, veal, venison, organ meats (heart, brain); duck; bonita, catfish, halibut, sole, tuna; abalone, crab, shrimp

**Dairy:** milk (whole, 2%, nonfat, raw, *goat's,* half-and-half, sweet cream, sour cream, *buttermilk,* kefir; yogurt (regular, low fat, nonfat, plain, or flavored), frozen yogurt, ice cream (Ben & Jerry's, Dreyer's, Swensen's)

**Cheese:** blue, Camembert, cottage, Edam, goat, Gouda, kefir, Limburger

**Nuts and Seeds:** almonds (raw, roasted), almond butter, Brazils, coconut, hazelnuts, peanuts (raw, roasted), peanut butter, pecans, English walnuts; raw or roasted seeds (caraway, pumpkin, sunflower), sunflower seed butter

**Legumes:** beans (adzuki, black, garbanzo, Great Northern, kidney, *lima, navy,* pinto, red, soy), black-eyed peas, *lentils,* split peas; hummus; miso, soy milk, tofu

**Grains:** barley, corn, corn grits, corn tortillas, couscous, hominy grits, millet, oats, popcorn, quinoa, rye, triticale, whole wheat, wheat bran, wheat germ, flour tortillas, breads (corn, corn/rye, French, garlic, Italian, multigrain, oat, rice, rye, seven-grain, sourdough, sprouted grain, whole wheat), bagels, English muffins, crackers (oat, rye, saltines, wheat), pasta, udon noodles, Chinese rice noodles, cream of wheat

**Vegetables:** arugula, asparagus, broccoflower, broccoli, cabbage (green, napa, red), cauliflower, celery, cilantro, cucumber, garlic, lettuce (Boston, butter, endive, iceberg, red leaf, romaine), *onions (brown, white, yellow),* parsnips, bell peppers (green, red, yellow), chili peppers, pimientos, potatoes (purple, red, russet, White Rose, Yukon Gold), radish, daikon radish, sauerkraut, shallots, squash (banana, butternut, spaghetti, yellow [summer], zucchini), *tomatoes (canned, hothouse, vine-ripened),* turnips

**Vegetable Juices:** carrot, carrot/celery, celery, parsley, spinach, tomato, V-8

**Fruits:** apples (McIntosh, Pippin, Rome Beauty), apricots, bananas, berries (blackberries, blueberries, boysenberries, cranberries, raspberries), cherries, dates, figs (fresh, dried), grapefruit (red, white), kumquats, lemons, loquats, melons (cantaloupe, casaba, Crenshaw, honeydew, watermelon), oranges, peaches, *Fuju persimmons,* plums (black, purple, red), raisins, rhubarb

**Fruit Juices:** apple, apple cider, apple/apricot, apricot, red cherry, cranapple, cranberry, grape (purple, red, white), guava, lemon, orange, pear, pineapple, pineapple/coconut, prune, tangerine

**Vegetable Oils:** all-blend, *almond,* avocado, coconut, *corn, olive, peanut, safflower, soy, sunflower*

**Sweeteners:** *fructose, molasses, sorghum,* sugar (*brown, date, raw, refined cane*), syrup (barley malt, brown rice, *corn*), *saccharin, succonant*

**Condiments:** *catsup, mustard, mayonnaise, horseradish, fish sauce, oyster sauce, pesto sauce, soy sauce,* salsa, tahini, dill or sweet pickles, vinegar, salt, sea salt, Vege-Sal

**Salad Dressings:** *blue cheese, creamy Italian, French, ranch, creamy avocado, Thousand Island,* vinegar and oil, lemon juice and oil

**Desserts:** *custards, tapioca, puddings, pies, cakes, chocolate, desserts containing chocolate, sherbet* (*orange, raspberry*)

**Chips:** *bean, corn* (*blue, white, yellow*), *potato*

**Beverages:** *coffee;* tea (*black,* green, herbal [mint], Chinese oolong); mineral water, sparkling water; *wine* (*red, white*), *sake,* liqueurs, *champagne, gin, scotch, vodka, whiskey, beer; regular sodas*

## Stressful Foods

Have no more than once a month.

**Dairy:** *most ice creams*
**Nuts:** *black walnuts*
**Vegetable:** roasted garlic
**Vegetable Oil:** *canola*
**Sweeteners:** *aspartame, Equal, NutraSweet, Sweet'n Low*
**Condiments:** *margarine*
**Beverages:** *Pepsi, diet sodas*
**Other:** *broiled and charbroiled foods and fish (e.g., broiled shrimp, charred toast)*

## Scheduling Meals

Breakfast, lunch, and dinner can be light to heavy. During times of stress or illness, breakfast should be a heavy meal.

*Breakfast:* 9–11 A.M. Light, moderate, or heavy; dense protein, nuts, seeds, cheese, grain, legumes, and vegetables. Fruit occasionally.

*Lunch:* 11:30 A.M.–2 P.M. Light, moderate, or heavy; dense protein, nuts, seeds, cheese, grain, legumes, vegetables, and occasionally fruit.

*Dinner:* 7–8 P.M. Light, moderate, or heavy; dense protein, nuts, seeds, cheese, grain, legumes, vegetables, and occasionally fruit.

## Snacks (optional)

*Midmorning or midafternoon:* fruit, vegetables, grain, nuts, seeds, dairy, protein

*Evening:* (9 P.M.–2 A.M.) sweets, fruit, vegetables, grain, nuts, seeds, dairy

## Sample One-Week Menu

DAY 1
*Breakfast:* sweet potato and peas
*Lunch:* turkey, mashed potato, and green beans
*Dinner:* tuna or orange roughy, beets, and peas

DAY 2
*Breakfast:* oatmeal w/butter and pine nuts
*Lunch:* Cornish game hen, wild rice, and carrots
*Dinner:* mahimahi, tossed salad, and green beans

DAY 3
*Breakfast:* steak and green beans
*Lunch:* salad of red leaf lettuce, tomatoes, English walnuts, tuna, and ricotta cheese
*Dinner:* pasta w/pesto sauce, steamed zucchini, and red bell peppers

DAY 4
*Breakfast:* chicken and acorn squash
*Lunch:* calamari, rice, and asparagus
*Dinner:* pork chop and peas

DAY 5: CLEANSE
Alternative of steamed vegetables all day
*Breakfast:* ginger tea or ginger and/or lemon juice in water
*Lunch:* watermelon including seeds and white part of rind
*Snack:* raw celery, cucumber, spinach, cabbage, or grapes, pears, nectarines, apple
*Dinner:* raw celery, cucumber, spinach, cabbage, jicama, or broccoflower; vegetable juice of carrot/celery, (parsley/cucumber/spinach) or fruit; apples (any) (cucumber), pears, nectarines, grapes
*Snack:* raw jicama, cucumber, apples, or grapes

DAY 6
*Breakfast:* beef patty and broccoli
*Lunch:* lamb chop, green beans, and potatoes
*Dinner:* rice, cucumber, and seaweed salad

DAY 7
*Breakfast:* cheese omelette w/onions and mushrooms
*Lunch:* chicken livers, sautéed onions, and peas
*Dinner:* lobster w/drawn butter and broccoli

# Alternative Menus

*(Foods in parentheses are optional.)*

## Breakfast
Hamburger patty and two eggs (barbecue sauce)
White or dark turkey and three-bean salad
Chicken breast, egg, and cheese (teriyaki or barbecue sauce)
Canadian bacon w/melted cheese or eggs
Ham and white or black beans or black-eyed peas
Cream of wheat w/milk
Grape-Nuts w/milk (tomato juice)

## Lunch
Chicken or shrimp stir-fry over rice
Chicken and noodles
Salad of tuna, egg, iceberg lettuce, and sweet pickle
Shredded vegetables such as green cabbage, zucchini, carrots, and chives w/sunflower or sesame seeds wrapped in flour tortilla with a dressing of sesame oil and lemon juice
Pinto beans and flour tortilla (salsa and/or guacamole)
Pasta w/vegetables and tofu
Split pea soup

## Dinner
Shark, baked potato, and a spinach salad with hard-boiled egg and a vinegar and oil dressing
Salmon and asparagus w/blue cheese dressing
Vegetarian chili, basmati rice, and cucumber salad
Meat loaf, rice, green beans w/onions and garlic, raw green bell peppers, and/or celery
Stir-fried onions, garlic, squash, carrots, and celery (rice)
Salad of lettuce, carrots, green onions, broccoli, and celery (garlic)
Yam (peas)

# Gallbladder

*The Gallbladder body type is symbolized by soapsuds. Like soap, bile is necessary to break down fats, and the digestion of fats is essential to all other functions. Reliable, loyal, and dependable, Gallbladder types are most fulfilled when they are being useful.*

FAMOUS PEOPLE: Bea Arthur, Maureen Stapleton, Jack Klugman, Harvey Korman

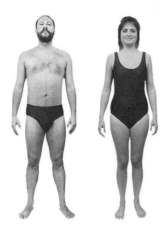

## GALLBLADDER
### Location and Function

The gallbladder is located on the right side of the abdomen, under the liver. It is a reservoir for bile (produced by the liver), which acts like soap in the breakdown and absorption of fats. Bile is necessary for assimilation of fat-soluble vitamins and for preventing putrefaction of intestinal contents.

## Psychological Profile

### Characteristic Traits

Placing a high value on peace and tranquillity, Gallbladder body types are generally patient, calm, and easygoing. Typically soft-spoken, they impress others as being kind, gentle, and congenial. Social harmony is a high priority, so they generally get along well with others. While Gallbladder types enjoy connecting with people, they are basically timid and shy, preferring to be around their families and close friends. A few Gallbladder types develop an outgoing nature, but the majority tend to be quiet and reserved around people unless they know them well.

With a general lack of experience in expressing emotions or connecting on an emotional level, Gallbladder types are reluctant to venture into new social situations, but they will go if someone takes them. Relating best to what can be physically seen and touched and deriving a great deal of personal fulfillment from being useful, they feel comfortable nurturing others. Much of their satisfaction comes from making themselves useful to those around them.

Task oriented, Gallbladder types would rather undertake a task or project that is well defined and already laid out for them than generate one on their own. Careful, practical, and dependable, they show comparatively little interest in leadership positions. They're not interested in standing out or making waves—or, for that matter, doing anything that might wind up being disruptive.

### Motivation

Gallbladder types process information and make decisions by taking in information, letting it digest, and then seeing how it feels. They prefer life to be steady and consistent, structured and dependable. Because the feel safe around what is known, their changes are usually gradual. While open-minded, Gallbladder types are generally skeptical about the myriad of claims, assertions, and changing perceptions that permeate the sociocultural environment. Nevertheless, they are open to new ideas that make good sense or can be validated.

Typically cautious, their views lean toward the traditional, conservative, or conventional. Not especially intuitive or individualistic, Gallbladder types tend to rely on external standards to guide their thinking or action. They have a tendency to follow what they think they should do rather than trust their intuition or feelings. They are relatively slow to accept new ideas and typically prefer to stay with the tried and true.

When they feel frightened or intimidated, Gallbladder types try to control their environment by closing down and withdrawing or by acting out. They have a tendency to control others in a manipulative, dominating, restrictive manner, usually through persuasion. This is often a defense against being controlled by someone else. Gallbladder types can also be quite persevering, even stubborn, in their attempts to get others to do what they think is important or to fully appreciate their beliefs and convictions.

## "At Worst"

When stressed, usually from physical imbalances, Gallbladder types become overwhelmed and their mental acuity is impaired. Feeling lethargic, they find it hard to concentrate. Consequently routine tasks are not done efficiently, and anything that requires focused thought is difficult. In this state they have trouble understanding what others are communicating and have to ask them to explain the same thing several different ways before they can begin to grasp it.

Emotionally, Gallbladder types can get into a state of depression, feeling low, melancholy, or generally frustrated. Because expressing anger doesn't fit their picture of how they should be, they often suppress their anger, holding it in as resentment or bitterness. It's easy for them to fall into the victim role, feeling they are at the mercy of their circumstances. When they feel impatient, picky, or emotional, they don't want to be around people, unless it's someone who will support them. Being basically self-contained, they prefer to withdraw from their own feelings, disconnecting from people and situations.

Because Gallbladder types have difficulty dealing with emotions—theirs as well as others'—they're apt to suppress them. This may take the form of denying their existence or of responding to negative emotions with stock words of reassurance or by prescribing some ethical rule that the other person should follow. These "shoulds" come from what they have been taught rather than from their own experience, so they may come across as rigid or dogmatic.

## "At Best"

When they find themselves in problematic situations they can do nothing about, Gallbladder types are able

### RECOMMENDED EXERCISE

Exercise for Gallbladder body types helps clear the mind and is most beneficial when it provides a sense of doing something useful. Useful, productive activities such as gardening, yard work, and cleaning windows or carpets are ideal. Walking, skiing (snow or water), treadmill, bicycling, rubberband exercises, Callanetics, swimming, and rebounding are good if they're enjoyable.

to turn their concerns over to a higher power, get into a meditative state, and allow their intuition to come forth. From here they are able to allow new awarenesses, solutions, and opportunities to become apparent, enabling them to be expansive, creative, and even adventurous—able to embrace new ideas and concepts.

Connecting with their quiet inner strength, Gallbladder types are able to take personal responsibility for themselves, knowing that there are no victims in this world and that everyone chooses their own experiences. By staying connected to their feelings and inner knowing, they are able to express their true nature, which is steady and dependable.

Gallbladder types are altruistic and are at their best when they are being of service to those in their world. They are conscientious, practical, dependable, and task oriented. Their strengths include hard work, orderliness, common sense, and persistence. They are careful, steady, and reliable, with good stamina and follow-through. They can be depended upon to get things done in a timely manner and are excellent support people. They are also calm, congenial, and considerate. They like to fit in with those around them and generally get along well with others. Being self-contained, they're not easily swayed by outside circumstances and are generally true to themselves.

## Dietary Profile

### Main Focus

- ▶ Meals should be high in fat, low in protein.
- ▶ Oils or seeds as fats with salads are necessary to digest raw vegetables.
- ▶ Reduce breads.
- ▶ Potatoes are an excellent carbohydrate source.
- ▶ Have largest meal at lunch.

## Dietary Emphasis

- From 20 to 40 percent of your calories are to come from fats.
- Best fat sources: butter; safflower, avocado, or olive oil; sesame seeds, sunflower seeds, and avocados.
- From 25 to 35 percent of your calories are to come from protein.
- From 0 to 30 percent of your calories are to come from dense protein.
- Best sources of the three amino acids threonine, isoleucine, and cystine: sesame seeds, ricotta cheese, and trout.
- Caloric intake: 1,500 to 1,800 calories a day for women and 1,700 to 2,000 calories a day for men. If you are engaging in intense exercise (competition type) or heavy labor, increase calories.
- Drink a minimum of 64 ounces of water a day. Drink water before and after meals, not with meals.
- Occasional desserts are best as an evening snack.
- Avoid fruit for lunch and midafternoon snack.
- Eat more cooked than raw vegetables.
- Eat beans, grains, chicken soup, arugula, nuts, and seeds.
- Watercress is a liver stimulant.
- Dense protein, including fish, supports the immune system.

## For Weight Loss

- Fat: 25 to 30 percent of daily calories.
- Dense protein: 15 to 30 percent of daily calories.
- Reduce breads, crackers, dairy, and fruit (including fruit juice and dried fruit).
- Eliminate sugar.
- Snacks are optional.
- If fats fall below 20 percent of calories, weight loss will be inhibited.
- May include midafternoon and evening snacks.

## For Weight Gain

- Dense protein: 15 to 30 percent of daily calories.
- Include breads and dairy.

### RECOMMENDED CUISINE

Homestyle cooking, Mexican, Italian, Thai, and Chinese.

## Healthy Foods List

There is no need to sacrifice delicious and filling foods to maintain a healthy Gallbladder body type. The following lists will help you focus on foods that support your health, and avoid foods that can stress your system.

*You'll notice that some foods are printed in italics; these foods take more energy to assimilate and could be ones you will want to avoid when you are in a sensitive state due to any physical or emotional stresses.*

Be sure to read Chapter 3, "Implementing the Body Type Diet," for lots of important information about how to use these many foods to gain their full benefit.

### Ultra-Support Foods

Foods to include in 3 to 7 meals a week, listed by category.

**Dense Protein:** beef broth, buffalo, veal; chicken broth, Cornish game hen; bass, catfish, flounder, haddock, herring, perch, sardines in oil, red snapper, orange roughy, trout; crab, eel, octopus

**Dairy:** goat's milk, buttermilk, kefir, yogurt (regular, plain, or vanilla), butter

**Cheese:** cream, mozzarella, Muenster, Parmesan, ricotta, Romano

**Nuts and Seeds:** coconut (raw), hazelnuts (raw or dry-roasted), macadamias (raw), pine nuts (raw), water chestnuts; sesame seeds (raw or dry-roasted), sesame seed butter

**Legumes:** beans (adzuki, black, lima, pinto), black-eyed peas, split peas

**Grains:** couscous, millet, rice (white basmati, Japanese, wild), rice cakes (unsalted), sesame rice cakes

**Vegetables:** artichokes, arugula, bamboo shoots, cooked green beans, yellow wax beans, broccoli, brussels sprouts, carrots, cauliflower, cucumbers, eggplant, garlic, kohlrabi, leeks, red leaf lettuce, mushrooms, okra, olives (green, ripe), onions (chives, brown, green, red, Vidalia, white, yellow), parsley, parsnips, peas, potatoes (all varieties), pumpkin, rutabaga, spinach, squash (acorn, banana, butternut, spaghetti), Swiss chard, turnips, watercress, yams

**Fruits:** apples (all varieties), berries (blackberries, cranberries, gooseberries), dates, figs (Black Mission), grapefruit (white, red), guavas, kiwi, mangoes, papayas, plums (black, purple, red), pomegranates, stewed or dried prunes, raisins, tangelos, watermelon

**Fruit Juices:** apple, grapefruit

**Vegetable Oils:** all-blend, avocado, corn, safflower, sesame, soy, sunflower

**Sweetener:** stevia

**Beverages:** herbal teas (peppermint, chamomile), Kombucha tea

## Basic Support Foods

Foods to include in 1 to 2 meals a week.

**Dense Protein:** beef, beef liver, liverwurst, lamb, venison, organ meats (brain, heart); beef or turkey bacon, chicken, chicken livers, duck, turkey; anchovy, bonita, cod, halibut, mackerel, mahimahi, salmon, sardines in tomato sauce, shark, sole, swordfish, tuna; abalone, calamari (squid), clams, lobster, mussels, oysters, scallops, shrimp; eggs

**Dairy:** milk (whole, 2%, low fat, raw), half-and-half, sweet cream, sour cream, yogurt (regular, low fat, plain, and flavored), *frozen yogurt,* ice cream (Ben & Jerry's, Dreyer's, Swensen's)

**Cheese:** American, blue, Brie, Camembert, cheddar, Colby, cottage, Edam, feta, goat, Gouda, kefir, Limburger, Monterey Jack, Swiss

**Nuts and Seeds:** raw or dry-roasted, unsalted nuts—almonds, *almond butter,* Brazils, cashews, cashew butter, hazelnuts, macadamia butter, pistachios, peanuts, *peanut butter,* pecans, walnuts (black, English); raw or dry-roasted seeds (caraway, pumpkin, *sunflower*), *sunflower seed butter*

**Legumes:** beans (garbanzo, Great Northern, navy, soy), *lentils;* hummus; miso, soy milk, *tofu*

**Grains:** *amaranth, barley, corn, corn grits,* blue corn, *corn tortillas, hominy grits, oats,* oat bran, popcorn, quinoa, rice (brown basmati, *short or long grain brown*), rice bran, salted rice cakes, *popcorn rice cakes, rye, triticale, wheat bran,* raw or toasted wheat germ, refined wheat flour, flour tortillas, breads (*corn, corn/rye,* French, garlic, Italian, rice, rye, sourdough, sprouted grain, white, *oat*), bagels, croissants, English muffins, crackers (oat, rye, saltines), *pasta, udon noodles,* Chinese rice noodles, cream of rice, *cream of rye, cream of wheat*

**Soups:** chicken vegetable, vegetable, clam chowder, bean with ham, beef vegetable, cream of broccoli, chili, asparagus, pumpkin, egg drop, corn chowder, miso

**Vegetables:** asparagus, avocados, raw green beans, beets, bok choy, cabbage (green, red, napa), celery, cilantro, corn, greens (beet, *collard,* mustard, turnip), hominy, jicama, *kale,* lettuce (Boston, butter, endive, *iceberg,* romaine), snow pea pods, bell peppers (green, yellow, red), chili peppers, pimientos, radish, daikon radish, sauerkraut, *seaweed (dulse, nori, wakame),* shallots, squash (yellow [summer], *zucchini*), sprouts (*alfalfa, mung bean, clover, radish, sunflower*), sweet potatoes, taro root, tomatoes (canned, hothouse, vine-ripened)

**Vegetable Juices:** carrot, celery, carrot/celery, parsley, spinach/parsley/celery, spinach, tomato, V-8

**Fruits:** *apricots,* bananas, berries (blueberries, boysenberries, raspberries, *strawberries*), *cherries, grapes (black, green, red),* kumquats, lemons, limes, loquats, melons (cantaloupe, *casaba,* Crenshaw, honeydew), *nectarines, oranges, peaches,* pears, persimmons, pineapples, rhubarb, tangerines

**Fruit Juices:** apple cider, apple/apricot, apricot, cherry (black, red), cranapple, cranberry, grape (purple, red, white), guava, lemon, orange, papaya, pear, pineapple, pineapple/coconut, prune, tangerine, watermelon

**Vegetable Oils:** *almond,* coconut, *flaxseed,* olive, *peanut*

**Sweeteners:** *fructose, honey, molasses, sorghum; sugar (brown, date, raw, refined cane);* syrup (barley malt, *brown rice,* corn); *saccharin, succonant*

**Condiments:** Braggs Liquid Aminos, brewer's yeast, *mustard, horseradish, barbecue sauce, pesto sauce, soy sauce;* salsa, tahini, dill or *sweet pickles,* salt, sea salt, Vege-Sal

**Salad Dressings:** blue cheese, French, ranch, creamy Italian, creamy avocado, Thousand Island, vinegar and oil, lemon juice and oil

**Desserts:** *custards, tapioca, puddings, pies, chocolate, desserts containing chocolate, sherbet (orange, raspberry)*

**Chips:** *bean, corn (blue, white, yellow), potato*

**Beverages:** *coffee;* tea (*black,* orange pekoe, Japanese, Chinese oolong); mineral water, sparkling water; *wine (red, white), champagne, sake,* liqueurs, *beer, barley malt liquor, gin, scotch, vodka, whiskey; root beer, regular sodas*

## Stressful Foods

Have no more than once a month.

**Dense Protein:** *pork, pork bacon, pork sausage, ham; sardines in mustard or chili*
**Dairy:** *nonfat milk, nonfat plain or flavored yogurt, most ice creams*
**Nuts and Seeds:** *all roasted, salted*
**Legumes:** *kidney* or *red beans*
**Grains:** *buckwheat, polished rice, whole wheat, breads (multigrain, seven-grain, whole wheat), whole wheat crackers*
**Vegetables:** *broccoflower, seaweed (arame, hijihki, kelp)*
**Vegetable Oil:** *canola*
**Sweeteners:** *maple syrup, aspartame, Equal, Nutra-Sweet, Sweet'n Low*
**Condiment:** *mayonnaise*
**Desserts:** *cakes, cookies*
**Beverages:** *diet sodas*

## Scheduling Meals

Gallbladder body types shouldn't feast or sacrifice. They need a moderate amount of food at every meal. Schedule your meals as follows:

*Breakfast:* 7–8 A.M. Moderate, with fruit, grain, vegetables, protein, dairy, nuts, and/or seeds.
*Lunch:* 12–2 P.M. Moderate to heavy, with protein, legumes, dairy, grain, and/or vegetables. Avoid fruit.
*Dinner:* 6–7 P.M. Moderate, with protein, legumes, dairy, vegetables, grain, and/or fruit.

### Snacks (optional)
*Midmorning:* (10–11 A.M.) fruit, grain, protein, dairy
*Midafternoon:* (4–5 P.M.) protein, nuts, seeds, grain, dairy, vegetables
*Evening:* (at least ½ hour after dinner) seeds, nuts, dairy, vegetables, fruit, grain, desserts

## Sample One-Week Menu

All snacks are optional.

DAY 1
*Breakfast:* corn bread and butter
*Lunch:* lamb chops, potato, and asparagus
*Snack:* celery w/cream cheese
*Dinner:* stir-fried or steamed broccoli, cauliflower, and carrots
*Snack:* orange

DAY 2
*Breakfast:* yam w/butter
*Lunch:* turkey, pickled beets, carrots or carrot salad
*Snack:* almonds
*Dinner:* split pea soup and sesame seed crackers
*Snack:* regular, plain, or vanilla yogurt

DAY 3
*Breakfast:* grapefruit and Grape-Nuts w/apple juice
*Lunch:* halibut, rice, tomato, cilantro or parsley
*Snack:* carrots
*Dinner:* vegetable beef soup
*Snack:* popcorn w/butter

DAY 4
*Breakfast:* corn tortilla w/avocado
*Lunch:* liver w/red onions and green peas
*Snack:* mozzarella or Muenster cheese and sesame seed crackers
*Dinner:* baked potato w/butter, ricotta cheese, and/or sour cream
*Snack:* pecans

DAY 5: CLEANSE
*Breakfast:* egg drop soup (chicken broth, stir in egg, serve w/green onion)
*Lunch:* chicken noodle soup (fresh or frozen—not canned)
*Dinner:* vegetable soup (potato, celery, onions, garlic, tomato, carrots)

DAY 6
*Breakfast:* applesauce and hazelnuts
*Lunch:* roast beef, potatoes, carrots, and onions
*Snack:* sunflower seeds
*Dinner:* carrots, onions, and chicken broth w/celery and rice
*Snack:* pumpkin pie

DAY 7
*Breakfast:* omelette w/onion, bell pepper, and mozzarella cheese
*Lunch:* trout (coated with cornmeal), rice, and a salad of romaine lettuce and carrots w/vinegar and oil dressing

*Snack:* deviled egg
*Dinner:* stir-fried broccoli, carrots, onions, yellow squash, and pea pods w/rice
*Snack:* blackberries w/sour cream

## Alternative Menus

*(Foods in parentheses are optional.)*

### Breakfast

Grapefruit or grapefruit juice, then couscous or cream of rice w/butter
Chicken livers and sourdough toast w/butter
Onion bagel, egg, and cream cheese
Cooked millet w/parsley and butter
Oatmeal or basmati rice w/butter
Couscous and cooked parsley (butter)
Egg and cheese omelette and corn tortilla
Eggs and onions

### Lunch

Turkey patty, green beans, and onions
Teriyaki chicken, rice, broccoli, carrots, and onions
Yellowtail tuna, asparagus, and pasta
Chopped blanched spinach, garlic, parsley, beaten egg, milk, and Colby cheese baked in a moderate oven (Parmesan cheese on top)
Salmon w/green onions and lemon juice, and green peas
Shrimp, rice, and coleslaw w/vinegar and oil
Beef Stroganoff
Meat loaf, potatoes, and a salad of romaine lettuce, tomatoes, and cucumber
Tuna-stuffed tomato, lettuce, and avocado

### Dinner

Black beans and rice w/onions
Green pea soup w/carrots and celery
Chicken livers and celery w/cream cheese
Pinto beans, corn bread w/avocado and/or cream cheese
Navy beans (w/onions) and corn bread w/butter
Chicken, broccoli, parsley, rice, and butter
Pasta, tomato sauce, and olives (w/beef, chicken, or turkey)
Stew of ground turkey, tomatoes, zucchini, and pinto beans
Egg and avocado (cheese)
Clam chowder

# Gonadal

*The Gonadal body type is symbolized by the male/female sign. Sexuality is expressed through the gonads and is associated with pleasure and being playful. Highly emotional, this type brings a light, playful, spontaneous quality to all aspects of life.*

FAMOUS PEOPLE: Marilyn Monroe, Al Pacino, Jennifer Lopez, Robert DeNiro

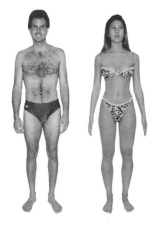

## GONADAL
### Location and Function

The gonads are reproductive glands—such as the ovaries and testes. They serve the function of reproduction and the secretion of hormones.

## Psychological Profile

### Characteristic Traits

While Gonadal body types generally have fine symmetrical features, it's their strong sexual energy that makes them exceptionally physically attractive. Beauty is of vital importance to them, whether it's in their personal appearance or their environment or the beauty they see in everyone and everything.

Oriented primarily through their emotions, Gonadal types are extremely sensitive to the emotional needs of others. Family is of utmost importance to them because they often link their personal identity with their intimate relationships. Highly emotional and physically expressive, Gonadal types quickly show their anger and hurt as well as their affection, nurturing, and joy. Their nature is to be playful, as it's through play that they are able to access their inner joy. Because they don't handle stress well, playtime is essential for maintaining a positive outlook.

Social interaction, whether at parties or family gatherings or with customers and coworkers, allows Gonadal types to bring out the best in people. They have a special ability to recognize and appreciate the feelings of others, and being sensitive and caring, they offer emotional support to those who need it. They derive much of their gratification simply from harmonious interactions. Being more people- than task-oriented, Gonadal types thrive on substantial human contact.

### Motivation

Gonadal types are inspired by beauty and see it as an undeniable aspect of God that exists in everything. For Gonadal types, beauty is a person's essence. This is apparent in the way Gonadal types look, in the expression of their talents, and in the kindness they show to others.

Gonadal types nurture by helping others recognize and express their inner beauty. They want others to see what they see, so they enjoy enhancing others' physical appearance or making their environment more beautiful. Emotionally sensitive, they feel others' pain and do whatever they can to assist them.

Being results oriented, Gonadal types want to see the physical effects of their actions. They tend to prefer the big picture to the details and like to see their efforts quickly making a difference. With the idea in their mind of what they want to create, they often jump enthusiastically into a project without fully considering what they need to do to finish it. Their level of maturity will dictate how well or even whether the project gets completed.

For Gonadal types, self-worth is often associated with how their accomplishments make them appear to others. This search for self-worth can lead them to be very conscientious, even to the point of perfectionism. While their basic nature is not especially industrious, they have the ability to apply themselves to a project with great determination when they feel it is relevant to their life. The desire to establish a sense of identity can lead them to be quite focused on business while still maintaining their emotional focus in their personal lives.

Basing their identity on their family's and friends' responses and expectations of them, Gonadal types may deny their own self-expression or fall into self-sacrifice. Their personal insecurity tends to make them overly concerned about their physical appearance. They are usually the first to follow fashion trends and group activities, since they often rely on others for personal validation.

## "At Worst"

When frustrated or exhausted or when life gets difficult, Gonadal types often become stubborn and self-centered. Highly reactive to those around them, they may cry, yell, or explode in anger and may be impatient, irritable, and difficult to deal with. It is easy for them to harbor bad feelings when a situation has been unpleasant and they haven't openly expressed their displeasure. If they have learned to "control" their emotions and hold back their impulses, they tend to manifest their negative tendencies as secret hostility and resentment or victim syndrome.

For male Gonadal types, self-worth is often associated with how much in control of their families they appear to be to their friends. This can lead to macho behavior, which is an immature attempt to display masculine strength by dominating or controlling someone else. Depending on their degree of development, they may be more concerned about getting credit for work than about doing the job, and on getting it done as soon as possible rather than making sure it's done right. They look for shortcuts and generally choose the easiest way to completion rather than the best way. Preferring to get started right away and learn what they need to know only when they need to know it,

they often do not take enough time for preparation or deliberation about the details.

## "At Best"

Gonadal types are at their best once they have found their personal identity. By creating and maintaining a safe environment, they become free to express themselves fully. Able to see the beauty in everything, especially themselves, they bring it out so that everyone else can see it. The real purpose of their nurturing is to bring forth and allow other people to express the beauty that is their essence. Sharing the inspiration beauty brings them makes beholding the beauty an emotional experience.

Emotions ignite the creative spark in the Gonadal body type. To Gonadal types, creativity is an experience, rather than a mental process, and they must let go of the mind to access the creative source. Their creativity comes when they bring magic into their lives through adventure and fun and feeling unlimited. However, creativity is a receptive state that requires a safe, protected environment. Gonadals need this kind of nurturing environment to be light, spontaneous, and playful.

Gonadal types recognize their feelings as the activating energy that leads them back to their magical essence—God—their creative source. Accessing the magical child within allows the dream or make-believe to become real. Gonadal types nurture by creating an atmosphere or environment where people enjoy being themselves and can have fun, which releases the creative energy in everyone around them.

## RECOMMENDED EXERCISE

Gonadal body types do well with vigorous exercise, especially in the morning. Its benefit is initially emotional, then physical. Exercise gives a sense of accomplishment and gets energy moving. Callanetics, NordicTrack exercise, exercises that work and develop the upper body, aerobic dance or jogging 2 times a week, massage for legs, and walking are all very helpful for the maintenance of the Gonadal body type. Exposure to sunlight is also very important.

## Dietary Profile

### Main Focus

- Listen and pay attention to your emotions without judgment. Honor what your body is telling you. If you do this, you may eat what you want.
- Have a light breakfast.
- Have a heavier dinner.
- Eat salads, particularly for lunch.

### Dietary Emphasis

- From 20 to 35 percent of your calories are to come from fat.
- Best fat sources: nuts (almonds, Brazils, cashews, hazelnuts, macadamias, pecans, walnuts), seeds (pumpkin, sunflower), oils (avocado, olive, safflower, sesame), and butter.
- From 20 to 35 percent of your calories are to come from protein.
- From 0 to 30 percent of your calories are to come from dense protein.
- Best sources of the three amino acids threonine, isoleucine, and cystine: sesame seeds, peanuts, and turkey.
- Caloric intake: 1,500 to 1,800 calories a day for women and 1,700 to 2,000 calories a day for men. If you are engaging in intense exercise (competition type) or heavy labor, increase calories.
- Drink a minimum of 64 ounces of water a day. Drink water before and after meals, not with meals.
- Occasional desserts are best as an evening snack.
- Avoid fruit for dinner (also for lunch if sensitive).
- Mix cooked and raw vegetables.
- Eat green leafy vegetables, seaweed, potatoes, and tomatoes.
- Eat cottage cheese, fish, turkey, and brown basmati rice.

### For Weight Loss

- Fats: 20 to 30 percent of daily calories.
- Reduce sugars, including fruit.
- Avoid breads.

---

**RECOMMENDED CUISINE**

Mexican, Italian, seafood, Chinese, Japanese, Thai, Indian, Moroccan, Continental, French, English, or Irish 1 to 2 times a week.

---

- Minimize grain at dinner.
- Avoid spices.
- May include snacks, particularly midmorning.

### For Weight Gain

- Dense protein: 10 to 30 percent of daily calories.
- Increase food intake.
- Animal protein builds muscle mass, especially with exercise.

## Healthy Foods List

There is no need to sacrifice delicious and filling foods to maintain a healthy Gonadal body type. The following lists will help you focus on foods that support your health, and avoid foods that can stress your system.

*You'll notice that some foods are printed in italics; these foods take more energy to assimilate and could be ones you will want to avoid when you are in a sensitive state due to any physical or emotional stresses.*

Be sure to read Chapter 3, "Implementing the Body Type Diet," for lots of important information about how to use these many foods to gain their full benefit.

### Ultra-Support Foods

Foods to include in 3 to 7 meals a week, listed by category.

**Dense Protein:** beef broth (as a base), beef liver, buffalo; chicken broth, chicken livers, Cornish game hen, turkey; catfish, cod, flounder, haddock, herring, mackerel, mahimahi, perch, red snapper, yellowtail tuna; mussels

**Dairy:** *buttermilk,* yogurt (plain, strawberry, raspberry, spiced apple), butter

**Cheese:** low-fat or nonfat cottage, cream, feta, kefir, Muenster, Parmesan, ricotta, Romano, Swiss

**Nuts and Seeds:** Brazils, hazelnuts, macadamias (raw, roasted), salted peanuts (raw, roasted), pecans, pine nuts (raw, roasted), walnuts (black, English), water chestnuts; raw or roasted seeds (caraway, pumpkin, sesame, sunflower)

**Legumes:** beans (black, lima, garbanzo, Great Northern, kidney, navy, red, soy), black-eyed peas, split peas

**Grains:** corn, couscous, rice (brown basmati, short grain brown), focaccia (Italian bread), vegetarian flour tortillas, bran muffins, oat bran bagels, pasta (all varieties), udon noodles, Chinese rice noodles, cream of rice, cream of rye

**Vegetables:** green beans, broccoli, carrots, cucumber, garlic, White Rose potatoes, seaweed (arame, dulse, kelp, nori, wakame)

**Vegetable Juices:** carrot/celery/cucumber

**Fruits:** bananas, cantaloupes, dates, nectarines, pineapples, raisins, strawberries

**Fruit Juices:** cranraspberry, mango, orange/pineapple

**Vegetable Oils:** all-blend, *almond,* avocado, canola, corn, olive, safflower, sesame, *soy, sunflower*

**Sweetener:** stevia

**Condiment:** sea salt

**Beverage:** herbal iced tea

## Basic Support Foods

Foods to include in 1 to 2 meals a week.

**Dense Protein:** *lean beef,* lamb, pork, ham, bacon, sausage, veal, venison, organ meats (heart, brain); chicken, duck; anchovy, bass, bonita, halibut, orange roughy, salmon, sardines, shark, sole, swordfish, trout, tuna; abalone, calamari (squid), clams, crab, eel, lobster, octopus, oysters, scallops, shrimp; eggs

**Dairy:** milk (whole, low fat, nonfat, raw), half-and-half, sweet cream, sour cream, kefir, flavored yogurt, ice cream (Ben & Jerry's, Dreyer's, Swensen's)

**Cheese:** American, blue, Brie, Camembert, cheddar, Colby, Edam, *goat,* Gouda, Limburger, low-fat Monterey Jack, part-skim mozzarella

**Nuts and Seeds:** almonds (raw, roasted), almond butter, cashews (raw, roasted), cashew butter, coconut, macadamia butter, unsalted peanuts in shell (raw, roasted), pistachios; sesame seed butter, sunflower seed butter

**Legumes:** beans (adzuki, pinto), *lentils;* hummus; miso, soy milk, tofu

**Grains:** amaranth, barley, buckwheat, corn grits, corn tortillas, hominy grits, millet, oats, popcorn, quinoa, rice (white basmati, long grain brown, Japanese, wild), rice bran, rice cakes, rye, triticale, whole wheat, wheat bran, wheat germ, refined wheat flour, breads (corn, corn/rye, French, garlic, Italian, oat, rice, rye, *sourdough*), bagels, croissants, English muffins, flour tortillas, sprouted wheat tortillas, whole wheat tortillas, crackers (oat, rye, saltines, wheat), cream of wheat

**Vegetables:** artichokes, asparagus, avocados, bamboo shoots, yellow wax beans, beets, bok choy, broccoflower, brussels sprouts, cabbage (green, napa, red), cauliflower, celery, cilantro, corn, eggplant, greens (beet, collard, mustard, turnip), jicama, kale, kohlrabi, leeks, lettuce (Boston, butter, endive, *iceberg,* red leaf, romaine), mushrooms, okra, olives (black, green, ripe), onions (*brown, red, Vidalia, white, yellow*), parsley, parsnips, *peas,* snow pea pods, bell peppers (green, red, yellow), chili peppers, pimientos, potatoes (purple, red, Yukon Gold), pumpkin, radish, daikon radish, rutabaga, sauerkraut, shallots, spinach, sprouts (alfalfa, clover, mung bean, radish, sunflower), squash (acorn, banana, butternut, spaghetti, yellow [summer], zucchini), *sweet potatoes,* Swiss chard, *tomatoes (canned, hothouse, vine-ripened),* turnips, watercress, *yams*

**Vegetable Juices:** carrot, carrot/celery, celery, parsley, spinach, tomato, V-8

**Fruits:** apples (Golden or Red Delicious, Gala, Granny Smith, Jonathan, McIntosh, Pippin, Rome Beauty), apricots, berries (blackberries, blueberries, boysenberries, cranberries, gooseberries, raspberries), cherries, figs (fresh, dried), grapes (black, green, red), grapefruit (white, red), guavas, kiwi, kumquats, lemons, limes, loquats, mangoes, melons (Crenshaw, watermelon), oranges, papayas, peaches, pears, persimmons, *plums (black, purple, red),* pomegranates, prunes, rhubarb, tangerines, tangelos

**Fruit Juices:** apple, apple cider, apple/apricot, apricot, black cherry, red cherry, cranapple, cranberry, grape (purple, red, white), grapefruit, guava, lemon, papaya, pear, pineapple, pineapple/coconut, prune, tangerine, watermelon

**Vegetable Oils:** coconut, *flaxseed, peanut*

**Sweeteners:** *fructose, honey, molasses, sorghum; sugar (brown, date, raw, refined cane),* syrup (barley malt, *brown rice, corn, maple),* saccharin, *succonant*

**Condiments:** catsup, Dijon mustard, mustard, horseradish, *barbecue sauce, pesto sauce, soy sauce,* salsa, tahini, pickles, vinegar, salt, Vege-Sal

**Salad Dressings:** *blue cheese, French, ranch, creamy Italian, creamy avocado, Thousand Island,* vinegar and oil, lemon juice and oil

**Desserts:** *custards, tapioca, puddings, pies, cakes, chocolate, desserts containing chocolate, sherbet (orange, raspberry)*

**Chips:** *bean, corn (blue, white, yellow), potato*

**Beverages:** *coffee;* tea (*black,* green, herbal, Japanese, Chinese oolong); mineral water, sparkling water; *white wine,* red wine, sake, liqueurs, *champagne, beer, barley malt liquor, gin, scotch,* vodka, *whiskey; root beer, regular sodas*

## Stressful Foods

Have no more than once a month.

**Dairy:** *goat's milk, frozen yogurt, most ice creams*
**Nuts and Seeds:** *peanut butter*
**Grains:** *polished rice,* breads (*multigrain, seven-grain, sprouted grain, whole wheat*)
**Vegetables:** *arugula, chives, green onions, russet potatoes*
**Fruits:** *melons (casaba, honeydew)*
**Fruit Juice:** *orange*
**Sweeteners:** *aspartame, Equal, NutraSweet, Sweet'n Low*
**Condiments:** *mayonnaise, margarine*
**Beverages:** *diet sodas*

## Scheduling Meals

Gonadal types can handle a varied amount of food at lunch and dinner, but if sensitive, avoid fruit, nuts, and seeds for lunch and dinner. Schedule your meals as follows:

*Breakfast:* 7–9 A.M. Light, with fruit, or moderate, with protein, nuts, seeds, grain, fruit, and/or dairy.
*Lunch:* 1–3 P.M. Light to heavy, with protein, legumes, grain, nuts, seeds, fruit, dairy, and/or vegetables.
*Dinner:* 8–12 P.M. Moderate to heavy, with protein, legumes, grain, vegetables, nuts, seeds, and/or dairy. Avoid fruit.

### Snacks (optional)
*Midmorning:* fruit, dairy
*Midafternoon:* grain, dairy, nuts, seeds, vegetables
*Evening:* fruit, grain, dairy, vegetables, protein, sweets (healthy may include nuts and seeds)

## Sample One-Week Menu

Snacks are optional.

DAY 1
*Breakfast:* banana and cashew butter
*Lunch:* turkey or chicken and a salad of Boston lettuce, spinach, radish, and tomato w/vinaigrette dressing
*Dinner:* fish taco—fish, cabbage, and lime juice, corn tortilla, and beans

DAY 2
*Breakfast:* tomato soup
*Lunch:* turkey quesadilla, corn tortilla, and avocado
*Dinner:* salmon, rice, and green beans

DAY 3
*Breakfast:* roasted, unsalted pumpkin seeds
*Snack:* apple
*Lunch:* egg salad and asparagus
*Snack: vanilla yogurt w/pecans*
*Dinner:* fillet of tuna, rice, and broccoli

DAY 4
*Breakfast:* cottage cheese and avocado
*Lunch:* manicotti and green beans
*Dinner:* roast turkey, potatoes, and broccoli

DAY 5: CLEANSE
*Breakfast:* (cantaloupe) grapefruit, apple (Golden or Red Delicious)
*Lunch:* steamed broccoli, carrots, bok choy, cauliflower and/or raw jicama, bell peppers (green or red), celery, carrots or vegetable juice—carrot/ celery, (parsley), (spinach)
*Dinner:* White Rose baked potato; steamed green beans, celery, cucumber, radishes, spinach, lettuce, red cabbage or carrot/celery/cucumber juice

DAY 6
*Breakfast:* raw sunflower seeds
*Lunch:* sushi
*Dinner:* beef, baked potato, and peas

DAY 7
*Breakfast:* seviche—fish, such as white fish, in lime juice with tomatoes, onions, jicama, and cilantro and vegetables
*Lunch:* tuna and a salad of romaine lettuce, red onion, radishes, red and green bell peppers, and feta cheese with creamy Italian dressing
*Dinner:* roast chicken, brown basmati rice, carrots, and celery

# Alternative Menus

*(Foods in parentheses are optional.)*

## Breakfast

Apple, banana, strawberries, or pineapple

Watermelon or cantaloupe

Cherries or nectarine

V-8 juice

Strawberry yogurt (w/pine nuts and sunflower seeds)

Eggs and turkey (apple)

Turkey, White Rose potatoes, and peas

Mussels, raw or steamed

Rice cakes and hummus

Cream of rice w/butter and nuts

Soft-boiled egg and avocado on a rice cake

Corn grits and bacon

## Lunch

Chicken, brown basmati rice, peas, tomatoes, and capers

Turkey and low-fat cheese on tortilla

Turkey breast sandwich w/sprouts, cucumber, Swiss cheese, and Dijon mustard

Fish, tomato sauce, and carrots, broccoli, yellow onions, or green beans w/rice

Salad of carrots, tomatoes, garbanzo beans, and cucumber w/creamy garlic dressing

Low-fat cottage cheese and a salad of cucumber, bell pepper, beets, and romaine lettuce w/oil and vinegar dressing

Salad of romaine lettuce, cucumber, bell pepper, shoestring beets, and turkey or chicken w/vinaigrette dressing

Tuna, cottage cheese, and red leaf lettuce

Japanese udon noodles with white fish and fish broth

Salmon and seaweed salad w/vinegar

## Lunch or Dinner

Tuna salad, avocado, lettuce, and tomato

Flour tortilla, pinto beans, and onions

Rice, black beans, and onions

Carrot/celery/cucumber juice and a baked potato

Angel-hair pasta w/garlic, shrimp, olive oil, and peas

Lentil soup w/carrots and onions

## Dinner

Turkey, potatoes, green beans, and mushrooms

Chicken, potatoes, carrots, and onions or peas

Cornish game hen and sweet potato or yam

Cornish game hen, rice, and green beans

Beef, Yukon Gold potatoes, and peas

Beefsteak or roast beef, zucchini, tomatoes, and a salad of raw spinach, celery, and carrots w/Italian dressing

Vegetable soup in turkey broth w/celery, carrots, and onions

Baked Yukon Gold potato w/yogurt, corn, and broccoflower or brussels sprouts

# Heart

*The Heart body type is symbolized by a heart. Huggable and approachable, Heart types set the beat by getting in step with their environment and then shifting it to their desires. Like the heart, they bring their own rhythm or music to their environment.*

FAMOUS PEOPLE: Elvis Presley, Elton John, Mae West, Sally Field

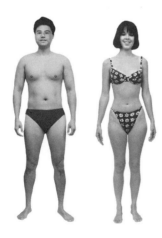

### HEART
### Location and Function

The heart is located on the left side of the upper chest, between the lungs. Its function is to circulate blood throughout the body.

## Psychological Profile

### Characteristic Traits

The body type that especially inspires hugs is the Heart. Distinguished by an approachability that is hard to define but easy to recognize, Heart types are typically soft, gentle, and giving. They project a sensitivity and caring that makes others feel at ease. Gentle and supporting, Heart types are usually easy to be around. Home and family are particularly important to them, and they tend to provide the glue that creates cohesiveness in their families.

While some Heart types are extroverted, most tend to be shy and cautious with strangers and in new situations. Very approachable, they are usually warm and receptive to others, yet passive when it comes to initiating relationships. People are drawn to them because of their sensitivity to others' needs.

Seeking the approval and acceptance of others, they can be very accommodating, going out of their way to avoid hurting anyone's feelings, striving to maintain peace and harmony, or gently guiding the situation to get their needs and desires met. Just as the heart is central to the body's circulatory system, the Heart type becomes central to the emotional dynamics of a group or gathering.

Highly emotional and strongly connected to their feelings, Heart types are sensitive, intuitive, and expressive. With a passive, accommodating, blending-in nature, Heart types are prone to stress and can easily get tense. Creative endeavors like music and art allow them to express their intuitive side. Other creative endeavors like painting, flower arranging, or computer graphics and cartoon creation promote a feeling of peace.

### Motivation

Heart types are worriers, especially the men, and they worry about everything. Worry is a means of protection—a belief that thinking about what could happen somehow makes it less threatening. Unfortunately, putting large amounts of emotional energy into a negative pattern can sometimes attract problems or at least create stress.

Heart types react to situations by exaggerating their worst fears, traits, and mistakes. They blow things out of proportion because their feelings are so amplified, and this puts them on an emotional roller coaster. Once they get caught in their emotions, it's hard for them to be objective and view anything from the outside.

In an attempt to create safety and stability, Heart types cover as many bases as possible mentally. When they become fatigued or when the next step becomes elusive, they go over and over the same material in their minds. This mental loop blocks intuition or creativity. Breaking the cycle can easily be accomplished by doing something physical, such as walking around the house or getting up for a drink of water.

Unsure of the value or effectiveness of what they have done, Heart types often seek outside approval and validation. Their belief is that if they do everything perfectly, they'll be safe. Consequently it's easy for them to get bogged down in details, spending too much time on a project. The desire to be thought well of often motivates them to be reliable, competent, and responsible.

## "At Worst"

When stressed, Heart types can easily become anxious, fearful, overemotional, and worried about everything. They can suffer from low self-esteem, reflected in the attitude "I'm not good enough." Caught in a feeling of failure, they amplify anything negative and make it worse, and they believe that what they see is the way it is.

Setbacks and criticism can cause Heart types to retreat within themselves, where they dwell excessively on negative experiences until they lose their motivation and eventually give up on life. They may become couch potatoes, eating junk food and expecting others to take care of them. Heart types often satisfy their senses, taking the easiest way and doing what is most convenient. Food and drugs are easy ways of sedating their emotions.

Emotionally oriented, Heart types often seek the approval of others as the basis of their self-approval. Not wanting to do anything that would make them stand out or appear to be in error, they are likely to "go with the flow" to gain acceptance, denying their feelings and intuition in the process. Since their self-worth is often connected with the way other people respond to them, they have a tendency to tell people what they want to hear or withhold information that could upset someone. They may then fail to follow through on agreements.

When Heart types are not at peace with themselves, their natural ability to influence others' moods can produce discord and conflict. Two Heart types in the same house, particularly boys, usually experience a need to establish their own identity and demonstrate some form of control. This is when they are apt to express opposite poles, such as positive or negative and introverted or extroverted. The result can be either balanced or destructive, harmony or chaos, positive or negative emotions and exchanges.

In an attempt to do what is best, protect themselves from harm, and control their environment, Heart types can become too persistent. This control element comes into play when they feel that their solution is what's best for another person. To get others to do what they want, they wear them down verbally until finally, to stop the nagging, others give in.

## "At Best"

Heart types at their best bring a gentle, harmonious, peaceful atmosphere into their environment. Their calm, positive, good-natured, supportive attitude is encouraging to others and helps them find the best in themselves.

When Heart types find their sense of self-worth within themselves rather than looking for it in the way others react to them, their positive qualities naturally surface. Once they have learned to open their hearts to themselves and nurture themselves, self-approval is easy and peace is the result.

Intuitive and emotionally sensitive, Heart types are extremely aware and considerate of the feelings of others. Loyal in relationships and family oriented, nurturing, and supportive, they are easy to talk to and readily listen to others, providing strength and comfort. By their very nature, they tend to draw out the best in those who associate with them.

The real gift of the Heart body type lies in their ability to manifest the spiritual principles of peace, harmony, and love in the practical, physical world.

### RECOMMENDED EXERCISE

Exercise is emotionally beneficial because it acts as a mood elevator and often provides an avenue for emotional connection with people. For weight loss, exercise a minimum of 20 minutes (up to an hour) 5 days a week; morning is the best time. Running, biking, brisk walking, isometric exercises, karate, and tennis may be done daily; yoga, stretching, or weight lifting, 1 to 2 times a week.

Good-natured, conscientious, and self-sufficient, they excel in what they set out to do, being particularly aware of the details. Sensitive and caring, they can be models of success in both business and personal relationships.

## Dietary Profile

### Main Focus

- Breakfast should be primarily fruit and/or grains.
- Have your largest meal at lunch.
- May include fruit for dessert after lunch but not after dinner.
- Include seeds, especially on salads.

### Dietary Emphasis

- From 25 to 40 percent of your calories are to come from fats.
- Best fat sources: butter, dense protein (chicken, fish, eggs, beef, pork, and lamb) and seeds (pumpkin, sesame, sunflower).
- From 20 to 35 percent of your calories are to come from protein.
- From 10 to 25 percent of your calories are to come from dense protein.
- Best sources of the three amino acids threonine, isoleucine, and cystine: quail, beef, and sesame and pumpkin seeds.
- Caloric intake: 1,500 to 1,800 calories a day for women and 1,700 to 2,000 calories a day for men. If you are engaging in intense exercise (competition type) or heavy labor, increase calories.
- Drink a minimum of 64 ounces of water a day. Drink water before and after meals, not with meals.
- Occasional desserts are best as an evening snack.
- Avoid honey and whole wheat bread.
- Avoid refined sugar, as it causes fatigue of muscles and the brain.
- Fruit for dessert after lunch acts as a digestive aid and often eliminates cravings for sweets.

### For Weight Loss

- Fat: 25 to 35 percent of daily calories.
- Eliminate all dairy and cheese except butter.
- Minimize carbohydrates and grains.
- Avoid wine; it inhibits weight loss.
- An evening snack is OK; a midafternoon snack is optional; no morning snack.

---

### RECOMMENDED CUISINE

Greek, German, seafood, English, Oriental, Chinese.

---

- Avoid eating potato or squash with dense protein.
- Soups and broths are nutritious and easy to digest.

### For Weight Gain

- Fat: 30 to 40 percent of daily calories.
- Emphasize dairy.

## Healthy Foods List

There is no need to sacrifice delicious and filling foods to maintain a healthy Heart body type. The following lists will help you will focus on foods that support your health and avoid foods that can stress your system.

*You'll notice that some foods are printed in italics; these foods take more energy to assimilate and could be ones you will want to avoid when you are in a sensitive state due to any physical or emotional stresses.*

Be sure to read Chapter 3, "Implementing the Body Type Diet," for lots of important information about how to use these many foods to gain their full benefit.

### Ultra-Support Foods

Foods to include in 3 to 7 meals a week, listed by category.

**Dense Protein:** beef, beef broth, beef liver, buffalo, lamb, pork, ham, bacon, sausage, veal, venison, organ meats (heart, brain); chicken, chicken broth, chicken livers, Cornish game hen, duck, turkey; anchovy, bass, bonita, catfish, cod, flounder, haddock, *halibut,* herring, mackerel, mahimahi, perch, orange roughy, salmon, sardines, shark, red snapper, sole, swordfish, trout, tuna; abalone, calamari (squid), clams, crab, eel, lobster, mussels, octopus, oysters, scallops, shrimp; eggs
**Dairy:** butter
**Cheese:** nonfat cottage, cream
**Nuts and Seeds:** almonds without skin, cashews (raw, roasted), cashew butter, pistachios; pumpkin seeds,

sesame seeds, sesame seed butter, raw sunflower seeds

**Legumes:** beans (adzuki, black, Great Northern, lima, navy, red, soy), black-eyed peas

**Grains:** amaranth, barley, *buckwheat,* oats, popcorn, quinoa, rice (all varieties), rice bran, rice cakes, rye, wheat germ, breads (oat, rice, rye), cream of rice, cream of rye, cream of wheat

**Vegetables:** beans (green, yellow wax), beets, broccoli, carrots, celery, onions (chives, brown, green, red, Vidalia, white, yellow), peas, snow pea pods, potatoes (all varieties), seaweed (arame, dulse, kelp, nori, wakame)

**Vegetable Juices:** carrot, carrot/beet, carrot/celery, celery, spinach

**Fruits:** apples (Red or Golden Delicious, Granny Smith, Jonathan, McIntosh, Pippin, Rome Beauty), apricots, berries (blackberries, blueberries, boysenberries, cranberries, gooseberries, raspberries, strawberries), dates, figs, grapes (black, green, red), grapefruit (red, white), guavas, kiwi, kumquats, lemons, limes, loquats, mangoes, nectarines, oranges, papayas, peaches, pears, pineapples, plums (black, red, purple), prunes, raisins, tangerines

**Fruit Juices:** apple, apple cider, apple/apricot, apricot, cranberry, grape (white, purple, red), grapefruit, guava, lemon, papaya, pear, pineapple, pineapple/coconut, prune, tangerine

**Sweeteners:** molasses, sorghum, barley malt powder, barley malt syrup, stevia

## Basic Support Foods

Foods to include in 1 to 2 meals a week.

**Dairy:** milk (whole, raw, goat's), half-and-half, sweet cream, sour cream, buttermilk, *kefir, yogurt (plain, flavored), ice cream* (Alta Dena, Ben & Jerry's, Dreyer's, Swensen's)

**Cheese:** American, blue, Brie, Camembert, cheddar, Colby, low-fat and regular cottage, Edam, feta, goat, Gouda, kefir, Limburger, Monterey Jack, mozzarella, Muenster, Parmesan, ricotta, Romano, Swiss

**Nuts and Seeds:** almonds (raw, roasted), almond butter, Brazils, coconut, hazelnuts, macadamias (raw, roasted), macadamia butter, peanuts (raw, roasted with or without salt), peanut butter, pecans, pine nuts (raw, roasted), walnuts (black, English), water chestnuts; roasted sunflower seeds, sunflower seed butter, nut milk

**Legumes:** *pinto beans,* lentils, split green peas; miso, soy milk, tofu

**Grains:** corn, corn grits, corn tortillas, couscous, hominy grits, millet, triticale, refined wheat flour, wheat bran, flour tortillas, breads (corn, corn/rye, French, garlic, Italian, *multigrain, seven-grain,* sourdough, white), bagels, croissants, English muffins, crackers (oat, rye, saltines, *wheat*), pasta, udon noodles, Chinese rice noodles

**Vegetables:** artichokes, avocado, bamboo shoots, bok choy, broccoflower, brussels sprouts, cabbage (green, napa, red), cauliflower, cilantro, cucumbers, *eggplant,* garlic, greens (beet, collard, mustard, turnip), hominy, jicama, kale, kohlrabi, leeks, lettuce (Boston, butter, red leaf, romaine), mushrooms, okra, olives (green, ripe), parsnips, bell peppers (green, red, yellow), chili peppers, pimientos, pumpkin, radish, daikon radish, rutabaga, sauerkraut, shallots, spinach, sprouts (alfalfa, clover, mung bean, radish, sunflower), squash (acorn, banana, butternut, spaghetti, yellow [summer], zucchini), sweet potato, Swiss chard, tomatoes, turnips, watercress, yams

**Vegetable Juice:** V-8

**Fruits:** bananas, cherries, melons (cantaloupe, casaba, Crenshaw, honeydew, *watermelon*), persimmons, pomegranates, rhubarb, tangelos

**Fruit Juices:** black cherry, red cherry, cranapple, orange

**Vegetable Oils:** all-blend, *almond,* avocado, coconut, *corn, flaxseed, olive, peanut, safflower, sesame, soy, sunflower*

**Sweeteners:** *fructose, sugar (brown, date, raw), syrup (brown rice, corn, maple), succonant*

**Condiments:** *mustard, mayonnaise, horseradish, barbecue sauce, pesto sauce, soy sauce, salsa, tahini,* vinegar, salt, sea salt, Vege-Sal

**Salad Dressings:** *blue cheese, French, ranch, creamy Italian, creamy avocado, Thousand Island,* vinegar and oil, lemon juice and oil

**Desserts:** *custards, tapioca, puddings, pies, cakes, chocolate, desserts containing chocolate, sherbet (orange, raspberry)*

**Chips:** *bean, corn (blue, white, yellow), potato*

**Beverages:** tea (*black,* green, herbal, Japanese, Chinese oolong); mineral water, sparkling water; *barley malt liquor, champagne, gin, scotch, vodka, whiskey; root beer, regular sodas*

## Stressful Foods

Have no more than once a month.

**Dairy:** *nonfat or low-fat milk, frozen yogurt, most ice creams*
**Legumes:** *garbanzo and kidney beans, hummus*
**Grains:** *whole wheat, sprouted grain bread, whole wheat bread*
**Vegetables:** *arugula, asparagus, corn, lettuce (iceberg, Bibb, endive), parsley*
**Vegetable Juices:** *parsley, tomato*
**Vegetable Oil:** *canola*
**Sweeteners:** *honey, refined cane sugar, saccharin, aspartame, Equal, NutraSweet, Sweet'n Low*
**Condiments:** *catsup, margarine*
**Beverages:** *coffee; wine (red, white), sake, liqueurs, beer; diet sodas*

## Scheduling Meals

### Healthy

Light meals aren't on the menu; go for moderate to heavy. Schedule your meals as follows:

*Breakfast:* 7–8 A.M. Light to moderate, with grain, fruit, dairy, and/or limited protein.
*Lunch:* 12–2 P.M. Heavy, with protein, dairy, grain, and/or vegetables. Fruit for dessert.
*Dinner:* 7–9 P.M. Moderate, with grain, vegetables, protein, dairy, nuts, seeds, and/or legumes. Avoid fruit.

### Snacks (optional)
*Midmorning:* (10 A.M.) fruit
*Midafternoon:* (3 P.M.) fruit, vegetables, grain, protein, dairy, nuts, or seeds
*Evening:* fruit, sweets, or dairy

### Sensitive

Adjust your intake as follows:

*Breakfast:* Moderate, with grain and/or fruit.
*Lunch:* Moderate, with grain, vegetables, legumes (beans, tofu), and/or limited protein (fish, eggs). Avoid fruit.
*Dinner:* Early. Moderate to heavy, with grain, vegetables, protein (fowl, beef, lamb), nuts, seeds, and/or legumes.

## Sample One-Week Menu

Snacks are optional.

DAY 1
*Breakfast:* oatmeal w/banana or blueberries
*Lunch:* steak and green beans
*Dinner:* beef, chicken, or vegetable soup
*Snack:* almonds

DAY 2
*Breakfast:* fresh mango, grapefruit, or cantaloupe
*Lunch:* roast turkey, carrots, and bell peppers
*Dinner:* salmon or red snapper, rice, and broccoli

DAY 3
*Breakfast:* corn tortilla w/butter
*Lunch:* shrimp sautéed in butter and garlic, stir-fried vegetables of zucchini, carrots, and onions, and rice
*Snack:* almonds, pecans, cashews, Brazils, and hazelnuts
*Dinner:* salad of spinach, water chestnuts, slivered almonds and sesame seeds and/or raw sunflower seeds w/creamy Italian or balsamic vinaigrette

DAY 4
*Breakfast:* peach or apricots, fresh or frozen
*Lunch:* roast chicken, broccoli, carrots, and apple
*Dinner:* sole, rice, carrots, cauliflower, and onions

DAY 5: CLEANSE
*Breakfast:* ginger tea, apple or grapes (black, green, or red)
*Lunch:* steamed zucchini, green beans, and/or yellow squash
*Dinner:* steamed chard and/or spinach

DAY 6
*Breakfast:* blueberry pancakes w/butter
*Lunch:* tuna (fillet, canned, or Japanese sashimi and seaweed) and a salad of tomato, avocado, and onions w/balsamic vinaigrette
*Snack:* pumpkin seeds
*Dinner:* chicken vegetable soup and salad of red leaf lettuce, jicama, bell pepper, and peas

DAY 7
*Breakfast:* bagel w/cream cheese and lox
*Lunch:* egg drop or wonton soup and egg foo yung

*Dinner:* lamb, pasta, and a salad of romaine lettuce, cucumbers, mushrooms, tomatoes, and onion with blue cheese or lemon juice and oil dressing

## Alternative Menus

*(Foods in parentheses are optional.)*

**Breakfast**
Scrambled eggs w/broccoli
Eggs and potato
Eggs and corn tortilla w/butter
Stewed prunes and an apple
Oatmeal w/apple
Cream of wheat (w/raisins)
Potato and kefir cheese (w/butter)
Kefir

**Lunch**
Turkey on flour tortilla (w/salsa)
Halibut and green beans
Broiled or grilled fish, pasta, and peas
Meat loaf and artichokes (potatoes)

**Lunch or Dinner**
Quail, rice, and red cabbage
Split pea soup
Eggs and steamed spinach w/lemon juice

**Dinner**
Chicken, rice, and a beet salad
Egg drop soup
Omelette or scrambled eggs w/green beans, onions, and mushrooms
Chicken, beef, lamb, or duck, sunflower or sesame seeds, beans, and mushrooms

# Hypothalamus

*The Hypothalamus body type is symbolized by a traffic signal. Hypothalamus types have an intense sense of responsibility and are therefore cautious about their decisions. They gather data extensively and focus exclusively on what is at hand.*

FAMOUS PEOPLE: Christopher Reeve, Meg Ryan, Meredith Baxter-Birney, Anthony Robbins

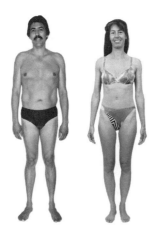

**HYPOTHALAMUS**
**Location and Function**

The hypothalamus is located at the center of the brain base, in front of the thalamus and the posterior pituitary. It controls visceral activities, such as water balance, temperature, and sleep.

## Psychological Profile

### Characteristic Traits

Characterized by phases, Hypothalamus body types totally immerse themselves in an activity or endeavor, often to the point of becoming crusaders. However, once they complete what they need to do, they switch to the next subject that catches their interest. These phases encompass all facets of reality, including relationships, inner probings, travel to unfamiliar places, and career changes.

It's not unusual for Hypothalamus men to focus on business, retire, devote themselves to family and home, then abandon retirement to repeat the cycle. They seem most at home in the financial world, often as stockbrokers or financial consultants. Money problems are common, and they often experience the extremes of abundance and subsistence. Hypothalamus women tend to have a better sense of money management.

With a deep, innate curiosity about the nature and function of things, Hypothalamus types are comfortable in the world of concepts and ideas. Their basic strengths include logic, decisiveness, commitment, and determination, traits that are essential to professional success, especially in the business world. Generally quick thinking and able to see the big picture, Hypothalamus types tend to work through steps one to three of a project, then leap ahead to steps nine and ten, delegating the intermediate steps to others.

### Motivation

Hypothalamus types move through different phases as a means of finding themselves. By immersing themselves in what interests them, they are able to travel to their inner depths and connect integral parts of their being, thereby learning to rely on their internal guidance rather than conventional standards and opinions. This self-integration is the key to their fulfillment. Although they may not stay focused on an experience or activity for long, while absorbed in something they experience it fully.

The inherent nature of Hypothalamus types is self-contained and independent. Carried to the extreme, it may appear as a difficulty with self-disclosure. This behavior pattern usually forms in childhood because of a suppressive family background. Many grew up in homes where their parents were either very critical or overly protective. Sensitive and fearful of failing, making mistakes, or otherwise losing their parents' support or approval, they often felt obliged to inhibit their self-expression. Their natural urges toward exploration of their inner and outer worlds thus subdued, they may have developed (at least in the company of others) a habit of self-restraint. This is why, if they are to realize their full potential, they must be around people with whom they can feel safe. The more they're able to experience external support, the more open they'll be about their thoughts and feelings and the more they'll be able to embrace the changes that can enable them to realize their multifaceted nature.

## "At Worst"

At times Hypothalamus types have difficulty trusting their intuition. They may struggle with a problem for too long, trying to solve it logically, without loosening the reins of the intellect to create a space for the solution to appear. In addition, they may become stuck in a mental loop and fail to move outside themselves. Being focused mentally, they sometimes need other people to serve as sounding boards, particularly if they're to get in touch with their emotions. Focused inward mentally, they may be unable to see what others are mirroring back and remain within the limitations of their own thinking.

Frequently, Hypothalamus types seem to expect that outside forces will intervene and take charge of their lives, assuming that things will magically fall into place without their having to do anything. This is often the case when it comes to managing money. Hypothalamus types may become so focused on the situation in front of them, such as how to help their children get what they want, that they fail to consider the long-term effects of not setting financial boundaries. While they may be very good at managing other people's money, Hypothalamus men often fail to do their own financial planning.

Intimate relationships are often a major challenge. Hypothalamus women often have difficulty maintaining their identity and self-expression, and men have difficulty dealing with problems and sharing their emotions. Unresolved emotional stress is usually manifested initially as depression. Alcohol and drugs are commonly used to avoid facing what often seem like insoluble problems. Work can also be a means of escape, as can finding ways of neglecting an unfulfilling relationship.

## "At Best"

Mentally adept, Hypothalamus types are good at analyzing things objectively. Decision making comes naturally, since they are inclined to understand or relate to things through judging them. They are effective at handling projects because they can easily grasp what needs to be done, devise an appropriate plan for accomplishing it, and see the job through responsibly. Typically, when embarking on a new project, they study the written instructions conscientiously (while other types bypass them) and learn as much as they can before scrupulously following the plan they have developed.

Hypothalamus types thoroughly investigate a subject before taking action. Then they handle whatever obstacles arise and, if necessary, redo things later on to achieve their desired results. They are generally receptive and flexible enough to change their approach as situations change or if they become aware of a better way of reaching their goals. Hypothalamus types are happiest when they can become creatively absorbed in their current challenge, whether professional or personal.

With active, inquiring minds, Hypothalamus types are proficient not only in acquiring but also in applying new knowledge. Receptive, sensitive, and intuitive, they are comfortable in the world of concepts and ideas. At times they throw themselves into life with intensity, willing to follow their enthusiasm wherever it may lead. While their curiosity drives them to experience the world with immediacy and passion, their caution and need to be physically safe hold them back. How well they're able to balance these aspects is reflected in the degree of their aliveness. It's when they dance with life that they excel.

---

### RECOMMENDED EXERCISE

Exercise is physically beneficial for Hypothalamus body types. It facilitates physical integration by providing a way to connect with the physical body. It gives the mind a rest and allows centering to occur. Ideally, exercise 20 minutes every other day (e.g., walking, dancing, singing, Callanetics, tennis, basketball, biking, and low-impact aerobics). Exercise works best when recreational; otherwise it becomes a low priority.

One of their special gifts is the capacity to get the insights or solutions they require simply by raising a question to themselves and then waiting for the answer to come to them. When they're able to join this innate receptivity or intuitiveness to their inborn tenacity, their success in any endeavor is virtually assured.

## Dietary Profile

### Main Focus

- Have a late breakfast with fruit followed by protein.
- Avoid fruit for lunch and dinner.
- Lunch on raw vegetables, salads, nuts, and seeds.
- Make dinner a cooked meal with steamed vegetables.
- Emphasize vegetables, fruit, cheese, nuts, and soups.

### Dietary Emphasis

- From 25 to 30 percent of your calories are to come from fats.
- Best fat sources: avocados, seeds (pumpkin, sunflower, and sesame), tahini, and nuts (almonds, pecans, Brazils, coconut, macadamias, pistachios, and dry-roasted cashews).
- From 20 to 35 percent of your calories are to come from protein.
- From 0 to 25 percent of your calories are to come from dense protein.
- Best sources of the three amino acids threonine, isoleucine, and cystine: turkey, tuna, and pumpkin seeds.
- Caloric intake: 1,500 to 1,800 calories a day for women and 1,700 to 2,000 calories a day for men. If you are engaging in intense exercise (competition type) or heavy labor, increase calories.
- Drink a minimum of 64 ounces of water a day. Drink water before and after meals, not with meals.
- Occasional desserts are best as an evening snack.
- To detoxify system, drink herbal tea or hot water with lemon upon rising. Wait 2 to 3 hours before eating breakfast.
- Raw vegetables are best assimilated at lunch.
- Cooked vegetables are best for dinner.
- Broccoli, zucchini, and yellow squash should always be eaten raw.
- Eat more raw vegetables than cooked.
- Rotate foods.

### For Weight Loss

- Dense protein: 15 to 25 percent of daily calories.
- Protein and fruit for breakfast at least 2 times a week.
- Limit dairy, cheese, frozen yogurt, fried foods, alcohol, caffeine, diet sodas, and breads with yeast.
- Limit snack to evening.
- May skip lunch and have light snack at midafternoon or when hungry.
- Adhere to time schedule for meals: breakfast, 9–10 A.M.; lunch, 1–2 P.M.; dinner, 6:30–9 P.M.

### For Weight Gain

- Fat: 35 percent of daily calories. Emphasize dairy, avocados, nuts, and seeds.
- Dense protein: 15 to 25 percent of daily calories.
- Consume protein and fruit for breakfast.
- Increase quantity of food and include snacks.
- Exercise is essential to build muscle weight.

## Healthy Foods List

There is no need to sacrifice delicious and filling foods to maintain a healthy Hypothalamus body type. The following lists will help you focus on foods that support your health, and avoid foods that can stress your system.

*You'll notice that some foods are printed in italics; these foods take more energy to assimilate and could be ones you will want to avoid when you are in a sensitive state due to any physical or emotional stresses.*

Be sure to read Chapter 3, "Implementing the Body Type Diet," for lots of important information about how to use these many foods to gain their full benefit.

---

**RECOMMENDED CUISINE**

Mexican, Thai, Chinese, Greek, Italian, French. Basically simple menus with grains, noodles, salads, soups, and legumes.

## Ultra-Support Foods

Foods to include in 3 to 7 meals a week.

**Dense Protein:** turkey; tuna; calamari (squid), clams, crab, lobster, mussels, oysters; eggs

**Cheese:** cheddar, Colby, Monterey Jack, mozzarella, Romano, raw goat cheese

**Nuts and Seeds:** cashews (roasted, unsalted), macadamias, macadamia butter, seeds (caraway, pumpkin, sunflower), sunflower seed butter

**Legumes:** beans (adzuki, pinto)

**Grains:** popcorn, rice (white or brown basmati, long or short grain brown or white), *wheat bran, wheat germ,* breads (French, multigrain, seven-grain), semolina pasta

**Vegetables:** asparagus, fresh green beans, broccoli, carrots, *cabbage* (green, napa, red), cauliflower, corn, garlic, leeks, mushrooms, peas, snow pea pods, bell peppers (green, red, yellow), pimientos, potatoes (White Rose, russet), pumpkin, sauerkraut, Swiss chard

**Vegetable Juice:** carrot

**Fruits:** *bananas,* dates, figs (fresh, dried), grapes (black, green, red), *grapefruit (white, red),* oranges, papayas, pineapples, prunes, raisins, strawberries; dried fruits

**Fruit Juices:** (morning) *unfiltered raw apple,* grape (purple, red, white), orange, pear

**Vegetable Oils:** *canola, olive, safflower*

**Sweetener:** stevia

**Beverages:** decaf coffee

## Basic Support Foods

Foods to include in 1 to 2 meals a week.

**Dense Protein:** *beef,* beef broth, beef liver, buffalo, lamb, *ham, pork, bacon, sausage,* venison, veal, organ meats (heart, brain); chicken, chicken broth, chicken livers, Cornish game hen, duck; anchovy, bass, bonita, catfish, cod, flounder, haddock, halibut, herring, mackerel, mahimahi, perch, roughy, salmon, sardines, shark, red snapper, sole, swordfish, trout; abalone, eel, octopus, scallops, shrimp

**Dairy:** milk (*whole,* 2%, *low fat, nonfat,* raw, raw goat's), half-and-half, sweet cream, sour cream, kefir, yogurt (plain or flavored), ice cream (Alta Dena, Baskin 31 Robbins, Ben & Jerry's, Breyer's, Dreyer's, Häagen-Dazs, Swensen's)

**Cheese:** American, blue, Brie, Camembert, cottage, cream, Edam, feta, raw goat's milk, Gouda, kefir, Limburger, Muenster, Parmesan, ricotta, Swiss

**Nuts and Seeds:** *almonds,* almond butter, Brazils, cashew butter, coconut, hazelnuts, peanuts, peanut butter, pecans, pine nuts, pistachios, walnuts (black, English), water chestnuts; sesame seeds, sesame seed butter

**Legumes:** beans (black, garbanzo, kidney, Great Northern, lima, navy, red, soy), lentils, black-eyed peas, split peas; hummus; miso, soy milk, tofu

**Grains:** amaranth, barley, buckwheat, corn, corn tortillas, couscous, hominy grits, millet, oats, quinoa, rice (Japanese, *polished,* wild), rice bran, rice cakes, *triticale, wheat,* refined wheat flour, flour tortillas, breads (corn, Italian, garlic, oat, sourdough, sprouted grain, *white, whole wheat*), croissants, English muffins, crackers (oat, saltines, *whole wheat*), pasta (corn, whole wheat), udon noodles, Chinese rice noodles, cream of rice, *cream of wheat*

**Vegetables:** artichokes, *arugula,* avocados, bamboo shoots, yellow wax beans, beets, bok choy, broccoflower, brussels sprouts, celery, cilantro, cucumber, eggplant, greens (beet, collard, mustard, turnip), hominy, jicama, kale, kohlrabi, lettuce (Boston, endive, iceberg, red leaf, romaine), okra, olives (green, ripe), onions (chives, brown, green, red, Vidalia, white, yellow), parsley, parsnips, chili peppers, potatoes (red, *Yukon Gold*), radish, daikon radish, rutabaga, *sauerkraut,* seaweed (arame, dulse, kelp, nori, wakame), shallots, spinach, sprouts (alfalfa, mung bean, clover, radish, sunflower), squash (acorn, banana, butternut, spaghetti, yellow [summer], zucchini), sweet potatoes, tomatoes, turnips, *watercress,* yams

**Vegetable Juices:** carrot/celery, celery, parsley, spinach, tomato, V-8

**Fruits:** apples (Golden or Red Delicious, Granny Smith, Jonathan, McIntosh, Pippin, Rome Beauty), apricots, berries (blackberries, blueberries, boysenberries, cranberries, gooseberries, raspberries), cherries, guavas, kiwi, kumquats, *lemons,* limes, loquats, mangoes, melons (casaba, Crenshaw, honeydew, watermelon), nectarines, *peaches,* pears, persimmons, *plums (black, purple, red),* pomegranates, rhubarb, tangelos, tangerines

**Fruit Juices:** (morning) apple cider, apple/apricot, apricot, black cherry, red cherry, cranapple, cranberry, *grapefruit,* guava, *lemon,* papaya, pineapple, pineapple/coconut, prune, tangerine

**Vegetable Oils:** all-blend, *almond*, avocado, coconut, *corn, flaxseed, peanut, sesame, soy, sunflower*

**Sweeteners:** *fructose, honey, molasses, sorghum, sugar (brown, date, raw, refined cane), syrup (bar-*ley malt, brown rice, *corn, maple), succonant*

**Condiments:** *catsup, mustard, horseradish, barbecue sauce, pesto sauce, soy sauce,* salsa, tahini, vinegar, salt, sea salt, Vege-Sal

**Salad Dressings:** *Blue cheese, French, ranch, creamy Italian, creamy avocado, Thousand Island,* vinegar and oil, lemon juice and oil

**Desserts:** *custards, tapioca, puddings, pies, cakes, milk chocolate, desserts containing milk chocolate, sherbet (orange, raspberry)*

**Chips:** *bean, corn (blue, white, yellow), potato*

**Beverages:** *coffee;* tea (*black,* green, herbal, Japanese, Chinese oolong); mineral water, sparkling water; *wine (red, white), sake, beer, barley malt liquor, champagne, liqueurs, gin, scotch, vodka, whiskey;* root beer, diet sodas, regular sodas

## Stressful Foods

Have no more than once a month.

**Dairy:** *pasteurized goat's milk, buttermilk, frozen yogurt, most ice creams*

**Cheese:** *pasteurized goat*

**Nuts and Seeds:** *raw cashews*

**Grains:** *rye, rye bread, rye crackers, bagels, cream of rye*

**Vegetable:** *butter lettuce*

**Fruit:** *cantaloupes*

**Fruit Juice:** *filtered, pasteurized apple juice*

**Sweeteners:** *saccharin, aspartame, Equal, Nutra-Sweet, Sweet'n Low*

**Condiments:** *mayonnaise, margarine*

**Dessert:** *dark chocolate*

## Scheduling Meals

### Healthy

Hypothalamus types should avoid heavy meals. Schedule your meals as follows:

*Breakfast:* 9–10 A.M. Light, with protein, dairy, and/or fruit.

*Lunch:* 1–2 P.M. Moderate, with grain, raw vegetables, legumes, dairy, nuts, and/or seeds. Avoid fruit.

*Dinner:* 6:30–9 P.M. Moderate, with protein, dairy, legumes, cooked or steamed vegetables, and/or grain. Raw vegetables, as in salads, may be eaten with meat and pasta. Avoid fruit.

### Snacks (optional)

*Midmorning:* grain, vegetables, fruit, dairy, nuts, seeds, protein, and/or legumes

*Midafternoon:* (4 P.M.) dairy, nuts, seeds, grain, and/or vegetables

*Evening:* (10 P.M.–1 A.M.) protein, dairy, vegetables, grain, nuts, seeds, sweets

### Sensitive

Adjust your intake as follows:

*Breakfast:* Light to moderate, with fruit, protein, dairy, and/or grain.

*Lunch:* Moderate, with protein, dairy, and/or vegetables.

*Dinner:* Moderate, with grain, dairy, legumes, and/or vegetables.

## Sample One-Week Menu

DAY 1

*Breakfast:* grapes or white grape juice, then chicken breast

*Lunch:* pasta w/raw broccoli and Italian dressing

*Snack:* raw carrots and sunflower seeds

*Dinner:* steak, potatoes, and a salad of spinach, potatoes, and green onions w/balsamic vinegar and olive oil

DAY 2

*Breakfast:* orange, then mushroom and egg omelette

*Lunch:* tomato, avocado, and onion w/balsamic vinegar and oil over Boston lettuce and couscous

*Dinner:* split pea soup and French bread w/butter

DAY 3

*Breakfast:* bananas, then cottage cheese

*Lunch:* falafel, rice, and a salad of green leaf lettuce, feta cheese, onions, and Greek salad and bell pepper with olive oil and vinegar dressing

*Dinner:* salmon, basmati rice, and asparagus

*Snack:* kefir

DAY 4

*Breakfast:* cantaloupe, then a salad of chicken, grapes, walnuts, and celery

*Lunch:* bean burrito and a salad of red leaf or romaine lettuce, tomato, onion, and mushrooms

*Dinner:* fillet of tuna and basmati rice w/leeks, snow pea pods, and bell peppers

DAY 5: CLEANSE

*Breakfast:* watermelon whole w/seeds and white part of rind

*Lunch:* raw carrots, bell pepper, jicama, celery with olive oil and vinegar and/or juice of carrot or carrot/celery (parsley) (spinach)

*Dinner:* steamed broccoli and/or cauliflower, green beans, corn (no butter)

DAY 6

*Breakfast:* grapes, then hard-boiled eggs

*Lunch:* salad of romaine lettuce, alfalfa sprouts, cherry tomatoes, and pumpkin seeds w/ranch dressing

*Dinner:* teriyaki chicken rice bowl and vegetables such as broccoli, carrots, celery, snow pea pods, bamboo shoots w/soy sauce

DAY 7

*Breakfast:* orange juice, cheese omelette

*Lunch:* orange roughy and green beans

*Dinner:* turkey, White Rose potatoes, and green beans

# Alternative Menus

*(Foods in parentheses are optional.)*

## Breakfast

Grapefruit and eggs

Apples, applesauce, or unfiltered apple juice and turkey

Grapes or apples and lobster

Cherries or blackberries and lobster

Apples and mussels

Grapes and oysters

Pineapple chunks or pineapple juice and chicken

Cherries and duck

Apple, then ham or pork chops

Pineapple and cottage cheese

## Lunch

Pasta w/pesto sauce and raw carrots

Salmon, cauliflower, and raw broccoli

Salmon and a salad of cucumber, spinach, and green peas

Bean burrito w/avocado

Three-bean salad on red leaf lettuce

Chef's salad of turkey, romaine lettuce, alfalfa sprouts, and cherry tomatoes with ranch dressing

## Dinner

Chicken, spinach, and red potatoes

Cashew chicken, water chestnuts, snow pea pods, and rice

Rainbow trout, pasta, and raw broccoli

Halibut and asparagus

Red snapper, pasta, and asparagus

Rice and beans (cheese enchilada w/avocado, salsa)

Scrambled eggs w/broccoli

Lentils, onions, and peppers (rice, beans, or cauliflower)

Stir-fried mushrooms, onions, carrots, celery, red peppers, and pasta

Bean soup

Chicken noodle soup

## Snacks

Yogurt and pecans

Cottage cheese and pineapple (tomato)

Raisins and nuts (oatmeal)

Macadamia nuts and apricots

Potato, lettuce, and/or avocado

Peanuts and raisins

Almonds and dried cherries

Celery w/peanut butter

Cottage cheese w/pineapple

# Intestinal

*The Intestinal body type is symbolized by a funnel. Intestinal types accept everything that comes in and then discern what to keep and what to release. Constant new experiences are vital to their continued growth and expansion.*

FAMOUS PEOPLE: Tom Hanks, Cybill Shepherd, Matthew Perry, Suzanne Somers

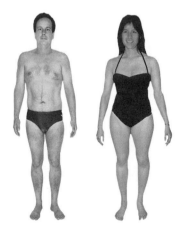

**INTESTINAL**
**Location and Function**

The intestines are located in the lower abdomen. Their function is to digest and absorb food, other nutrients, and water.

## Psychological Profile

### Characteristic Traits

Sensitive and extremely emotional, Intestinal body types are typically gentle, loving, and compassionate. Relationships are of utmost importance to them, particularly family and close friends. With their extreme sensitivity, they are exceedingly concerned about feelings. When they're not sure how to deal with an uncomfortable situation, their tendency is to internalize it. Being acutely aware of the stress that unresolved issues create for them personally as well as in their relationships, they have a strong need to clear the air.

Intestinal types have high standards and self-expectations. With their strong desire to do things right, they need to understand everything they encounter. Consequently, they are very good at responding to problems objectively and analytically. Responsible, orderly, methodical, and attentive to detail, Intestinal types are extremely capable.

Intestinal types are also imaginative, and their active imaginations often escape into the creative world of daydreams. By nature free spirits, they are typically a bit unconventional in their thinking and rarely bound by tradition. They're likely to be artistically inclined.

### Motivation

Creative and expansive, Intestinal types enjoy working with others. They are inspired by group association and interaction with other people. Therefore they generally function best when they can connect with others. Their inspiration often comes from the emotional boost of being around people who are positive and enjoy what they are doing. For Intestinal types, inspiration is a process that occurs within, not the kind that comes from a sales meeting or rally. With their strong emotional energy, they are good at motivating others and providing support wherever needed. They are often an inspiration themselves, as they can enliven a room by their presence alone.

While they enjoy working with others, Intestinal types are highly capable and can just as easily work alone, often preferring to figure things out by themselves. Being open to new or unconventional ideas, not limited by tradition, and being stimulated by personal growth, they are able to let their creativity soar and develop new ways of dealing with problems.

Intestinal types need variety and change to gain life experiences. They are intellectually curious, and mental stimulation satisfies their need to expand. Since expansion is essential in their lives, feelings of being restricted or held back are strong motivations for change. Change is not easy, however, because their sensitivity and feelings of insecurity in the world often cause an internal conflict. To feel safe, Intestinal types often gather all the information they can find on a new subject and analyze it in detail until they fully understand it. Gathering information and thoroughly analyzing whatever comes their way is another way of balancing their strong emotional responses. But having to explore all options before making a decision can be restrictive and can conflict with their need to expand. The analysis process alone can delay the implementation of beneficial changes in their lives. With limited real-life experience, Intestinal types need to rely more heavily on their free spirit, openness, and willingness to explore nonconventional areas.

## "At Worst"

Intestinal types often restrict their experiences and relationships by prejudging future situations based on past ones when things didn't go as planned. Also, once they have intellectual knowledge, they often shut out new information or insights by saying, "I already know it." In this way they discourage others from openly discussing any limiting behavior they may inadvertently be expressing.

With their emotions so close to the surface, Intestinal types can be overly sentimental, easily crying or laughing or swinging to the opposite extreme of being abrasive. When they let people push their buttons, their soft-spoken demeanor quickly changes into suspicion and contentiousness. Prone to worry, they get caught up in negative emotions when physically stressed. Fatigue alone is often enough to trigger depression or pessimism. Not knowing how to deal with their emotions, they often retreat into fantasy or denial. They have a natural tendency to become suspicious and challenge all new information, especially if it can't be proven. Lack of courage to face the fear of the unknown is common and can cause them to be skeptical and pessimistic, especially when they get stuck in worry and all the negatives that accompany it.

Because of a fear of loss or rejection, Intestinal types tend to get too attached to their families. With low self-esteem, they often find themselves in physically or emotionally abusive relationships and stay in them too long, lacking the courage to speak out or make a change. Since confrontation is difficult, they often avoid it at all costs.

Change is difficult for Intestinal types to initiate or sustain without external support because of their tendency to procrastinate, their pessimism, and their tendency to be hard on themselves. Needing outside validation to establish their self-worth, they make negative assumptions about others' opinions of them and then get upset (wallowing in self-pity) or self-absorbed or adopt the victim role, wanting to be rescued. Their pessimism often translates into a distrust of people in authority and even of the world in general.

## "At Best"

Intestinal types have a good sense of humor and can be a lot of fun to be around. They can fill a room with their joy and vivaciousness. Dependable and reliable, they are able to get things done and will work until the job is finished. Idealistic and altruistic, they particularly enjoy helping others.

Good with people and in organizations, Intestinal types genuinely like everybody. They are excellent support people or coordinators, as they inspire others to do their best and provide the cohesiveness needed to see things through. Having learned to trust and listen to their strong intuitive nature, they are able to assess situations and projects quickly and accurately, easily making the best decisions.

Their strong intuitive side attracts them to opportunities for new settings, situations, and people and also draws them to nontraditional experiences. They have fun with physical expression and are active, enjoying

---

### RECOMMENDED EXERCISE

Exercise relieves emotional stress and aids digestion. Ideally, Intestinal types should do some form of exercise at least 5 days a week. However, not all exercises are beneficial on a daily basis. Maximum weekly frequency for each activity is as follows: walking—5 times; swimming—daily; Callanetics—twice; biking—twice; stretching—twice; low-impact aerobics—twice. Most exercise should be moderate, with no heavy weight lifting. Intestinal types can become exhausted with morning or evening exercise; the best time is between 11 A.M. and 4 P.M., for 20 minutes to 1 hour.

whatever experience shows up. Self-sufficient and introspective, they take care of themselves, setting limits and establishing boundaries for what other people can expect from them. This way they protect their energies from becoming depleted. Self-nurturing often comes through personal growth.

Once Intestinal types are able to express their creative energies effectively by keeping the channel to their intuitive side open and learning to observe their emotions and let them pass, they seem to be intuitively connected to the universe and are able to flow with life.

## Dietary Profile

### Main Focus

▶ Expand emotionally, mentally, and/or spiritually, primarily through creativity and relationships.
▶ Make lunch your largest meal.
▶ Avoid breads containing yeast.
▶ Rotate foods and food combinations.

### Dietary Emphasis

▶ From 20 to 35 percent of your calories are to come from fats.
▶ Best fat sources: sesame seeds, tahini, butter, fish (halibut, orange roughy, salmon, shark, swordfish, lobster, shrimp), olive oil, sesame oil, beef, chicken, turkey, and cream.
▶ From 20 to 40 percent of your calories are to come from protein.
▶ From 0 to 30 percent of your calories are to come from dense protein. Sensitive may increase dense protein to 40 percent of calories.
▶ Best sources of the three amino acids threonine, isoleucine, and cystine: chicken, turkey, and halibut.
▶ Caloric intake: 1,500 to 1,800 calories a day for women and 1,700 to 2,000 calories a day for men. If you are engaging in intense exercise (competition type) or heavy labor, increase calories.
▶ Drink a minimum of 64 ounces of water a day. Drink water before and after meals, not with meals.
▶ Occasional desserts are best as an evening snack.
▶ Eat legumes and squash.
▶ Balance cooked and raw vegetables.
▶ Raw vegetables are best at dinner.
▶ Rebuild body with protein and vegetables.

### For Weight Loss

▶ Fat: 15 to 30 percent of daily calories.
▶ Dense protein: 15 to 30 percent of daily calories.
▶ When body is exhausted, as is often the case with chronic excess weight gain, focus primarily on protein and vegetables, particularly for breakfast and lunch.
▶ Limit carbohydrates.
▶ Eliminate alcohol, bread, yeast, mayonnaise, and caffeine.
▶ Avoid lentils, dried peas, corn, bananas, dried fruit, and sweets.
▶ Limit fruit and fruit juice.
▶ Drink plenty of water.
▶ Snacks are OK to maintain blood sugar levels. Choose different forms of protein such as string cheese, protein bars, pumpkin seeds, sunflower seeds, turkey, or chicken.
▶ Insufficient protein results in sugar cravings and hunger.

### For Weight Gain

▶ Fat: 20 to 40 percent of daily calories.
▶ Dense protein: 15 to 30 percent of daily calories.
▶ Increase food quantity.

## Healthy Foods List

There is no need to sacrifice delicious and filling foods to maintain a healthy Intestinal body type. The following lists will help you focus on foods that support your health, and avoid foods that can stress your system.

*You'll notice that some foods are printed in italics; these foods take more energy to assimilate and could be ones you will want to avoid when you are in a sensitive state due to any physical or emotional stresses.*

Be sure to read Chapter 3, "Implementing the Body Type Diet," for lots of important information about how to use these many foods to gain their full benefit.

---

**RECOMMENDED CUISINE**

Mexican, Italian, home-style cooking, seafood

## Ultra-Support Foods

Foods to include in 3 to 7 meals a week, listed by category.

**Dense Protein:** chicken, turkey

**Dairy:** *raw whole milk,* yogurt (plain or flavored), plain kefir, butter

**Cheese:** low-fat white cheddar

**Nuts and Seeds:** cashews (unsalted, dry roasted), cashew butter, peanuts (unsalted, dry roasted), *peanut butter, pecans,* walnuts (black, English); *roasted and unsalted seeds (pumpkin, sesame, sunflower), sesame seed butter, sunflower seed butter*

**Legumes:** beans (black, lima, pinto), lentils

**Grains:** amaranth, *corn, corn grits, hominy grits,* millet, rice (brown or white basmati, *long or short grain brown,* Japanese, polished, *wild*), rice bran, rice cakes, popcorn rice cakes, rye, whole wheat, whole wheat tortillas, breads (corn, whole wheat), cream of rice, cream of rye, cream of wheat

**Vegetables:** artichokes, *beets,* broccoli, *brussels sprouts,* cabbage (green, napa, red), *corn, cucumbers,* garlic, jicama, red leaf lettuce, mushrooms, *onions (all varieties),* peas, snow pea pods, potatoes (all varieties), pumpkin, seaweed (arame, dulse, kelp, nori, wakame), spinach, squash (acorn, butternut), sweet potatoes, yams

**Fruits:** apples (Golden or Red Delicious), bananas, berries (*blueberries,* strawberries), cantaloupes, dates, grapes (black, red), dried pineapple, black plums, raisins

**Fruit Juices:** apple, apple cider, cranapple, cranberry, cranberry concentrate

**Sweeteners:** sorghum, *molasses,* date sugar, brown rice syrup, stevia

**Condiments:** pickles (dill, sweet)

**Beverages:** seltzer water

## Basic Support Foods

Foods to include in 1 to 2 meals a week.

**Dense Protein:** *beef,* beef broth, beef liver, buffalo, *lamb, pork, ham, bacon, sausage,* veal, venison, organ meats (heart, brain); chicken broth, chicken livers, *Cornish game hen,* duck; anchovy, bass, bonita, catfish, cod, flounder, haddock, halibut, herring, mackerel, mahimahi, perch, orange roughy, salmon, sardines, shark, red snapper, sole, swordfish, trout, yellowtail tuna; abalone, calamari (squid), clams, crab, eel, *lobster,* mussels, octopus, oysters, scallops, shrimp; *eggs*

**Dairy:** milk (*whole, low fat, nonfat,* goat's), half-and-half, sour cream, sweet cream, buttermilk, flavored kefir, *frozen yogurt, ice cream* (Ben & Jerry's, Dreyer's, Swensen's), Ice Bean, Rice Dream

**Cheese:** American, blue, Brie, Camembert, cheddar, Colby, cottage, cream, Edam, feta, goat, Gouda, kefir, Limburger, Monterey Jack, mozzarella, Muenster, Parmesan, ricotta, Romano, Swiss

**Nuts and Seeds:** *almonds (raw, roasted), almond butter, Brazils,* raw cashews, *coconut,* hazelnuts, macadamias (raw, roasted), macadamia butter, *raw peanuts,* pine nuts (raw, roasted), *pistachios,* water chestnuts; *raw seeds (sesame, sunflower), raw or roasted caraway seeds*

**Legumes:** beans (adzuki, garbanzo, Great Northern, kidney, navy, red, *soy*), black-eyed peas, split peas; hummus; miso, *soy milk, tofu*

**Grains:** *barley, buckwheat,* blue corn, *corn tortillas,* couscous, oats, oat flour pancakes, popcorn, quinoa, triticale, wheat bran, wheat germ, refined wheat flour, *flour tortillas,* breads (*corn/rye, French,* garlic, *Italian, multigrain,* rice, *rye, sevengrain, sourdough, sprouted grain, white), bagels, croissants,* English muffins, crackers (Carr's table water, oat, oriental rice, rye, saltines, sesame seed, whole wheat), pasta (plain, *spinach, beet*), udon noodles, Chinese rice noodles

**Vegetables:** asparagus, *avocados,* bamboo shoots, beans (green, yellow wax), bok choy, broccoflower, carrots, cauliflower, celery, cilantro, eggplant, greens (beet, collard, mustard, turnip), kale, kohlrabi, leeks, lettuce (Boston, butter, curly leaf, endive, romaine), okra, olives (black, green, ripe), parsley, parsnips, *bell peppers (green, red, yellow), chili peppers, pimientos,* radish, daikon radish, rutabaga, sauerkraut, shallots, sprouts (alfalfa, mung bean, clover, radish, sunflower), squash (banana, spaghetti, yellow [summer], zucchini), Swiss chard, *tomatoes* (canned, hothouse, vine-ripened), turnips, watercress

**Vegetable Juices:** carrot, carrot/celery, celery, parsley, spinach, tomato, V-8

**Fruits:** apples (Jonathan, Rome Beauty, McIntosh, Pippin, Granny Smith), berries (blackberries, boysenberries, cranberries, gooseberries, raspberries), cherries, figs (fresh, dried), green grapes, grapefruit (red, white), guavas, kiwi, kumquats, lemons, limes, loquats, mangoes, melons (casaba, Crenshaw, *honeydew, watermelon*), nectarines, *oranges,* papayas, peaches, pears, persimmons, pineapples, plums (purple, red), pomegranates, prunes, rhubarb, tangelos, tangerines

**Fruit Juices:** *apple/apricot,* apricot, black cherry, red cherry, grape (purple, red, white), grapefruit, guava, lemon, papaya, pear, pineapple, pineapple/coconut, prune, tangerine, watermelon

**Vegetable Oils:** all-blend, *almond,* avocado, coconut, corn, flaxseed, olive, peanut, safflower, sesame, *soy,* sunflower

**Sweeteners:** *honey, sugar (brown, raw, refined cane),* syrup (barley malt, *corn),* succonant

**Condiments:** *catsup, mustard, horseradish, barbecue sauce, pesto sauce, soy sauce, salsa,* tahini, vinegar, salt, sea salt, Vege-Sal

**Salad Dressings:** *blue cheese, French, ranch, creamy Italian, creamy avocado, Thousand Island,* vinegar and oil, lemon juice and oil

**Desserts:** *custards, tapioca, puddings, pies, cakes, chocolate, desserts containing chocolate*

**Chips:** *bean, corn (blue, white, yellow),* potato

**Beverages:** *coffee;* tea (*black,* blends—Bigelow and *Constant Comment,* green, herbal—peppermint and raspberry, Japanese, Chinese oolong); *mineral water, sparkling water;* wine *(red, white), sake, beer, barley malt liquor, champagne, liqueurs, gin, scotch, vodka, whiskey; root beer, regular sodas*

## Stressful Foods

Have no more than once a month.

**Dense Protein:** *tuna*
**Nuts and Seeds:** *raw pumpkin seeds*
**Grain:** *tomato pasta*
**Vegetables:** *arugula, iceberg lettuce*
**Fruit:** *apricots*
**Fruit Juice:** *orange*
**Vegetable Oil:** canola
**Sweeteners:** *fructose, maple syrup, saccharin, aspartame, Equal, NutraSweet, Sweet'n Low*
**Condiments:** *margarine, mayonnaise*
**Dessert:** *sherbet (orange, raspberry)*
**Beverages:** *diet sodas*

## Scheduling Meals

### Healthy

Intestinal types should avoid heavy meals. Schedule your meals as follows:

*Breakfast:* 8–9 A.M. Light to moderate, with fruit juice, fruit, or dairy.

*Lunch:* 12–2 P.M. Moderate, with grain, protein, dairy, legumes, cooked vegetables, and/or seeds. Raw vegetables may be eaten with protein (e.g., Caesar salad with chicken). Avoid fruit.

*Dinner:* 7–9 P.M. Moderate, with higher fat, dairy, legumes, protein, raw vegetables, and/or seeds. Avoid fruit.

### Snacks (optional)

*Midmorning:* (10–11 A.M.) fruit, dairy, vegetables, nuts, seeds

*Midafternoon:* (3–4 P.M.) fruit or grain

*Evening:* (10 P.M.–2 A.M.) nuts, seeds, vegetables, grain, protein, fruit, sweets

### Sensitive

Increase your intake as follows:

*Breakfast:* Moderate to heavy, with vegetables, protein, seeds, and/or grain. Avoid fruit.

*Lunch:* Moderate to heavy, with protein, cooked vegetables, and/or grain.

*Dinner:* Light to moderate, with vegetables, legumes, dairy, protein, and/or grain.

*Snacks:* Same as above for healthy.

## Sample One-Week Menu

DAY 1
*Breakfast:* oatmeal w/raisins
*Lunch:* halibut, pasta, and green beans
*Dinner:* Chili relleno and beans

DAY 2
*Breakfast:* strawberries or red grapes
*Lunch:* pork chops, rice, and yellow squash
*Dinner:* yams, green beans, and raw carrot sticks

DAY 3
*Breakfast:* cottage cheese w/pineapple
*Lunch:* mahimahi, rice, and broccoflower
*Dinner:* manicotti w/red sauce

DAY 4
*Breakfast:* peaches or pears
*Lunch:* pot roast, red potatoes, and carrots
*Dinner:* butternut squash and a salad of romaine lettuce, mushrooms, and eggs w/balsamic vinegar

DAY 5: CLEANSE

*Breakfast:* unfiltered apple juice and/or apples

*Lunch:* steamed cauliflower, squash, collards and/or kale or raw cucumber and/or carrot/celery juice

*Snack:* steamed collards, Swiss chard, or kale and/or carrot/celery juice

*Dinner:* steamed zucchini or other squashes, raw and/or carrot/celery juice

*Snack:* steamed squash (all) and/or carrot/celery juice

DAY 6

*Breakfast:* yam and peas

*Lunch:* salmon, rice, and asparagus

*Dinner:* broccoli quiche and tomatoes

DAY 7

*Breakfast:* cheese omelette w/broccoli

*Lunch:* turkey w/cranberry sauce, potato w/gravy, and cauliflower

*Dinner:* pumpkin soup and a salad of spinach, beets, sesame seeds, onions, and jicama with vinegar and oil

## Alternative Menus

*(Foods in parentheses may be omitted.)*

### Breakfast

Grapefruit

Cream of rice w/walnuts, sunflower seeds, and apple

Banana, raisins, and pumpkin seeds

Eggs, snow peas, bamboo shoots, and celery (chicken)

Chicken livers and Swiss chard

Halibut and asparagus

Spinach quiche

### Lunch

Lamb, pasta, and peas (onions)

Catfish, rice, and asparagus

Ham, yam, and green beans

Chicken and coleslaw

Chicken Marsala (cream sauce w/mushrooms) and pasta

Chicken cacciatore over spaghetti squash

Beef or chicken fajita

Lamb chops, red potatoes, peas, and romaine salad

Tamale, rice, and beans

### Dinner

Grilled swordfish and broccoli (baked potato)

Cheese omelette

Turkey and angel-hair pasta w/garlic, butter, and broccoli

Salad of spinach, cheese, and eggs

Split pea soup

# Kidney

*The Kidney body type is symbolized by a bowline knot. This unique knot takes hold when under pressure and relaxes when the pressure subsides. Procrastinating until sufficient pressure builds enables Kidney types to move further than they ever imagined.*

FAMOUS PEOPLE: Kathy Rigby, Kristi Yamaguchi, Scott Hamilton, Brad Pitt

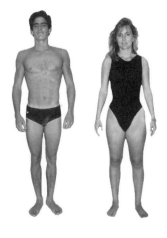

**KIDNEY**
**Location and Function**

The kidneys are located in the lower back near the lower ribs, about four inches on each side of the spine. Their function is to filter blood and secrete urine.

## Psychological Profile

### Characteristic Traits

Kidney body types are known for their procrastination. Pressure produces the stimulation they need to get busy and start a job. Ideally, successful completion then propels them to the next level. Realistically, too much procrastination causes them to fall behind, so their acceleration only brings them up to where they should be.

Relationships are of paramount importance to Kidney types, whether with family, children, or friends. In touch with their emotions, sensitive, and expressive, Kidney types are exceptionally good at helping others become more aware of their feelings and communicate them effectively. Being good listeners, they typically respond to the words of others accurately and objectively rather than emotionally. They can look at a problem, size it up, and break it down, laying out the best approach to its solution.

Willing and supportive, kidney types may find that their friends frequently call them and ask for assistance in dealing with their problems. Being generally optimistic and positive, Kidney types are usually nonjudgmental and look for the good qualities in people. They excel when working with others, particularly in a service or teaching capacity.

Kidney types need new experiences, options, and challenges. Highly creative and easily bored with conventional, routine, or repetitive activities, they are often drawn toward new, unproven ideas and technologies.

### Motivation

Needing the stimulation of new concepts and projects, Kidney types find the routine, day-to-day stuff boring. When they don't really want to do something, they procrastinate, begin to feel tired, and have a hard time getting motivated. Craving variety, they welcome new ventures with extreme enthusiasm. Once they get started, they tend to work in spurts, giving their all until they either complete the task or collapse, too tired to work any longer. When motivated, they are persistent and tenacious; they jump right in and go for it, even getting things done ahead of schedule.

Kidney types control by controlling their environment. Needing to sift through a wide range of life experiences to find their purposes and ideals, in their sorting process they put things in "boxes" as a way of controlling and handling them. In their attempt to control outcomes, they need everything to look perfect. Unknowns are unnerving because they bring up the fear of not being able to handle a situation perfectly.

Unsure of themselves, Kidney types are fearful of making wrong decisions. In reality, since their life is about experience, the only wrong decision is no decision because it causes them to miss opportunities or stay in situations too long. Kidney types often find themselves torn between wanting enough time to make the best decision and wanting to be in control, where they are forced to make quick decisions. Being in leadership roles minimizes unknowns and adds to their sense of power and importance. Deadlines force them to make a decision or accept someone else's decision. When situations become too uncomfortable or they feel trapped, Kidney types venture into unknown areas, which forces them to excel and move beyond their previous limits.

Another reason Kidney types have such a hard time making decisions is that they have a hard time letting go. Being quite tenacious, they tend to dwell on a situation for days on end. This often comes from their need to get the essence, fullness, or lesson of the experience before they can release it. Ironically, the essence of an experience usually doesn't come until they are able to let it go.

## "At Worst"

Kidney types can be lazy, irresponsible, and lackadaisical. They can procrastinate too much and get stuck. Fearful of making a mistake or being inadequate, they may avoid taking any action. Lacking self-esteem, they may stay in abusive or codependent relationships. Being too hard on themselves or impatient often results in their being impulsive or irrational. Their self-defeating and self-destructive behavior can affect all aspects of their lives. Lacking self-confidence and knowledge of what they really want, they easily succumb to peer pressure, drugs, and/or alcohol.

When their fear surfaces, the underlying pessimist appears, and they get caught in negative thought patterns: "You know my luck" or "What if . . . ?" Being exceptionally good at visualization, they may create negative situations through what they focus on. Basically fearful, they may impose their own limits on themselves. Unresolved emotional stress tends to affect them physically, resulting in excess weight gain or restrictive health problems.

Kidney types are bored by routine, but without structure they procrastinate. Seeking approval, they overcommit or overextend themselves, making promises they can't keep or exhausting themselves trying to do it all. When they spread themselves too thin, their health eventually suffers or they lose significant opportunities by not prioritizing and following through on important projects. They spend an excessive amount of time getting ready to do something. By not handling tasks efficiently, they allow the pressure to build until they are forced to act. They then react to situations emotionally, either with directionless activity or with a lackadaisical attitude fueled by fear.

## "At Best"

Sensitive and expressive, Kidney types are in touch with their emotions. They love people and have a special gift for helping others connect with their feelings and communicate them. With their ability to listen and hear what a person is truly saying, as well as to see viable, practical solutions, Kidney types make excellent mediators, counselors, and teachers. They are especially gratified by serving others in ways that make significant differences in their lives.

Having developed their self-confidence to the point where they are no longer compelled to hold themselves back, Kidney types can be capable of making quick decisions and acting on their feelings. They are able to take advantage of new experiences, focusing on those that have a purpose or embody an ideal. They are extremely adaptable and are happiest when they are open to multiple experiences and free to choose among several options. Of particular importance are experiences with people.

Creative and intuitive, Kidney types are good at seeing and implementing practical solutions. Extremely visual, they are good at visualizing expected results and outcomes before they happen. By making conscious choices and pushing through the fear that holds them back, they find that the world opens up

---

### RECOMMENDED EXERCISE

Exercise allows movement in life and gets energy moving through the body. Yoga, stretching, Callanetics, tennis, running, and walking are best. Although Kidney body types may have difficulty getting motivated, exercise 4 times a week is important for the alleviation of stress.

and supports them, allowing them to experience the fullness of life. Having learned to balance their feelings with their mind, and their receptive feminine side with their active masculine side, Kidney types are able to visualize what they want and make it happen. They are able to move beyond any limitation and help others do the same. Being firmly connected with God or their spiritual source gives them the courage to know and speak their truth.

## Dietary Profile

### Main Focus

- Have a heavy lunch with protein, no fruit.
- Have a light dinner without dense protein.
- Olive oil once a day builds the immune system.
- Rotate foods.
- Eat bananas and vegetables.

### Dietary Emphasis

- From 20 to 35 percent of your calories are to come from fats.
- Best fat sources: olive oil, almonds, peanuts, butter, and dairy (cheese and yogurt).
- From 25 to 40 percent of your calories are to come from protein.
- From 0 to 30 percent of your calories are to come from dense protein.
- Best sources of the three amino acids threonine, isoleucine, and cystine: beef, tuna, and shrimp.
- Caloric intake: 1,500 to 1,800 calories a day for women and 1,700 to 2,000 calories a day for men. If you are engaging in intense exercise (competition type) or heavy labor, increase calories.
- Drink a minimum of 64 ounces of water a day. Drink water before and after meals, not with meals.
- Occasional desserts are best as as evening snack.
- Minimize refined grains.
- Eat the following foods only in these combinations. Together they are Basic Support Foods, while alone they are Stressful:
  Eggs with tomato, salsa, or catsup
  Tuna with lettuce
  Turkey with cranberry sauce
- Salsa and other spicy foods stimulate the lymphatics.

### For Weight Loss

- Fat: 20 to 30 percent of daily calories.
- Dense protein: 10 to 30 percent of daily calories.
- Rotate foods, eating as many different foods as possible.
- Have a light breakfast (heavy if sensitive or protein deficient).
- May include midafternoon snack.
- Observe the following intervals between meals: 4 to 6 hours between breakfast and lunch, 5 to 7 hours between lunch and dinner, and 3 to 4 hours between lunch and a midafternoon snack.
- Decrease carbohydrates.
- Use visualization to create and hold a mental picture of yourself at your ideal weight.

### For Weight Gain

- Fat: 30 to 35 percent of daily calories.
- Protein: 30 to 45 percent of daily calories.
- Dense protein: 25 to 30 percent of daily calories.
- Increase quantity of food, emphasizing protein and carbohydrates.
- When at ideal weight or above (though not when underweight), creamy foods, such as ice cream, cream pie, and cheese cake, as well as all foods containing sugar and fat, will quickly increase weight.

## Healthy Foods List

There is no need to sacrifice delicious and filling foods to maintain a healthy Kidney body type. The following lists will help you focus on foods that support your health, and avoid foods that can stress your system.

*You'll notice that some foods are printed in italics; these foods take more energy to assimilate and could be ones you avoid when you are in a sensitive state due to any physical or emotional stresses.*

Be sure to read Chapter 3, "Implementing the Body Type Diet," for lots of important information about how to use these many foods to gain their full benefit.

### RECOMMENDED CUISINE

Mexican, Thai, Chinese, Italian, seafood, or Indian.

## Ultra-Support Foods

Foods to include in 3 to 7 meals a week, listed by category.

**Dense Protein:** beef; salmon, trout, *tuna; crab, lobster,* scallops
**Dairy:** sour cream, butter
**Cheese:** *blue,* feta
**Nuts and Seeds:** *almonds* (raw, roasted), peanuts (raw, roasted), peanut butter, pine nuts (raw, roasted), *walnuts (black, English)*
**Legumes:** beans (black, garbanzo, kidney, lima, navy, pinto); hummus
**Grains:** couscous, rice (white or brown basmati, Chinese or Japanese white), refined wheat breads (*dill/rye,* French, Italian, sourdough, white), croissants, pasta
**Vegetables:** avocados, green beans, cabbage (green, napa, red), *carrots,* cucumbers, *eggplant, garlic, iceberg lettuce,* cooked onions, peas, snow pea pods, yellow bell peppers, potatoes (purple, Yukon Gold), radishes, daikon radishes, sweet potatoes, *cherry tomatoes, tomatoes* (canned, hothouse, vine-ripened), *yams*
**Fruits:** *apples* (all varieties), bananas, cantaloupes, grapefruit (white, red), *kiwi,* lemons, limes, loquats, *oranges,* peaches, raspberries
**Sweeteners:** stevia
**Beverages:** tea (Good Earth, peppermint, spearmint)

## Basic Support Foods

Foods to include in 1 to 2 meals a week.

**Dense Protein:** beef broth, beef liver, *buffalo, lamb, pastrami, pepperoni, pork, ham, bacon, sausage,* veal, venison, organ meats (heart, brain); chicken, chicken broth, chicken livers, Cornish game hen, *duck,* turkey; *anchovy,* bass, bonita, catfish, cod, flounder, haddock, halibut, herring, mackerel, mahimahi, perch, orange roughy, sardines, shark, red snapper, sole, swordfish, ahi tuna; abalone, calamari (squid), clams, eel, mussels, octopus, oysters, *shrimp; eggs*
**Dairy:** milk (nonfat, raw, *goat's*), half-and-half, sweet cream, *buttermilk,* kefir, yogurt (low fat or nonfat flavored), *frozen yogurt, ice cream* (Ben & Jerry's, Dreyer's, Swensen's)
**Cheese:** American, Brie, Camembert, cheddar, Colby, cottage, *cream,* Edam, goat, Gouda, kefir, Limburger, Monterey Jack, mozzarella, Muenster, Parmesan, ricotta, Romano, Swiss
**Nuts and Seeds:** almond butter, *Brazils,* cashews (raw, roasted), cashew butter, coconut, hazelnuts, *macadamias (raw, roasted), macadamia butter,* pecans, pistachios, water chestnuts; raw or roasted seeds (caraway, pumpkin, sesame, sunflower), sesame seed butter, sunflower seed butter
**Legumes:** beans (adzuki, Great Northern, red, soy), *split peas;* miso, soy milk, tempeh, tofu
**Grains:** amaranth, barley, *buckwheat, corn, corn grits, corn tortillas,* millet, *oats,* oat bran, popcorn, quinoa, rice (long or short grain brown, wild), rice bran, rice cakes, rye, triticale, *whole wheat,* wheat bran, wheat germ, white flour, flour tortillas, breads (*corn, corn/rye,* English toasting, *multigrain,* rye, *seven-grain,* sprouted grain), bagels, English muffins, crackers (oat, rye, saltines, wheat), vegetable pasta, udon noodles, cream of rice, cream of rye, cream of wheat
**Vegetables:** artichokes, *arugula, asparagus,* bamboo shoots, yellow wax beans, *beets,* bok choy, broccoflower, *broccoli, brussels sprouts, cauliflower,* celery, cilantro, *corn,* greens (beet, collard, mustard, turnip), jicama, kale, kohlrabi, leeks, lettuce (butter, endive, red leaf, romaine), *mushrooms,* okra, olives (black, green, ripe), *raw onions* (chives, brown, green, red, Vidalia, white, yellow), *parsley,* parsnips, *bell peppers (red, green),* chili peppers, pimientos, potatoes (*red, russet,* White Rose), pumpkin, rutabaga, sauerkraut, seaweed (arame, dulse, kelp, nori, wakame), shallots, spinach, sprouts (alfalfa, clover, *mung bean,* radish, sunflower), squash (acorn, banana, butternut, spaghetti, yellow [summer], *zucchini*), Swiss chard, taro leaves, turnips, *watercress*
**Vegetable Juices:** carrot, carrot/celery, celery, parsley, spinach, tomato, V-8
**Fruits:** apricots (*fresh* and unsulfured dried), berries (blackberries, *blueberries,* boysenberries, *cranberries,* gooseberries, *strawberries*), cherries, dates, figs (fresh, dried), grapes (black, green, red, white), guavas, kumquats, *mangoes,* melons (casaba, Crenshaw, *honeydew, watermelon*), nectarines, *papayas,* pears, persimmons, pineapples, plums (black, purple, red), pomegranates, *prunes,* raisins, rhubarb, tangelos, tangerines
**Fruit Juices:** (rotate) apple, apple cider, apple/apricot, apricot, black cherry, cherry, cranapple, cranberry, grape (purple, red, white), grapefruit, guava,

lemon, *orange,* papaya, pear, pineapple, pineapple/coconut, *prune,* tangerine

**Vegetable Oils:** all-blend, almond, avocado, coconut, *corn,* flaxseed, olive, peanut, safflower, sesame, soy, sunflower

**Sweeteners:** *fructose, honey, molasses, sorghum,* sugar (brown, *raw, refined white*), syrup (*barley malt, corn*)

**Condiments:** *catsup, mustard, Miracle Whip, barbecue sauce, pesto sauce, soy sauce,* salsa, tahini, sweet or dill pickles, vinegar, salt

**Salad Dressings:** *blue cheese, French, Italian, ranch, Roquefort,* creamy avocado, *creamy Italian, Thousand Island,* vinegar and oil, lemon juice and oil

**Desserts:** custard, tapioca, sherbet (orange, raspberry)

**Chips:** *bean,* corn (*white, yellow*)

**Beverages:** tea (*black,* herbal, Japanese); mineral water, sparkling water; *wine (red, white), sake, beer, barley malt liquor, champagne, gin, scotch, vodka, whiskey; root beer, regular sodas*

## Stressful Foods

Have no more than once a month.

**Dairy:** *milk (whole, low fat), plain yogurt, most ice creams*

**Legumes:** *black-eyed peas, lentils*

**Grains:** *polished white rice, breads (buckwheat, oat, raisin, whole wheat)*

**Vegetable Oil:** *canola*

**Sweeteners:** *date sugar, syrup (brown rice, maple), saccharin, aspartame, Equal, NutraSweet, Sweet'n Low, succonant*

**Condiments:** *mayonnaise, horseradish, margarine*

**Desserts:** *chocolate, desserts containing chocolate*

**Chips:** *blue corn, potato*

**Beverages:** *coffee; diet sodas*

**Other:** *blue/green algae, acidophilus*

## Scheduling Meals

### Healthy

Kidney body types should begin and end the day with a light meal. Schedule your meals as follows:

*Breakfast:* 8–9 A.M. Light to moderate, with light protein (dairy, eggs, nuts, seeds) and vegetables, legumes, grain, and/or fruit.

*Lunch:* 12–2 P.M. Heavy, with dense protein, dairy, nuts, seeds, legumes, vegetables, and/or grain. Avoid fruit.

*Dinner:* 6–8 P.M. Light, with light protein (eggs, dairy, cheese, nuts, seeds), vegetables, legumes, grain, and/or fruit. Avoid dense protein.

### Snacks (optional)

*Midmorning:* (10 A.M.) fruit

*Midafternoon:* (4–5 P.M.) grain and butter

*Evening:* (10 P.M.–2 A.M.) protein, nuts, seeds, dairy, vegetables, grain, fruit, sweets

### Sensitive

Adjust your intake as follows:

*Breakfast:* Heavy, with dense protein and/or vegetables.

*Lunch:* Heavy, with dense protein, legumes, vegetables, and/or grain.

*Dinner:* Light, with vegetables, legumes, and/or vegetable juices. Avoid fruit.

## Sample One-Week Menu

DAY 1

*Breakfast:* banana and peanut butter

*Lunch:* Cornish game hen, white or brown basmati rice, and artichoke hearts w/olive oil vinaigrette

*Dinner:* cucumber, tomato, red onion, and feta cheese w/Italian dressing made with olive oil

DAY 2

*Breakfast:* low-fat yogurt w/almonds, sunflower seeds, and pineapple

*Lunch:* salmon, cabbage, onions, and peas

*Dinner:* vegetarian chili

DAY 3

*Breakfast:* potato and broccoli w/butter and cheese

*Lunch:* chicken breast, rice, and green beans

*Dinner:* French onion soup

DAY 4

*Breakfast:* chicken soup

*Lunch:* shark and a salad of red leaf lettuce, cucumber, and avocado w/lemon juice and oil

*Snack:* tortilla w/butter

*Dinner:* yellow and zucchini squash w/onion

DAY 5: CLEANSE

*Breakfast:* grapefruit or papaya

*Snack:* grapefruit or papaya

*Lunch:* raw jicama and/or spinach or steamed kale, or Swiss chard

*Dinner:* steamed green beans, broccoli, carrots, and/or asparagus

DAY 6

*Breakfast:* cottage cheese w/walnuts and banana

*Lunch:* sea bass and brown rice w/salsa and olive oil

*Dinner:* tuna and a salad of butter lettuce and celery w/olive oil and vinegar dressing

DAY 7

*Breakfast:* cheese omelette w/salsa

*Lunch:* beef, red potatoes, and carrots

*Dinner:* stir-fried tofu, bean sprouts, mushrooms, almonds, garlic, and onions over rice

## Alternative Menus

*(Foods in parentheses are optional.)*

### Breakfast

Oatmeal w/strawberries

Cream of rice w/banana

Bananas, kiwi, green apples, red apples, or orange

Kefir w/banana and pecans

Whey protein powder smoothie w/kiwi and banana

Cantaloupe

White basmati rice cooked in beef or chicken broth

Oat bran toast w/butter, banana, and orange juice

English muffin w/butter, peach, and tea

Chicken and green beans

Salmon and peas

### Lunch

Tuna, avocado, lettuce, tomato, and sunflower seeds

Shrimp, Indian rice, and vegetables

Trout, rice, and brussels sprouts

Broiled steak and a salad of romaine lettuce, radish, and onion

Beef or lamb and broccoli or peas

Steak or chicken, potatoes, and green beans

Liver and onions, broccoli, and peas

Chicken, potatoes, and broccoli

### Dinner

Steamed carrots, pea pods, green beans, and flour tortilla w/cheese

Salad of red leaf lettuce, sprouts, onion, garbanzo beans, spinach, and sunflower seeds w/Italian dressing

Waldorf salad

Salad of butter lettuce, yellow bell peppers, chives, and radish w/olive oil and lemon juice

Lentils and green beans

Baked eggplant, tomato sauce, and ricotta cheese

Fish taco

Baked potato (w/cream cheese) and beans

Baked potato w/sour cream and olive oil and broccoli

Apples and peanut butter or cheese

# Liver

*The Liver body type is symbolized by a food processor. Converting and processing sugars and protein is like putting the pieces together and fitting them into the flow of the day or project and continuation of life are key elements. Loyal and stable, this body type excels at helping with whatever needs to be done.*

FAMOUS PEOPLE: Princess Diana, John Bradshaw, Bette Midler, Alec Baldwin

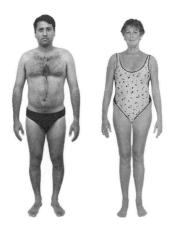

## LIVER
### Location and Function

The liver is located on the upper right side of the abdomen, just below the diaphragm. It produces bile and converts most sugars into glycogen, which it stores for later use.

## Psychological Profile

### Characteristic Traits

Liver body types are family oriented and extremely loyal. Consistent and reliable, they can always be counted on to carry out their duties and obligations. Faithful and dependable, supportive and caring, Liver types are known for being there through thick and thin.

The basic nature of Liver types is kind, patient, and considerate. People oriented, they function well in most social situations. Needing to be needed, they enjoy giving of themselves and being there for others. Teaching gives them the ultimate sense of fulfillment because it enables them to give to others and experience themselves as being important and valuable.

Liver types are tough and resilient. They have a great deal of physical endurance and are able to see a job through to its completion. They enjoy seeing the physical results of their efforts. They have a strong sense of commitment, perseverance, and orderliness. They derive a great deal of enjoyment from the actual doing of their tasks or creative projects.

Known for their good organizational skills, Liver types are attentive to detail and have the ability to view problems systematically as well as from a broad perspective. Moreover, if they see a problem as irreparable, they have little difficulty putting it out of their mind rather than worrying about it.

### Motivation

With an intense desire to experience all that life has to offer, Liver types have a strong need to know how and why things work. They enjoy physical activity that involves doing something constructive or accomplishing an objective. This allows them to put ideas into a form that can be seen, felt, or experienced.

Liver types make good teachers. Their own learning is usually done in a step-by-step manner, mastering each step along the way. Once they learn something, they really know it—it becomes integrated into their being. Teaching a subject allows them to learn it well and to interact with and assist others. They have an intense desire to help others by giving them the guidance they themselves didn't receive. Their goal is to help their students avoid some of the predictable pitfalls of life.

Especially when young, Liver types tend to follow their heart's desire and often go along with group activities without considering the consequences. This "do it first, think about it later" attitude leads to a certain impulsivity or rashness of behavior. Having made sufficient errors in judgment, many later resort to taking a safe observer role rather than striking out on their own to explore uncharted territories. Liver types with self-esteem issues run the risk of becoming codependent in their relationships.

Being much better at nurturing others physically and emotionally than at identifying and taking care of their own needs, Liver types often hold an unconscious belief that "If I take care of someone else, they'll take care of me." The basis of this belief is in part the fact that outside support is often a vital motivator for them in making major personal changes. Often coming from backgrounds where they were deprived of nurturing support or emotional intimacy, however, they may have developed a protective barrier that creates emotional distance from others, thus preventing them from getting the support they desire. Fortunately, lack of support is just as effective as a motivating force.

## "At Worst"

Better at nurturing others than taking care of their own needs, Liver types may shy away from relationships that could offer them the emotional support they were deprived of in early life. With low self-esteem and lack of functional role models, loyalty, and strong family ties, they often find themselves trapped in codependent relationships. To deal with this situation, they often transfer their need to care for their family to work and become workaholics.

Substance abuse is another means of escaping emotional pain. Liver types often use alcohol to take the edge off their emotions. It makes them less aware of their problems, allows them to relax with their friends, and releases their self-control. Unfortunately, alcohol can also release their suppressed anger, leading to emotional outbursts or violent behavior.

When in control, Liver types tend to be rather soft-spoken and restrained and to have difficulty locating and expressing negative feelings, especially anger. When they keep their emotions pent up, they often become depressed or addicted in an attempt to drown their feelings with excess food or alcohol. Liver types are capable of blocking their emotions and continuing to function in the world without emotional involvement. Liver males in particular often learn to hide behind an "I don't need anybody" attitude. Ultimately, this emotional suppression erupts in a fit of anger that can be just as surprising to themselves as to others.

## "At Best"

Once they are able to connect with their personal higher power, Liver types have a sense of self-sufficiency. They project a real "can do" attitude and are capable of handling things efficiently and effectively. They are naturally creative and have a knack for putting things together. When free of emotional turmoil, they can access their excellent organizational skills and provide stability to their work and family. At their best, they can express their emotions in a positive manner, turning anger into laughter and hurt into creativity.

Having learned the hard way, Liver types are excellent teachers. Patient and genuinely concerned about others, they often impart their knowledge to others in the concrete form of showing them how to do something or the more abstract form of introducing them to new concepts and ideas. Teaching is ultimately their most rewarding endeavor.

Liver types have a strong need to be efficient in their work and find that job satisfaction is far more important than monetary reward. If they don't have the authority to do what they feel is necessary to be effective, they seek work where their ideals and efforts are more appreciated. They have the courage to move on when they feel they're in a rut.

When they are in tune with life, Liver types seem to know what needs to be done and how to organize it so that all necessary tasks are completed by day's end. They have a sense about people, places, and things that allows them to pick up on what's going on, gives them insight into the basic nature of those around them, and often allows them to predict others' behavior.

## Dietary Profile

### Main Focus

- ▸ Rotation and variety of foods are important.
- ▸ Get emotional support from others, preferably more than one person; group support is great.

### RECOMMENDED EXERCISE

For Liver body types, exercise has the physical benefit of burning calories. Exercise is best when there is fluidity of movement, such as in dance, Jazzercise, Callanetics, tai chi, walking, backpacking, and downhill skiing. Exercise machines, weights, and bicycling are helpful.

- Make lunch your largest meal.
- Exercise helps your emotional state besides cleansing your body.

## Dietary Emphasis

- From 15 to 35 percent of your calories are to come from fats.
- Best fat sources: butter, cheese, cottage cheese, fish, and chicken.
- From 20 to 40 percent of your calories are to come from protein.
- From 10 to 25 percent of your calories are to come from dense protein.
- Best sources of the three amino acids threonine, isoleucine, and cystine: ground sirloin, turkey, and chicken.
- Caloric intake: 1,500 to 1,800 calories a day for women and 1,700 to 2,000 calories a day for men. If you are engaging in intense exercise (competition type) or heavy labor, increase calories.
- Drink a minimum of 64 ounces of water a day. Drink water before and after meals, not with meals.
- Reduce alcohol, especially grain alcohol.
- Food is best assimilated when eaten in combinations.
- Garlic supports the immune system.
- Include more raw than cooked vegetables.
- Raw foods are generally supportive to the system.
- Eat vegetables, fruits, protein (eggs, poultry, fish); moderate dairy.
- Occasional desserts are best as an evening snack.

## For Weight Loss

- Fat: 15 to 30 percent of daily calories.
- Protein: 25 to 40 percent of daily calories.
- Dense protein: 20 to 25 percent of daily calories.
- May snack midafternoon and evening.
- Eliminate salt.
- Avoid chocolate, sodas, and alcohol.
- Exercise daily.
- Get emotional support; weight loss groups are often successful.

## For Weight Gain

- Fat: 25 to 35 percent of daily calories.
- Protein: 25 to 40 percent of daily calories.
- Dense protein: 20 to 30 percent of daily calories.

---

### RECOMMENDED CUISINE

Seafood, Chinese, Japanese, Thai, Indian, Italian, Mexican, English, German, Irish, and home-style foods (like meat and potatoes) prepared with gravies and sauces. Spicy foods, such as jalapeño peppers and curry, stimulate the lymphatic system.

## Healthy Foods List

There is no need to sacrifice delicious and filling foods to maintain a healthy Liver body type. The following lists will help you focus on foods that support your health, and avoid foods that can stress your system.

*You'll notice that some foods are printed in italics; these foods take more energy to assimilate and could be ones you will want to avoid when you are in a sensitive state due to any physical or emotional stresses.*

Be sure to read Chapter 3, "Implementing the Body Type Diet," for lots of important information about how to use these many foods to gain their full benefit.

### Ultra-Support Foods

Foods to include in 3 to 7 meals a week, listed by category.

**Dense Protein:** beef broth, beef liver, buffalo; chicken (white), chicken broth, chicken livers; anchovy, bass, catfish, flounder, haddock, halibut, herring, mahimahi, orange roughy, sardines, red snapper, sole, trout; clams, eel, mussels; octopus, oysters, scallops
**Dairy:** *yogurt (plain or flavored low fat)*, butter
**Cheese:** Brie, Camembert, cheddar, Colby, low-fat cottage, feta, low-fat Monterey Jack
**Nuts and Seeds:** Brazils, coconut, hazelnuts, pine nuts; seeds (pumpkin, sesame)
**Legumes:** beans (adzuki, Great Northern, kidney, navy, lima, red, soy), black-eyed peas
**Grains:** amaranth, buckwheat, couscous, millet, quinoa, white or brown basmati rice, cream of rice
**Vegetables:** asparagus, beets, cabbage (green, napa, red), celery, cucumber, eggplant, garlic, greens (beet, collard, mustard, turnip), jicama, kale, kohlrabi, okra, ripe black olives, peas, potatoes

(red, russet, White Rose, Yukon Gold), pumpkin, rutabaga, sprouts (alfalfa, clover, mung bean, radish, sunflower), squash (butternut, spaghetti), Swiss chard, turnips, watercress

**Fruits:** cranberries, cherries, guavas, kiwi, limes, mangoes, melons (cantaloupe, casaba, Crenshaw, honeydew, watermelon), pomegranates, rhubarb

**Fruit Juices:** (mix with carbonated water) red cherry, pineapple/coconut

**Vegetable Oils:** all-blend, almond, avocado, corn, olive, safflower, sesame, soy

**Sweetener:** stevia

**Beverage:** Berry Calistoga water

## Basic Support Foods

Foods to include in 1 to 2 meals a week.

**Dense Protein:** *bacon,* beef, lamb, veal, venison, organ meats (heart, brain); chicken (dark), Cornish game hen, duck, *turkey;* bonita, cod, mackerel, perch, salmon, shark, swordfish, tuna; calamari (squid), crab, lobster, shrimp; eggs

**Dairy:** *milk (low fat, nonfat, raw, goat's), sweet cream, sour cream, buttermilk,* kefir, *frozen yogurt, ice cream* (Ben & Jerry's, Dreyer's, Swensen's)

**Cheese:** American, blue, cream, Edam, goat, Gouda, kefir, Limburger, mozzarella, Muenster, Parmesan, ricotta, Romano, Swiss

**Nuts and Seeds:** almonds, almond butter, cashews, cashew butter, hazelnuts, macadamias, macadamia butter, peanuts, peanut butter, pecans, pistachios, walnuts (black, English), water chestnuts; seeds (caraway, sunflower), sesame seed butter, sunflower seed butter

**Legumes:** beans (black, garbanzo, pinto), lentils, split peas; hummus; miso, soy milk, tofu

**Grains:** barley, corn, corn tortillas, corn grits, hominy grits, millet, oats, air-popped popcorn, rice (long or short grain brown, Japanese, wild), rice bran, rice cakes, rye, triticale, wheat bran, wheat germ, refined wheat flour, *flour tortillas,* breads (corn, corn/rye, French, garlic, Italian, multigrain, oat, rice, rye, seven-grain, sourdough, sprouted grain, white, *whole wheat*), bagels, croissants, English muffins, pasta (durum, semolina, vegetable, herbed—garlic, basil), udon noodles, Chinese rice noodles, Nutri-Grain, granola, cream of rye, cream of wheat

**Vegetables:** artichokes, avocados, bamboo shoots, beans (green, yellow wax), bok choy, broccoflower, broccoli, *brussels sprouts,* carrots, cauli-flower, cilantro, corn, hominy, leeks, *lettuce (Boston, butter, endive, iceberg, red leaf, romaine),* mushrooms, green olives, onions (chives, brown, green, red, Vidalia, white, yellow), parsley, parsnips, snow pea pods, bell peppers (green, red, yellow), chili peppers, pimientos, radishes, daikon radishes, sauerkraut, seaweed (arame, dulse, kelp, nori, wakame), shallots, *spinach,* squash (acorn, banana, *yellow [summer], zucchini*), sweet potatoes, tomatoes, yams

**Vegetable Juices:** carrot, carrot/celery, celery, parsley, spinach, tomato, V-8

**Fruits:** apples (Red or Golden Delicious, Gala, Granny Smith, Jonathan, McIntosh, Pippin, Rome Beauty), apricots, bananas, berries (blackberries, blueberries, boysenberries, gooseberries, raspberries, strawberries), dates, black Mission figs, grapes (black, green, red), grapefruit (red, white), kumquats, lemons, loquats, nectarines, *oranges, papayas,* peaches, pears, Fuyu persimmons, plums (black, red, purple), *pineapples,* prunes, raisins, tangelos, tangerines

**Fruit Juices:** apple, apple cider, apple/apricot, apricot, black cherry, cranapple, cranberry, grape (purple, red, white), grapefruit, guava, lemon, *orange, papaya,* pear, *pineapple,* prune, tangerine, watermelon

**Vegetable Oils:** coconut, flaxseed, peanut, sunflower

**Sweeteners:** *fructose, honey, molasses, sorghum, sugar (brown, date, raw, refined cane), syrup (barley malt, brown rice, corn, maple), succonant*

**Condiments:** *catsup, mustard, horseradish, barbecue sauce, pesto sauce, soy sauce,* salsa, tahini, pickles

**Salad Dressings:** *blue cheese, French, ranch, creamy Italian,* creamy avocado, *Thousand Island,* vinegar and oil, lemon juice and oil

**Desserts:** *custards, tapioca, puddings, pies, cakes, sherbet (orange, raspberry)*

**Chips:** *bean, corn (blue, white, yellow)*

**Beverages:** *coffee;* tea *(black, green,* herbal, Japanese, Chinese oolong); mineral water, sparkling water; *wine (red, white), sake, beer, barley malt liquor, champagne, gin, scotch, vodka, whiskey; root beer*

## Stressful Foods

Have no more than once a month.

**Dense Protein:** *pork, ham, sausage; abalone*

**Dairy:** *milk (whole, 2%), half-and-half, high-fat yogurt, most ice creams*

**Grains:** *whole wheat, Grape-Nuts*
**Vegetable:** *arugula*
**Vegetable Oil:** *canola*
**Sweeteners:** *saccharin, aspartame, Equal, NutraSweet, Sweet'n Low*
**Condiments:** *mayonnaise, margarine, salt, Braggs Liquid Aminos, MSG*
**Desserts:** *chocolate, desserts containing chocolate*
**Chips:** *salted potato chips*
**Beverages:** *regular and diet sodas*

## Scheduling Meals

### Healthy

Liver types should progress through the day from light to heavy meals. Schedule your meals as follows:

*Breakfast:* 6–9 A.M. Light, with grain, dairy, protein, vegetables, legumes, and/or fruit or fruit juice.
*Lunch:* 12–2 P.M. Heavy, with protein, dairy, nuts, seeds, legumes, grain, vegetables, and/or limited fruit.
*Dinner:* 6–9 P.M. Moderate to heavy, with legumes, grain, protein, dairy, and/or vegetables.

### Snacks (optional)
*Midmorning:* (10 A.M.) vegetables, grain
*Midafternoon:* (3:30–4 P.M.) vegetables, grain, fruit, dairy, protein, nuts, seeds
*Evening:* (9 P.M.–2 A.M.) fruit, vegetables, grain, dairy, limited protein; sweets 1 hour or more after dinner

### Sensitive

Adjust your intake as follows:

*Breakfast:* Moderate to heavy, with grain, dairy, protein, vegetables, legumes, and/or fruit or fruit juice.
*Lunch:* Light to moderate, with protein, dairy, nuts, seeds, legumes, grain, vegetables. Avoid fruit.
*Dinner:* Moderate, with legumes, grain, protein, dairy, and/or vegetables. Avoid fruit.

## Sample One-Week Menu

Snacks are optional.

DAY 1
*Breakfast:* eggs, rice, and onions
*Lunch:* chicken livers w/sautéed onions and pickled beet and onion salad

*Snack:* jicama and carrots
*Dinner:* halibut, coleslaw, and red potatoes

DAY 2
*Breakfast:* oatmeal w/cinnamon
*Lunch:* fillet of tuna, pasta, and asparagus w/butter, lemon, and garlic sauce
*Snack:* apple
*Dinner:* salad of spinach, raw carrots, bean sprouts, mushrooms, and hard-boiled egg w/ranch dressing

DAY 3
*Breakfast:* carne asada (beef) burrito w/salsa
*Lunch:* red snapper w/lemon, basmati rice, and peas
*Snack:* macadamia nuts
*Dinner:* couscous, eggplant w/olive oil, and pine nuts

DAY 4
*Breakfast:* potato w/sour cream
*Lunch:* chicken breast, brown basmati rice, onion, and mushrooms
*Snack:* grapefruit or kiwi
*Dinner:* steak and broccoli

DAY 5: CLEANSE
*Breakfast:* asparagus (steamed or canned), squash (any)
*Lunch:* steamed broccoflower, cauliflower, and/or squash (any)
*Dinner:* steamed broccoflower, cauliflower, peas, green beans, squash (any)

DAY 6
*Breakfast:* rice and stir-fried vegetables—asparagus, celery, mung bean, mushrooms, red bell peppers with soy sauce
*Lunch:* roasted turkey breast, green beans, and cranberries
*Snack:* almonds
*Dinner:* salad of sprouts, avocado, tomatoes, and cabbage w/avocado dressing

DAY 7
*Breakfast:* corn grits and butter
*Lunch:* liver and onions and potatoes
*Snack:* string cheese
*Dinner:* rice and stir-fried vegetables, such as broccoli, bok choy, carrots, snow pea pods, w/chicken or shrimp

## Alternative Menus

*(Foods in parentheses may be omitted.)*

### Breakfast

Chicken and cheese omelette (w/sour cream and/or salsa)

Cottage cheese w/Parmesan cheese

Hamburger and peas

Eggs, brown basmati rice, and red onion

Chicken breast and rice or asparagus

Cream of rice w/banana, peaches, or blueberries

Raisin bran w/low-fat milk

Apple, papaya, or pineapple/papaya juice

### Lunch

Sirloin steak, potato, and asparagus

Spinach lasagna

Tuna, tomato, and salad of celery, apples, and nuts w/creamy avocado dressing

Chicken breast, cauliflower, and broccoli

Grilled chicken, corn or flour tortilla, and a salad of lettuce, avocado, and tomato

Chicken breast and a salad of spinach, carrots, cucumbers, mushrooms, broccoli, and red peppers w/rice vinegar

Salmon or trout, rice, and stir-fried carrots, broccoli, cauliflower, and cabbage

### Lunch or Dinner

Miso soup and California roll or sushi

Steak and potato w/butter and chives

Tuna, rice, and asparagus

Shark, zucchini, and rice

Butternut soup (chicken breast)

Steak; salad of red leaf lettuce, cucumber, snow pea pods, red bell pepper with vinegar and oil; and corn

Codfish, carrots, green beans, brussels sprouts, and rice

Cheese enchilada w/corn tortilla, rice, and beans

Lentil soup (ground beef, jicama)

Black beans and rice

Beef liver, broccoli, carrots, and cauliflower

# Lung

*The Lung body type is symbolized by a hot-air balloon. Air creates buoyancy and is necessary for life. Nurturing and creative, Lung types give life to their world by expressing positive, supportive emotions, enabling them to make the most of the moment.*

FAMOUS PEOPLE: Cameron Diaz, Harrison Ford, John Denver, Jacqueline Kennedy Onassis

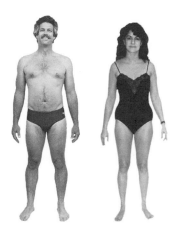

## LUNG
### Location and Function

The lungs are located in the lateral cavities of the chest. They are separated from each other by the heart. Their function is to provide oxygen to the blood through respiration.

## Psychological Profile

### Characteristic Traits

Lung body types are generally sensitive, caring, idealistic, even-tempered, and mild-mannered. Emotional by nature, they tend to breathe in others' emotions, which can cause their own to snowball, or they go to the opposite extreme of suppressing their own and discounting others' emotions. In an attempt to avoid being driven entirely by emotions, they have a tendency to become too analytical and suppress them altogether.

Systematic in their thought processes, Lung types like to think things through before taking any action. They like to understand what's taking place and feel sure about their choices before making any changes, which often inhibits their spontaneity.

Lung types are naturally creative as well as very practical. Being quite imaginative and gifted at working with their hands, they can take abstract ideas and translate them into physical forms. Having a well-developed sense of style, they can express these talents through drawing, sculpturing, design, or construction. With a good sense of rhythm and timing, they also tend to express their nurturing and creativity through music or dance.

### Motivation

Lung types have a strong need to nurture and be nurtured. This often leads them into service-oriented vocations where they can be expressive and establish emotional connections. They tend to value relationships more than personal achievements. It's easy for them to become caretakers or rescuers of those in need, often losing touch with their own needs in the process. Between their sense of responsibility and their fear of change, Lung types are prone to stay in relationships much longer than is beneficial for them and may at times find it difficult to let go and get on with their lives.

Idealistic, Lung types basically have a high regard for peace. Not only do they work for peace in the outside world, but they do everything they can to establish it in their personal relationships. Even when a relationship has ended in divorce, they often do everything they can to restore it to at least friendship status.

Lung types are persistent and loyal, particularly in their attempts to right wrongs or effect necessary reforms. It's not unusual for them to devote a great deal of energy to helping the underdog. In social situations, they are the ones who dance with the "wallflowers" and make sure no one is left out.

Creative expression is essential for a Lung type's personal fulfillment. The need for self-expression provides the motivation to grow, develop, and make changes. The Lung types' emotional sensitivity and drive to nurture others serve as catalysts for their creativity. Work that is methodical and requires care is more appealing to them than work that requires making quick decisions and that includes great responsibility because Lung types are not comfortable taking risks that involve other people.

## "At Worst"

Lung types often experience difficulty finding balance in their lives. Their attention is often too focused on a single aspect of life, such as work, at the expense of others, and they may ignore their personal needs for rest, relaxation, or play. Being overly concerned with the expectations of others, Lung types tend to take on more than they can realistically expect to accomplish. Even though they may be overwhelmed, they are still reluctant to back out of their commitments. Not wanting to decline openly, they then tend to withdraw, or get too busy.

Fearful of disapproval and rejection, with a strong need to please others, Lung types are often unsuccessful at pleasing themselves. Being extremely uncomfortable with conflict, they often accommodate others to avoid it and end up resentful or disappointed, sad or depressed. By making themselves less important than others, they can deepen their own self-doubts. It's usually their lack of confidence and other internal barriers that interfere with their self-acceptance and self-respect.

Strong-willed to the point of stubbornness and rigidity, Lung types may tend to operate from gut feelings rather than outside information. They have a tendency to become narrow-minded and get stuck in the rut of a routine. They often have difficulty organizing their time, planning, prioritizing, and making decisions. It's easy for them to fritter their time away socializing or puttering around on a project.

Lung types expend a great deal of time and energy serving humanity. They are particularly sensitive to the needs of those around them and will go to great lengths to fulfill those needs.

## "At Best"

Practical, efficient, and aware of things that need to be done, Lung types can accurately analyze the effect their actions have on others. Because they are tactful and indirect, rarely is their behavior perceived as pushy or offensive. They are honest, loyal, and can be trusted to honor their commitments while acting in the best interests of those they are serving.

Lung types are nurturing to others as well as to themselves. They are basically self-sufficient and tend to regenerate best through sleep. They are generally comfortable being alone, particularly since they need time to integrate and process information when making decisions. They have their own sense of direction and are not led by what everyone else is doing.

Lung types are known for being creative, imaginative, and often vocally expressive. They can be quite persuasive and can leave a lasting impression on people, which makes them effective as social reformers, speakers, or performers. They have an ability to connect with and activate others' emotional energy. By trusting their intuition and inner guidance, Lung types can be successful and influential in helping humanity.

## Dietary Profile

### Main Focus

- ► Have a heavy breakfast, emphasizing protein.
- ► Have a moderate lunch, emphasizing vegetables.
- ► Have a light dinner, with no fruit.
- ► Increase oxygen intake through exercise and deep breathing.
- ► Get sufficient sleep.

### Dietary Emphasis

- ► From 10 to 35 percent of your calories are to come from fat.
- ► Best fat sources: nuts (almonds, pine nuts, pecans, coconut, cashews), seeds, protein (beef, chicken, turkey, lamb, fish, eggs), olive oil, and butter.

### RECOMMENDED EXERCISE

Exercise is beneficial because it calms the mind and oxygenates the body. Walking, swimming, dancing, kick-boxing, Pilates, and lower-body exercises are particularly helpful.

- From 20 to 40 percent of your calories are to come from protein.
- From 0 to 35 percent of your calories are to come from dense protein.
- Best sources of the three amino acids threonine, isoleucine, and cystine: pine nuts, turkey, and chicken.
- Caloric intake: 1,500 to 1,800 calories a day for women and 1,700 to 2,000 calories a day for men. If you are engaging in intense exercise (competition type) or heavy labor, increase calories.
- Drink a minimum of 64 ounces of water a day. Drink water before and after meals, not with meals.
- Occasional desserts are best as an evening snack.
- Eating sweets between 8 and 10 P.M. may result in waking up around 3 to 4 A.M. Eating cheese or cheese and crackers often allows one to go back to sleep.
- May include nuts and seeds for snack, especially midmorning.
- Peppermint tea aids digestion and assimilation.
- Eat pine nuts, rice with steamed kale, collards, and Swiss chard.

## For Weight Loss

- Fats: 10 to 30 percent of daily calories.
- Dense protein: 15 to 35 percent of daily calories.
- Add lemon juice or a drop of peppermint oil to drinking water.
- Exercise.
- Reduce fruit; eliminate sugar.

## For Weight Gain

- Fats: 20 to 35 percent of daily calories.
- Dense protein: 30 to 35 percent of daily calories.
- Include fruit and grains.

## Healthy Foods List

There is no need to sacrifice delicious and filling foods to maintain a healthy Lung body type. The following lists will help you focus on foods that support your health, and avoid foods that can stress your system.

*You'll notice that some foods are printed in italics; these foods take more energy to assimilate and could be ones you will want to avoid when you are in a sensitive state due to any physical or emotional stresses.*

Be sure to read Chapter 3, "Implementing the Body Type Diet," for lots of important information about how to use these many foods to gain their full benefit.

## Ultra-Support Foods

Foods to include in 3 to 7 meals a week, listed by category.

**Dense Protein:** chicken, Cornish game hen, turkey; salmon, shark, swordfish, tuna; eggs
**Dairy:** butter
**Cheese:** cheddar, cottage, Monterey Jack
**Nuts and Seeds:** almonds, *cashews,* coconut, pecans, pine nuts
**Legumes:** Great Northern beans, split peas
**Grains:** amaranth, barley, blue corn, millet, oats, quinoa, rice (white or brown basmati, long or short grain brown, Japanese, polished, wild), rice bran, rice cakes, rye, breads (seven-grain, sprouted rice, sprouted rye), rice noodles, cream of rice, cream of rye
**Vegetables:** bamboo shoots, green beans, beets, bok choy, broccoli, brussels sprouts, cabbage (green, red, napa), carrots, cauliflower, celery, corn, eggplant, greens (beet, collard, mustard, turnip), kale, kohlrabi, leeks, lettuce (Boston, butter, endive, iceberg, red leaf, romaine), mushrooms, okra, olives (green, ripe), parsnips, peas, bell pepper (green, red, yellow), Yukon Gold potatoes, pumpkin, radishes, daikon radishes, rutabagas, sauerkraut, seaweed (arame, dulse, kelp, nori, wakame), spinach, sprouts (alfalfa, clover, mung bean, radish, sunflower), squash (acorn, banana, butternut, yellow [summer], spaghetti), Swiss chard, cherry tomatoes, turnips, watercress, yams
**Vegetable Juices:** *carrot,* carrot/celery, celery, spinach, tomato, V-8 (no salt)
**Fruits:** *apples (Red or Golden Delicious,* Granny Smith, Jonathan, McIntosh, *Pippin,* Rome Beauty), *apricots, bananas,* berries (*blackberries, blueberries,*

---

RECOMMENDED CUISINE

Chinese, Thai, Japanese (sushi), vegetable-style Mexican, Italian, soup, and salad.

boysenberries, cranberries, gooseberries, raspberries, strawberries), cherries, figs, *grapes* (*black, green*), guavas, kiwi, lemons, limes, loquats, *nectarines, persimmons,* pineapples, plums (red, purple, black), pomegranates, raisins, rhubarb, tangelos, tangerines

**Fruit Juices:** apple, black cherry, cranapple, cranberry, grape (purple, white), papaya, pineapple/coconut, pineapple, prune, tangerine

**Vegetable Oils:** flaxseed, olive

**Sweeteners:** honey, maple syrup, stevia

## Basic Support Foods

Foods to include in 1 to 2 meals a week.

**Dense Protein:** *beef,* beef broth, beef liver, buffalo, *lamb, pork, bacon, ham, sausage,* veal, venison, organ meats (heart, brain); chicken broth, chicken livers, duck; *anchovy,* bass, bonita, catfish, cod, flounder, haddock, halibut, herring, mackerel, mahimahi, perch, orange roughy, sardines, red snapper, sole, trout; abalone, calamari (squid), clams, crab, eel, lobster, mussels, octopus, *oysters,* scallops, shrimp

**Dairy:** *goat's milk, half-and-half, sweet cream, sour cream, buttermilk,* kefir, *plain yogurt, frozen yogurt, ice cream* (Ben & Jerry's, Dreyer's, Swensen's)

**Cheese:** American, blue, Brie, Camembert, Colby, *cream, Edam, feta, goat, Gouda,* kefir, Limburger, *mozzarella,* Muenster, Parmesan, ricotta, Romano, *Swiss*

**Nuts and Seeds:** almond butter, almond milk, Brazils, cashew butter, hazelnuts, macadamias, macadamia butter, *peanuts, peanut butter,* pistachios, *walnuts* (*black, English*), water chestnuts; seeds (caraway, pumpkin, sesame, sunflower), sesame seed butter, sunflower seed butter

**Legumes:** beans (adzuki, black, garbanzo, *kidney,* lima, navy, pinto, red, *soy*), lentils, black-eyed peas; hummus; miso, *soy milk, tofu*

**Grains:** corn, corn grits, *corn tortillas,* couscous, hominy grits, popcorn, triticale, refined wheat flour, *flour tortillas,* breads (corn, corn/rye, French, garlic, Italian, multigrain, oat, rye, seven-grain, sourdough, sprouted grain, white), bagels, croissants, crackers (oat, rye, saltines), pasta, udon noodles, *cream of wheat*

**Vegetables:** artichokes, asparagus, avocados, basil, yellow wax beans, *broccoflower,* cilantro, cucum-

bers, garlic, jicama, onions (all varieties), parsley, snow pea pods, chili peppers, pimientos, potatoes (purple, *red,* russet, White Rose), shallots, sweet potatoes, *tomatoes,* zucchini

**Vegetable Juice:** parsley

**Fruits:** dates, *red grapes,* grapefruit (red, white), kumquats, mangoes, melons (*cantaloupe,* casaba, Crenshaw, *honeydew,* watermelon), *oranges,* papayas, *peaches, pears,* prunes, rhubarb

**Fruit Juices:** apple cider, apple/apricot, apricot, *red cherry,* red grape, grapefruit, guava, lemon, *orange,* pear, prune, watermelon

**Vegetable Oils:** all-blend, almond, avocado, coconut, corn, *peanut,* safflower, sesame, *soy, sunflower*

**Sweeteners:** *fructose,* molasses, sorghum, sugar (*brown,* date, *raw, refined cane*), syrup (barley malt, corn, rice bran), *succonant*

**Condiments:** *catsup, mustard,* Dijon mustard, *horseradish, barbecue sauce, pesto sauce, soy sauce,* salsa, tahini, *pickles, vinegar, salt, sea salt,* Vege-Sal

**Salad Dressings:** blue cheese, *French, ranch,* creamy Italian, creamy avocado, *Thousand Island,* vinegar and oil, lemon juice and oil

**Desserts:** *custards, puddings, tapioca,* pies, *cakes, chocolate, desserts containing chocolate,* sherbet (orange, raspberry)

**Chips:** *bean,* corn (*blue, white, yellow*)

**Beverages:** *coffee;* tea (black, green, herbal—peppermint, Japanese, Chinese oolong); mineral water, sparkling water; *wine* (*red, white*), *sake, beer, barley malt liquor, champagne, gin, scotch, vodka, whiskey, tequila; root beer*

## Stressful Foods

Have no more than once a month.

**Dairy:** *milk, flavored yogurt, most ice creams*

**Grains:** *buckwheat, whole wheat, wheat bran, wheat germ, whole wheat bread, whole wheat crackers, English muffins*

**Vegetable:** *arugula*

**Vegetable Oil:** *canola*

**Sweeteners:** *aspartame, Equal, NutraSweet, Sweet'n Low*

**Condiments:** *mayonnaise, margarine*

**Beverages:** *regular or diet sodas*

**Others:** *French fries, fried foods*

## Scheduling Meals

Lung body types should start the day with a heavy meal and then reduce intake throughout the day, ending with a light dinner. Schedule your meals as follows:

*Breakfast:* 7–8 A.M. Heavy, with protein, grain, nuts, seeds, dairy, fruit, legumes, and/or vegetables.
*Lunch:* 12–2 P.M. Moderate, with grain, vegetables, legumes, dairy, nuts, seeds, protein, and/or fruit.
*Dinner:* 7–9 P.M. Light, with small portions of protein, legumes, vegetables, and/or grain. Avoid fruit.

### Snacks (optional)
*Midmorning* (10–11 A.M.) *or midafternoon* (4 P.M.): vegetables, protein, nuts, seeds, dairy, legumes, grain and/or fruit
*Evening:* (10 P.M.–2 A.M.) fruit, sweets, dairy, grain, nuts, seeds, protein, legumes, and/or vegetables

## Sample One-Week Menu

DAY 1
*Breakfast:* snapper, halibut, cod, shark, or swordfish and mixed vegetables
*Lunch:* Salad of pasta, peppers, tomatoes, green onions, and cucumbers and vinegar and olive oil
*Dinner:* bean soup

DAY 2
*Breakfast:* turkey, potatoes, peas and carrots, and yellow squash
*Lunch:* steamed cauliflower and broccoli w/pine nuts or almonds
*Dinner:* orange roughy, rice, and peas

DAY 3
*Breakfast:* omelette w/onions and mushrooms
*Lunch:* sushi/cucumber roll
*Dinner:* lamb, summer squash, and Swiss chard

DAY 4
*Breakfast:* cream of rice w/banana, peaches, or blueberries
*Lunch:* mixed vegetables and yams
*Dinner:* salmon, rice, and broccoli

DAY 5: CLEANSE
*Breakfast:* steamed kale or Swiss chard
*Snack:* raw Spanish black radishes
*Lunch:* steamed green beans, broccoli; and/or raw bell peppers, carrots, cucumbers, jicama; and/or carrot/celery juice
*Dinner:* steamed Swiss chard and/or kale and/or raw celery, salad w/butter leaf and/or red leaf lettuce w/celery, radishes, and sprouts

DAY 6
*Breakfast:* eggs, shrimp, onions, and white grain basmati rice
*Lunch:* pasta, vegetables, herbs, garlic, and onions
*Dinner:* baked potato w/flaxseed oil and broccoli

DAY 7
*Breakfast:* rice, steamed kale, and beef or lamb
*Lunch:* spinach salad w/pine nuts and olive oil and lemon juice
*Dinner:* lamb or beef and potatoes or rice

## Alternative Menus

*(Foods in parentheses are optional.)*

### Breakfast
Bran muffin and chicken
Eggs and green beans (flour tortilla)
Chicken, turkey, beef, or lamb and salad of butter lettuce, jicama, snow pea pods, cherry tomatoes with creamy Italian dressing
Rice and beans (avocado)
Chicken, spinach, and wild rice
Tuna and broccoli, brussels sprouts, or cauliflower
Quinoa and steamed vegetables such as broccoli, carrots, cauliflower, celery, or snow pea pods (sesame oil)
Couscous w/banana or strawberries and pine nuts
Raw almonds or pine nuts and apples, bananas, pears, or figs (orange juice or apple juice)

### Lunch
Tofu and rice
Chicken, broccoli, and carrots on rice
Corn, collard greens, kale, and carrots
Chicken or vegetable soup
Salad of butter lettuce, romaine, w/pine nuts and chicken or turkey
Tuna or egg salad w/Italian dressing

Spinach, beet greens, beets, and brown rice

Baked potato w/salsa, broccoli or carrots w/Braggs Liquid Aminos, and green or black bean juice

### Dinner

Baked potato with green onions and broccoli

Stir-fried shrimp, rice, water chestnuts, shiitake mushrooms, and green onions

Almond or cashew chicken and rice

Salmon loaf and steamed vegetables

Chicken, spinach, and wild rice (peas and carrots, yellow squash)

Pinto beans w/red and yellow peppers and onions (small beef tenderloin fillet)

Lentil soup

Chicken and rice soup

Chicken tortellini soup

Escarole and egg in chicken broth

# Lymph

*The Lymph body type is symbolized by ocean waves. Constant movement, fluidity, and variety through physical or mental activity provide the stimulation this body type needs to feel vibrant and alive. Fun-loving and playful, Lymph types are happiest when they are active.*

FAMOUS PEOPLE: Tom Cruise, Heather Locklear, Jane Fonda, Mikhail Baryshnikov

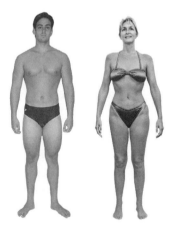

## LYMPH
### Location and Function

Lymph glands are located throughout the body. Large numbers of lymph nodes are in the groin, underarms, neck, and chest and behind the knees. Lymph helps the body eliminate toxins and waste. It flows throughout the body in the vessels of the lymphatic system.

## Psychological Profile

### Characteristic Traits

Lymph body types are physically strong and naturally well coordinated. Athletically inclined and usually health conscious, they often become professional athletes or personal trainers. Basically playful, they thrive on constant stimulation, variety, and change. Mentally quick and alert, Lymph types are stimulated by learning. Creative and artistic, they love to express themselves imaginatively, usually in areas associated with movement, such as dance, playing a musical instrument, or other forms of artistic or aesthetic expression.

Lymph types tend to be extremely beautiful or handsome. Their bodies are characterized by fine, well-sculpted features, broad shoulders, and easily definable muscles. They typically are quite conscientious about their dress and grooming, generally maintaining a striking appearance. Since physical attractiveness is usually a high priority, they tend to put a lot of energy into maintaining a youthful appearance.

Typically extroverted and sociable, Lymph types add stimulation and excitement to whatever they do. Romantically inclined, they tend to enter new relationships with great optimism. Sensitive and caring, charismatic and mentally focused, they can come on very strong, easily sweeping the objects of their attention off their feet.

### Motivation

Highly optimistic, when attracted to a potential mate, Lymph types are likely to throw themselves totally into the relationship. They tend to focus almost all their attention on the other person and on outward appearances rather than on what may be taking place below the surface. They can become so absorbed by idealized fantasies of the relationship's potential that they lose sight of what may be a much less promising reality. Also, wanting to be "up front," they're likely to reveal themselves more than may be appropriate during the earlier stages of a relationship.

In addition to putting themselves on the line, they're apt to put strain on the relationship by continually questioning the other person about his or her thoughts and feelings. They desperately need to be reassured that they're cared for, loved, and appreciated. Without such reassurances, unresolved or buried feelings of self-doubt and inadequacy surface. Emotional pain is the Lymph type's main motivation for change and personal growth, so relationships play an important role. Ultimately Lymph types need to learn to love themselves, but their tendency is to seek validation that they are lovable from outside sources.

Stagnation occurs when movement is missing, and this leads to depression. Variety and frequent changes (even if only minor sensory changes, such as the colors, smells, or textures of their immediate environment) can keep them from getting bored. Lymph types like to keep things active and lively and can experience a real lift when they change their place of residence, which they do much more often than most other types.

## "At Worst"

Lymph types are susceptible to boredom when they allow their lives to become too routine. Without stimulation and excitement, they become discouraged, lethargic, or depressed. While they are generally adept at handling details and not given to procrastination, they become distracted, inattentive, or inefficient when an endeavor begins to bore them.

When unable to express themselves sufficiently, Lymph types feel tense and restricted and their underlying feelings of inadequacy and rejection surface. In their need to feel secure, they give too much of themselves at the expense of their own needs. Needing reassurance, they fish for what they want to hear.

Without sufficient reassurance that they are loved, cared for, and appreciated in their significant relationship, their deep-seated feelings of distrust will be aroused. Such distrust or suspicion can end up becoming a self-fulfilling prophecy—for the urgency of their questioning may lead the other person to question the relationship's viability. The more Lymph types demand from their primary relationship, the harder it is for their partner to meet their expectations, and the partner often ends up feeling overwhelmed or "cornered" and reacts negatively. With the partner in an emotional straitjacket, the relationship is apt to lose its authenticity and go downhill. Because relationships are so important, female Lymph types tend to work too hard or too long on them, doing their best to make them succeed even after their limited potential has become fairly obvious. Men, on the other hand, have more of a tendency to get out as soon as a problem arises, as their fear of failure and need to excel in everything they do will not allow them to be the one who is rejected.

## "At Best"

Lymph types are conscientious, capable, mentally quick, and self-motivated. They are attentive to details and can organize logically and quickly learn whatever they are studying. Since Lymph types like a lot of activity and variety, they are stimulated by being on the front line and can handle the pressure of having a lot going on at once without feeling overloaded. With high personal expectations and a natural ability to excel at whatever they do, Lymph types are often entrepreneurs or heads of corporations. It's their openness to change and variety that puts Lymph types on the leading edge of technology. Sensitive and genuinely helpful, with good focus and a sense of direction, Lymph types are also excellent leaders and role models.

Health oriented, Lymph types at their best have a sense of well-being and relate well to the outside world. While they hold high expectations of themselves, they are rarely judgmental, generally accepting people for who and what they are. When they learn to truly love and accept themselves, Lymph types are free to love others unconditionally, without judgment and expectations, and their personal relationships then become rewarding and fulfilling.

Blessed with a naturally high energy level, Lymph types love to be active. In touch with their bodies, they connect with their intuitive side and their true self through exercise. Feeling connected and sure of themselves enables them to live in the moment, free to

### RECOMMENDED EXERCISE

Exercising at least 1 hour every other day is essential for Lymph body types because it activates the immune system. Lymphatic activation requires all-over movement, such as walking (although not necessarily vigorously) for 20 minutes 5 times a week. Variety is important. Sufficient vigorous exercise may be obtained in 15 minutes from activities such as hiking, bicycling, in-line skating, kickboxing, yoga, Callanetics, dancing, aerobics, stair-stepping, tennis, racquetball, swimming, diving, running, or weight training. When sensitive, reduce exercise and emphasize bodily movement with music, such as walking, floor exercises, or dancing. Be aware of your body and stop when the exercise begins to feel excessive. Running may be contraindicated if having difficulty maintaining weight.

express their spontaneity and enthusiasm for life. They thrive on excitement, welcome change, and enjoy the opportunity to add variety to life.

## Dietary Profile

### Main Focus

▶ Limit vegetables for lunch; salads are best at dinner.
▶ You are sensitive to chemicals and additives, so use only chemical-free chicken, turkey, and beef; organic fruits, vegetables, and grains are best.
▶ May use protein powders and/or protein bars with nuts.
▶ Snacks are often supportive; may be included in 6 meals.
▶ Emphasize nuts, seeds, and avocados.

### Dietary Emphasis

▶ From 20 to 35 percent of your calories are to come from fats.
▶ Best fat sources: sunflower seeds, almonds, pecans, avocados, butter, kefir, fish (especially salmon), chicken, turkey, and Cornish game hen. When rebuilding body, increase fats to 50 percent of caloric intake by including more fish (especially salmon), chicken, turkey, duck, goose, and kefir cheese.
▶ From 15 to 40 percent of your calories are to come from protein.
▶ From 0 to 30 percent of your calories are to come from chemical-free dense protein.
▶ Best sources of the three amino acids threonine, isoleucine, and cystine: pheasant, quail, and duck.
▶ Caloric intake: 1,500 to 1,800 calories a day for women and 1,700 to 2,000 calories a day for men. If you are engaging in intense exercise (competition type) or heavy labor, increase calories.
▶ Drink a minimum of 64 ounces of water a day. Drink water before and after meals, not with meals.
▶ Occasional desserts are best as an evening snack.
▶ Rotate foods.
▶ Eat carrots, rice (white basmati if sensitive), and adequate protein.
▶ Spicy foods (Thai spices, salsa, or cayenne pepper) stimulate lymphatic movement.

### For Weight Loss

▶ Dense protein: 20 to 25 percent of daily calories.
▶ Eliminate all dairy except butter.
▶ Reduce breads.
▶ If fat from appropriate sources falls below 20 percent of daily calories, weight loss will be inhibited.

### For Weight Gain

▶ Fat: 20 to 50 percent of daily calories.
▶ Protein: 15 to 45 percent of daily calories.
▶ Dense protein: 15 to 30 percent of daily calories.
▶ Add dairy.

## Healthy Foods List

There is no need to sacrifice delicious and filling foods to maintain a healthy Lymph body type. The following lists will help you focus on foods that support your health, and avoid foods that can stress your system.

*You'll notice that some foods are printed in italics; these foods take more energy to assimilate and could be the ones you will want to avoid when you are in a sensitive state due to any physical or emotional stresses.*

Be sure to read Chapter 3, "Implementing the Body Type Diet," for lots of important information about how to use these many foods to gain their full benefit.

### Ultra-Support Foods

Foods to include in 3 to 7 meals a week, listed by category.

**Dense Protein:** chemical-free beef, beef broth, beef liver, *bear, buffalo, venison,* organ meats (heart, brain); chemical-free chicken, chicken broth, chicken livers, Cornish game hen, *duck, quail, pheasant, rabbit,* turkey; *rattlesnake;* anchovy, catfish, cod, flounder, haddock, halibut, herring,

---

**RECOMMENDED CUISINE**

Frequently: Thai, Chinese, steamed vegetables.
Moderately: Mexican, Italian.

mackerel, mahimahi, *perch,* orange roughy, sardines, shark, red snapper, sole; *calamari (squid),* clams, crab, eel, lobster, mussels, octopus, oysters, scallops

**Dairy:** kefir, butter

**Cheese:** cheddar, ricotta

**Nuts and Seeds:** coconut, sunflower seeds

**Grains:** popcorn, rice (all varieties), rice bran, rice cakes, cream of rice

**Vegetables:** artichokes, asparagus, green beans, *broccoli,* carrots, celery, peas, spinach, Swiss chard, *yams*

**Fruits:** bananas, oranges, strawberries

**Sweetener:** stevia

**Beverage:** green tea

## Basic Support Foods

Foods to include in 1 to 2 meals a week.

**Dense Protein:** *lamb;* bass, bonita, salmon, swordfish, trout, tuna; abalone, *shrimp,* snails; eggs

**Dairy:** raw milk, goat milk, half-and-half, sweet cream, sour cream, buttermilk, *plain or flavored yogurt, ice cream* (Ben & Jerry's, Dreyer's, Swensen's)

**Cheese:** American, blue, Brie, Camembert, Colby, cottage, cream, Edam, feta, goat, Gouda, kefir, Limburger, Monterey Jack, mozzarella, Muenster, Parmesan, Romano, Swiss

**Nuts and Seeds:** *almonds, almond butter,* Brazils, *cashews, cashew butter,* hazelnuts, macadamias, macadamia butter, *peanuts, peanut butter,* pecans, pine nuts, pistachios, *walnuts (black, English),* water chestnuts; caraway seeds, sunflower seed butter

**Legumes:** beans (adzuki, black, garbanzo, Great Northern, kidney, lima, *navy,* pinto, red, *soy),* lentils, *black-eyed peas,* split peas; hummus; miso, soy milk, *tofu*

**Grains:** amaranth, barley, *buckwheat,* corn, corn grits, corn tortillas, couscous, hominy grits, *millet,* oats, oatmeal, quinoa, *rye,* triticale, wheat germ, refined wheat flour, flour tortillas, breads (corn, corn/rye, French, garlic, Italian, multigrain, oat, rice, *rye,* seven-grain, sourdough, sprouted grain, white), bagels, croissants, English muffins, crackers (oat, *rye,* saltine); pasta, udon noodles, Chinese rice noodles, *cream of rye,* cream of wheat

**Vegetables:** *avocado,* bamboo shoots, basil, yellow wax beans, beets, bok choy, brussels sprouts, cabbage (red, napa, green), *cauliflower,* cilantro, corn, cucumbers, eggplant, garlic, greens (beet, collard, mustard, turnip), jicama, kale, kohlrabi, leeks, lettuce (all varieties), mushrooms, okra, olives (green, ripe), onions (chives, brown, green, red, Vidalia, white, yellow), parsley, parsnips, snow pea pods, *bell peppers (green, red, yellow),* chili peppers, pimientos, potatoes (red, *russet,* Yukon Gold), pumpkin, radishes, daikon radishes, rutabaga, sauerkraut, seaweed (arame, dulse, kelp, nori, wakame), shallots, sprouts (alfalfa, clover, mung bean, radish, sunflower), squash (acorn, banana, butternut, spaghetti, yellow [summer], *zucchini),* sweet potatoes, *tomatoes* (vine-ripened), turnips, watercress

**Vegetable Juices:** carrot, carrot/celery, celery, parsley, spinach, *tomato,* V-8

**Fruits:** apples (all varieties), apricots, berries (blackberries, blueberries, boysenberries, cranberries, gooseberries, raspberries), cherries, dates, figs, grapes (black, green, red), grapefruit (red, white), guavas, kiwi, kumquats, lemons, limes, loquats, mangoes, melons (cantaloupe, *casaba, Crenshaw,* honeydew, *watermelon),* nectarines, papayas, peaches, pears, persimmons, pineapples, plums (black, purple, red), pomegranates, prunes, raisins, rhubarb, tangelos, tangerines

**Fruit Juices:** *apple, apple cider,* apple/apricot, apricot, black cherry, red cherry, cranapple, cranberry, grape (purple, red, white), grapefruit, guava, lemon, *orange,* papaya, pear, pineapple, pineapple/coconut, prune, tangerine, *watermelon*

**Vegetable Oils:** all-blend, *almond,* avocado, coconut, *corn, flaxseed, olive, peanut, safflower, sesame, soy, sunflower*

**Condiments:** *mustard, mayonnaise, horseradish, barbecue sauce, pesto sauce, soy sauce,* salsa, tahini, vinegar, paprika, Braggs Liquid Aminos, salt, sea salt, Vege-Sal

**Salad Dressings:** *blue cheese, French, ranch, creamy Italian, creamy avocado, Thousand Island,* vinegar and oil, lemon juice and oil

**Desserts:** *custards, tapioca, puddings, pies, cakes, chocolate, desserts containing chocolate, sherbet (orange, raspberry)*

**Chips:** *bean, corn (blue, white, yellow), potato*

**Beverages:** tea (black, herbal, Japanese, Chinese oolong); mineral water, sparkling water; *sake, wine* (red, white), *beer, barley malt liquor, champagne, gin, scotch, vodka, whiskey;* ginger ale, root beer

## Stressful Foods

Have no more than once a month.

**Dense Protein:** *chemical-fed beef, pork, bacon, ham, sausage, veal; chemical-fed chicken or turkey*

**Dairy:** *pasteurized milk, frozen yogurt, most ice creams*

**Nuts and Seeds:** *seeds (pumpkin, sesame), sesame seed butter*

**Grains:** *whole wheat, wheat bran,* wheat germ, *whole wheat bread, whole wheat crackers*

**Vegetables:** *arugula, broccoflower, White Rose potatoes, hothouse tomatoes*

**Vegetable Oil:** *canola*

**Sweeteners:** *fructose, honey, molasses, sorghum, sugar (brown, date, raw, refined cane), syrup (barley malt, brown rice, corn, maple), saccharin, aspartame, Equal, NutraSweet, Sweet'n Low, succonant*

**Condiments:** *catsup, margarine*

**Beverages:** *coffee, regular sodas, diet sodas*

## Scheduling Meals

### Healthy

Lymph types should eat lightly in the morning and progress from moderate to heavy during the day. Schedule your meals as follows:

*Breakfast:* 6–7 A.M. Light to moderate, with grain, nuts, seeds, vegetables, legumes, protein, and/or dairy. Eggs 2 times a week. Fruit or fruit juice alone 30 minutes before or 1 hour after breakfast, 2 times a week. Mix grains with fat such as nuts or butter.

*Lunch:* 12–2 P.M. Moderate to heavy, with grain, dairy, nuts, seeds, and/or protein. Avoid fruit. Minimize vegetables.

*Dinner:* 6–8 P.M. Moderate to heavy, with grain, protein, dairy, nuts, seeds, legumes, and/or vegetables. Avoid fruit.

### Snacks

*Midmorning or midafternoon* (optional): fruit, vegetables, protein, grain, nuts, seeds, dairy

*Evening:* sweets, fruit, vegetables, protein, grain, dairy, nuts, and seeds

### Sensitive

Adjust your intake as follows:

*Breakfast:* Heavy, with protein, nuts, seeds, grain, and/or vegetables.

*Lunch:* Light, with grain and/or vegetables.

*Dinner:* Moderate, with grain, vegetables, and/or legumes.

## Sample One-Week Menu

Snacks are optional.

**DAY 1**

*Breakfast:* spinach, potato, and onion omelette

*Lunch:* chicken soup—chicken broth, chicken, rice, celery, and carrots

*Snack:* macadamia nuts

*Dinner:* salmon fillet and green beans w/water chestnuts

*Snack:* banana

**DAY 2**

*Breakfast:* chicken, cheese, and corn tortilla

*Lunch:* manicotti and mixed nuts and seeds

*Dinner:* Cornish game hen, asparagus, and baby green salad w/sunflower seeds, roasted almonds, and balsamic vinaigrette

*Snack:* popcorn

**DAY 3**

*Snack:* orange

*Breakfast:* cream of rice w/almonds

*Snack:* protein powder w/fruit or fruit juice

*Lunch:* sushi—fish and rice

*Snack:* pecans

*Dinner:* red potatoes, avocado, carrots, and peas

*Snack:* apple and cheese

**DAY 4**

*Breakfast:* chicken sausages, walnuts, and green beans in flour tortilla

*Lunch:* rice, eggs, and mushrooms

*Snack:* cheese and sunflower seeds

*Dinner:* red snapper topped with crushed cashews and a salad of spinach, red peppers, onions, and snow peas w/creamy avocado dressing

DAY 5: CLEANSE

*Breakfast:* watermelon including seeds and white part of rind

*Snack:* watermelon

*Lunch:* soaked almonds and/or pumpkin seeds

*Snack:* soaked almonds and pumpkin seeds or raw carrots or vegetable juice, carrot/celery (parsley), carrot/celery (beet, beet tops) (broccoli)

*Dinner:* steamed cabbage, cauliflower, yams or raw jicama, cucumbers, lettuce, sprouts (avocado) and/or juice of carrot/celery (parsley)

DAY 6

*Breakfast:* bagel, cream cheese, and lox

*Lunch:* beans, rice, and corn tortilla

*Snack:* cottage cheese and tomatoes

*Dinner:* kabobs of shrimp, onions, bell peppers, and zucchini

*Snack:* dried cherries

DAY 7

*Breakfast:* turkey patty, potatoes, and Swiss chard

*Lunch:* spinach pasta, chemical-free chicken, and tuna and pasta with pesto sauce

*Dinner:* chicken pieces baked with Thai peanut sauce, steamed broccoli, and summer squash served on salad of spinach, red bell peppers, and pine nuts w/Thai peanut salad dressing

## Alternative Menus

*(Foods in parentheses may be omitted.)*

### Breakfast

Turkey sausage, sweet potato, and kefir

Salad of crab, celery, sunflower seeds, and peas

Eggs and bagel with cheese

Basmati or short grain brown rice (w/butter or tamari) and green beans

Steak and yams

Oatmeal w/sunflower seeds

Cream of wheat w/rice milk (banana later)

Pasta and peas

Potato and green beans (squash)

Baked Yukon Gold potato or yam w/butter

Smoked salmon, sliced onion, and tomato on oat bagel (capers)

Vegetable soup—carrot, onion, yam, cumin, coriander, pepper, and turmeric, brown rice, and raw cucumber

### Lunch

Matza ball soup w/noodles and rice

Salmon and/or crab, clams, or tuna and pasta

Sea bass or sole, and rice pilaf

Fish taco—flour tortilla, light fish fillet, avocado, lemon, shredded green cabbage—and rice

Pinto beans and rice w/sliced black olives and corn tortilla

Chicken and coleslaw w/chopped peanuts

Polenta, cashews, and melted cheese

### Dinner

Filet mignon w/crushed hazelnuts and a raw vegetable salad of avocado, basil, bok choy, cabbage, jicama, and tomatoes

Turkey patty and broccoli (asparagus)

Pheasant, carrots, peas, and rice

Rabbit and White Rose potatoes (carrots, broccoli, and onions)

Veal Parmesan, carrots, and peas

Scallops, pasta, and peas

Halibut, artichoke pasta, and spinach

Vegetable manicotti w/tomato sauce

Split pea soup and corn muffin or sourdough bread

Vegeburger w/tomatoes and cheese

Red snapper w/teriyaki marinade, rice pilaf, and corn

# Medulla

*The Medulla body type is symbolized by a metronome. Steady and consistent, medulla types persevere unwavering in their activities and beliefs. With an intense sense of responsibility, they will remain loyal indefinitely to a worthwhile cause.*

FAMOUS PEOPLE: Jane Seymour, Madonna, Ronald Reagan, George Clooney

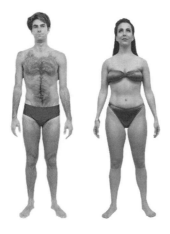

## MEDULLA
### Location and Function

The medulla oblongata is located in the brain stem between the pons and the spinal cord. It is an area of the brain that controls such vital functions as respiration and circulation.

## Psychological Profile

### Characteristic Traits

Medulla body types are characteristically steady, stable, and persistent. They love structure, order, consistency, and stability. Highly responsible, once they have committed to something they generally follow through, keeping their promises and agreements. Loyal, patient, and tenacious, they typically won't quit until the job is finished.

Endowed with strong, inquiring minds, Medulla types are drawn to things that appeal to their creativity. While open to new ideas and philosophies, they are typically cautious about getting into new situations. Conscientious, conservative, and generally conventional, they like to study subjects in depth. When they feel more secure, they may at times swing to the opposite extreme of flying by the seat of their pants.

Medulla types possess a sensitivity that is expressed in their responsiveness to others or protected with a hard exterior. Tending toward one of the two extremes, they are either quite sensitive to people around them or closed and self-centered. When sensitive to people, Medulla types have strong nurturing and/or healing qualities coupled with a depth of caring and compassion. Kind, gentle, and helpful, they are altruistic, with a strong desire to help people individually and the human race in general.

### Motivation

Medulla types generally start life with a strong physical energy that needs to be channeled. When it isn't, this energy reverses and leads to illnesses or environmental sensitivities. While their physical body is still strong, they are able to handle working long hours, smoking, and alcohol. They are able to drive themselves, particularly at work. Because their bodies are basically strong, when they are stressed they go into overdrive and become hyper, resulting in a surplus of nervous energy. This can cause them to become scattered and run around in circles, expending energy without focus.

Although physically strong, Medulla types are especially sensitive to chemicals, antibiotics, and pollutants. Many experience chronic health problems of a degenerative nature or environmental sensitivities after a period of prolonged chemical exposure (e.g., a hairdresser using bleaches and dyes) or physical trauma (e.g., intestinal parasites or food poisoning, or whiplash injury). The neck tends to be a particularly vulnerable area, with stiffness, rigidity, and muscle aching followed by chronic illness or diseases that involve muscle rigidity, such as Parkinson-like muscle spasms.

Being sensitive to their environment, Medulla types feel a need to control it to protect themselves. Control usually takes the form of mental exactness, wanting to know everything about an area before stepping into it. Being too detail oriented can cause them to become rigid in their thought processes and narrow-minded, afraid to step out into the world and let life take them where they need to go. Mental rigidity can also lead to an indecisiveness that prevents them from getting anything done or bringing things to completion.

Change triggers old fears and feelings of inadequacy. Fear of failure or lack of acceptance is the main impetus for change, so there is a tendency to avoid it at all costs. With such a strong desire for structure and stability, change is difficult. It usually occurs only after all the options on the current path have been exhausted. If Medulla types can't find a way of implementing change, life's challenges may cause them to give up, accept defeat, and become impotent—physically unable to move forward in life.

### "At Worst"

Medulla types can become stiff and rigid. Insisting on being precise, they can belabor a point. They can become narrow-minded and controlling by being too cautious and exacting. Afraid to make a move, they may limit themselves and those around them, resulting in a lack of growth, spontaneity, and movement. It's easy for them to become too serious or too intense, restricting freedom and expansion. By being too cautious, they become hard, heavy, and boring. By being too analytical, they take the fun out of life. Medulla types can be demanding, abrasive, and authoritarian when trying to get things done or get things to work their way. This inflexibility can manifest itself as obsessiveness in behavior or relationships and lead to food or substance addiction. When Medulla types are stuck in their development, their sensitivity can be directed inward, causing them to overfocus on their own desires and become self-centered and demanding. By being too dependent on structure and stability, Medulla types resist change, staying too long in circumstances that are clearly draining or detrimental.

Armored and controlling, Medulla types can be skeptical and pessimistic about everything new.

Intellectually exacting, they find it easy to rationalize their skepticism. Prone to indecisiveness and disorganization, Medulla types can find it almost impossible to get anything done. They can get caught up in their fears and beliefs, causing them to keep plugging dikes frantically rather than addressing real issues, or otherwise engage in impulsive or self-defeating behavior.

Medulla types may feel overly responsible for someone else but fail to take personal responsibility for their own destinies. They may consciously or unconsciously manipulate others to take over for them. By not truly knowing themselves, they can get caught up in appearances, looking to the outside world for approval or to take care of them and tell them what is accepted. By trying too hard to please others, they may neglect their own needs and emotional welfare.

### "At Best"

Medulla types are steady, persistent, and imaginative. When they are able to integrate their mental capability with their physical energy, they can accomplish almost anything. When self-confidence allows them to let go of their need to control, their love of structure, order, consistency, and stability provides them with the ability to be highly successful in both the business and professional worlds.

Medulla types are naturally consistent, responsible, and loyal. With their high level of perseverance and mental acuity, they can master any subject that piques their interest. Patient, caring, and committed, they will "go the extra mile" with a person until he or she fully understands a subject, making them excellent teachers. Having connected with their own intuitive process, they have a great deal of insight and perception, which allows them to see the value in leading technology or interpersonal work. Not only do they have the ability to figure things out through other than the accepted channels, they are able to teach these things to others. Willing to learn, they explore new areas and embrace change that reflects forward movement, integrating it into the established structure.

Medulla types take their relationships seriously and will do what is in the highest and best interest of everyone. Sensitive, kind, gentle, helpful, and compassionate, they effectively express their altruistic nature, helping people individually and the human race in general.

Having integrated their emotional and spiritual or intuitive sides with their strong physical and mental aspects, Medulla types are in step with life, changing and flowing with it, allowing it to change them. Flexible and self-confident, they are self-reliant; validating and appreciating themselves, they excel in thought and action.

## Dietary Profile

### Main Focus

- Eat vegetables, especially first bite each morning to activate digestion; then follow with other foods.
- Make lunch the largest meal between 10:30 A.M. and 3 P.M.
- May eat a large late dinner with protein between 9 and 11 P.M.
- Have no protein for dinner unless consumed after 9 P.M.
- You are sensitive to chemicals, so eat only chemical-free chicken, turkey, and beef; organic fruits, vegetables, and grains are best.

### Dietary Emphasis

- From 20 to 35 percent of your calories are to come from fats.
- Best fat sources: dense protein (chicken, turkey, Cornish game hen) and/or nuts.

---

### RECOMMENDED EXERCISE

Exercise is helpful to Medulla body types because it activates the immune system, but its benefit is primarily emotional: it relieves tension and moves stuck emotions. Activities requiring eye-hand coordination, such as tennis, racquetball, and volleyball, are recommended. As a means of relaxing and regaining personal equilibrium, try walking, biking, yoga, Callanetics, skating, skiing, dancing, and stretching—particularly in the afternoon or evening, since morning exercise often results in midafternoon fatigue. Regular exercise, like weight lifting and stair-stepping, builds muscle mass. Sustained exercise for 3 hours or more, such as dancing, walking, hiking, backpacking, or cross-country skiing 1 to 2 times per week, causes weight loss, as it acts to pull glucose out of muscles.

---

- From 20 to 35 percent of your calories are to come from protein.
- From 0 to 30 percent of your calories are to come from dense protein.
- Best sources of the three amino acids threonine, isoleucine, and cystine: ham, tuna, swordfish, salmon.
- Caloric intake: 1,500 to 1,800 calories a day for women and 1,700 to 2,000 calories a day for men. If you are engaging in intense exercise (competition type) or hard labor, increase calories.
- Drink a minimum of 64 ounces of water a day. Drink water before and after meals, not with meals.
- Occasional desserts are best as an evening snack.
- Follow food and time schedule: breakfast, 7–9 A.M.; lunch, 10:30 A.M.–3 P.M.; dinner, 6–8 P.M.; and/or late dinner, 9–11 P.M.
- Food rotation is important.
- Fruit often helps regulate bowels. Green beans and peas strengthen intestines.
- Have vegetables at every meal (especially breakfast), particularly green beans, celery, greens, peas, and soups.

### For Weight Loss

- Fat: 20 to 30 percent of daily calories.
- Best fat sources: dense protein (chicken, turkey, Cornish game hen), nuts, butter, ghee, kefir, yogurt, and cheese.
- May fast on apple juice and water up to 2 days a week, with walking or yoga to keep lymphatics moving.
- Working up a sweat for 3 hours or more activates weight loss.
- Medulla types build muscle easily. A 1-hour workout will build muscle, making weight loss in thighs difficult.
- Follow recommended food groups at designated meals.
- Emphasize vegetables.

### For Weight Gain

- Dense protein: 20 to 30 percent of daily calories.
- Adhere to eating schedules for recommended food groups.
- Emphasize nuts, seeds, dairy (may include ice cream), and vegetables.

## Healthy Foods List

There is no need to sacrifice delicious and filling foods to maintain a healthy Medulla body type. The following lists will help you focus on foods that support your health, and avoid foods that can stress your system.

*You'll notice that some foods are printed in italics; these foods take more energy to assimilate and could be ones you will want to avoid when you are in a sensitive state due to any physical or emotional stresses.*

Be sure to read Chapter 3, "Implementing the Body Type Diet," for lots of important information about how to use these many foods to gain their full benefit.

### Ultra-Support Foods

Foods to include in 3 to 7 meals a week, listed by category.

**Dense Protein:** beef broth, buffalo, pork, bacon, ham, sausage, veal; chemical-free chicken, chicken broth, turkey; anchovy, bass, cod, flounder, halibut, herring, mackerel, mahimahi, perch, orange roughy, salmon, sardines, shark, red snapper, sole, swordfish, trout, tuna; calamari (squid), clams, crab, eel, lobster, mussels, octopus, oysters, scallops

**Dairy:** kefir (peach, apricot)

**Cheese:** blue, extra-sharp cheddar

**Nuts and Seeds:** almonds, cashew butter, coconut, pine nuts; sesame seed butter, raw sunflower seeds

**Grains:** corn tortillas, couscous, rice (white basmati, Japanese), rye, pasta

**Vegetables:** acorn squash, carrots, *cauliflower,* celery, collard greens, green beans, red Swiss chard, yams

**Vegetable Juice:** carrot

**Fruits:** lemons, pears, persimmons, plums (black, purple, red), pomegranates, raisins, rhubarb, tangelos, tangerines

**Vegetable Oil:** *olive*

**Sweeteners:** *molasses, sorghum,* stevia

**Salad Dressing:** balsamic vinegar and *olive oil*

**Beverage:** herbal tea

### Basic Support Foods

Foods to include in 1 to 2 meals a week.

**Dense Protein:** beef, beef liver, lamb, venison, wild game, organ meats (heart, brain); Foster Farms or Zacky chicken or turkey, chicken livers, Cornish game hen, duck; bonita, *catfish,* haddock; abalone, shrimp; eggs

**Dairy:** milk (whole, 2%, low fat, raw, goat's), half-and-half, sweet cream, sour cream, buttermilk, yogurt (plain or *flavored*), frozen yogurt, *ice cream* (Ben & Jerry's, Dreyer's, Swensen's), butter

**Cheese:** American, Brie, Camembert, cheddar, Colby, cottage, cream, Edam, feta, goat, Gouda, kefir, Limburger, Monterey Jack, mozzarella, Muenster, Parmesan, ricotta, Romano, Swiss

**Nuts and Seeds:** almond butter, Brazils, cashews, hazelnuts, macadamias, macadamia butter, peanuts, peanut butter, pecans, pistachios, walnuts (black, English), water chestnuts; raw or roasted seeds (caraway, pumpkin, sesame), roasted sunflower seeds, sunflower seed butter

**Legumes:** beans (adzuki, black, garbanzo, Great Northern, kidney, lima, navy, pinto, red, soy), lentils, split peas, black-eyed peas; hummus; miso, soy milk, tofu

**Grains:** amaranth, *barley,* buckwheat, corn, corn grits, hominy grits, millet, oats, popcorn, quinoa, rice (brown basmati, long or short grain brown, *polished,* wild), rice bran, rice cakes, triticale, wheat bran, wheat germ, sprouted wheat, refined wheat flour, flour tortillas, breads (corn, corn/rye, French, garlic, Italian, *multigrain,* oat, pumpernickel, rice, rye, sourdough, *sprouted grain,* white), bagels, croissants, English muffins, crackers (oat, rye, saltines), udon noodles, rice noodles, cream of rice, cream of rye, cream of wheat

**Vegetables:** artichokes, *arugula,* asparagus, avocados, bamboo shoots, yellow wax beans, beets, bok choy, broccoflower, broccoli, brussels sprouts, cabbage (green, napa, red), cilantro, corn, cucumbers, eggplant, garlic, greens (beet, mustard, turnip), jicama, kale, kohlrabi, leeks, lettuce (Boston, butter, endive, iceberg, red leaf, romaine), mushrooms, okra, olives (green, ripe), onions (chives, brown, green, red, Vidalia, white, yellow), parsley, parsnips, peas, snow peas, bell peppers (green, red, yellow), chili peppers, pimientos, potatoes (red, russet, White Rose, Yukon Gold), pumpkin, radishes, daikon radishes, rutabaga, seaweed (arame, dulse, kelp, nori, wakame), sauerkraut, shallots, spinach, sprouts (alfalfa, clover, mung bean, radish, sunflower), squash (banana, butternut), Swiss chard, tomatoes, turnips, *watercress*

**Vegetable Juices:** carrot/celery, celery, spinach, parsley, lettuce, beet, tomato, V-8

**Fruits:** apples (Red or Golden Delicious, Granny Smith, Jonathan, McIntosh, Pippin, Rome Beauty), apricots, bananas, berries (blackberries, cranberries, gooseberries, raspberries), cherries, dates, figs, grapes (black, green, red), grapefruit (red, white), guavas, kiwi, kumquats, limes, loquats, mangoes, melons (cantaloupe, Crenshaw, honeydew, watermelon), nectarines, oranges, papayas, peaches, pineapples, prunes

**Fruit Juices:** apple, apple cider, apple/apricot, apricot, black cherry, red cherry, cranapple, cranberry, grape (red, purple, white), guava, grapefruit, lemon, orange, papaya, pear, pineapple, pineapple/coconut, prune, tangerine, watermelon

**Vegetable Oils:** all-blend, *almond,* avocado, coconut, *corn, flaxseed, peanut, safflower, sesame, soy, sunflower*

**Sweeteners:** *fructose, honey, sugar (brown, date, raw, refined cane), syrup (barley malt, corn, brown rice, maple), saccharin, succonant*

**Condiments:** *catsup, mustard, horseradish, mayonnaise, barbecue sauce, pesto sauce, soy sauce,* salsa, tahini, *vinegar,* salt, sea salt, Vege-Sal

**Salad Dressings:** *blue cheese, French, ranch, creamy Italian, creamy avocado, Thousand Island,* lemon juice and oil

**Desserts:** *custards, tapioca, puddings, pies, cakes, sherbet (orange, raspberry)*

**Chips:** bean, corn (*blue, white, yellow*), *potato*

**Beverages:** *coffee;* tea (*black,* green, Japanese, Chinese oolong); mineral water, sparkling water; *wine (red, white), sake, beer, barley malt liquor, champagne, gin, scotch, vodka, whiskey; root beer, regular sodas*

## Stressful Foods

Have no more than once a month.

**Dense Protein:** *chemical-fed chicken or turkey*
**Dairy:** *nonfat milk, most ice creams*

**Grains:** *whole wheat, bread (seven-grain, whole wheat), whole wheat crackers*
**Vegetables:** *squash (spaghetti, yellow [summer], zucchini), sweet potatoes*
**Fruits:** berries (*blueberries, boysenberries, strawberries*), *casaba melons*
**Vegetable Oil:** *canola*
**Sweeteners:** *aspartame, Equal, NutraSweet, Sweet'n Low*
**Condiment:** *margarine*
**Desserts:** *chocolate, desserts containing chocolate*
**Beverages:** *diet sodas*

## Scheduling Meals

Medulla body types can enjoy moderate to heavy meals throughout the day. Schedule your meals as follows:

*Breakfast:* 7–9 A.M. Moderate, with vegetables. May have fruit and protein, nuts, seeds, legumes, or grain if vegetables (even a few bites) are eaten first. Avoid dense protein.
*Lunch:* 10:30 A.M.–3 P.M. Heavy, with protein, dairy, nuts, seeds, legumes, grain, vegetables, and/or fruit.
*Dinner:* 6–8 P.M. Moderate, with vegetables, legumes, and/or grain. Avoid fruit. Avoid dense protein.
*Late dinner:* (optional) 9–11 P.M. Protein, nuts, seeds, dairy, legumes, vegetables, grain, fruit, and/or sweets.

### Snacks (optional)
*Midmorning:* fruit
*Midafternoon:* (3–5 P.M.) fruit, seeds, nuts, dairy, vegetables, grain
*Evening:* (1 hour after dinner) fruit

## Sample One-Week Menu

DAY 1
*Breakfast:* steamed kale, then oatmeal w/seeds and/or nuts
*Lunch:* salmon, rice, and cauliflower
*Dinner:* angel-hair pasta w/tomatoes, capers, black olives, and crushed red pepper

DAY 2
*Breakfast:* potato soup
*Lunch:* chemical-free turkey and broccoli
*Dinner:* brown basmati rice and green beans

DAY 3
*Breakfast:* spinach and eggs
*Lunch:* Cornish game hen, rice, and asparagus
*Dinner:* spinach salad, cooked White Rose potatoes, and corn

DAY 4
*Breakfast:* cooked mixed vegetables (carrots, peas, and green beans)
*Lunch:* swordfish, couscous, and peas
*Dinner:* Japanese cucumber rolls w/ginger and soy sauce

DAY 5: CLEANSE
*Breakfast:* juice of carrot/celery/beet (parsley/spinach)
*Snack:* juice of carrot/celery/beet (parsley/spinach)
*Lunch:* steamed broccoli, cauliflower, chard, greens (collard, mustard) w/onions, green peas, squash, zucchini
*Dinner:* steamed broccoli, brussels sprouts, cauliflower, squash, chard, peas, and/or salad w/red leaf lettuce, bell peppers, carrots, jicama, alfalfa sprouts

DAY 6
*Breakfast:* peas, then chicken and white basmati rice
*Lunch:* steak and tomatoes
*Dinner:* vegetable soup

DAY 7
*Breakfast:* couscous, eggs, mushrooms, and red leaf lettuce
*Lunch:* fillet of tuna and pasta w/mushrooms, peas, and pesto sauce
*Dinner:* lentils w/sautéed onions and sliced tomatoes

## Alternative Menus

*(Foods in parentheses are optional.)*

### Breakfast
Raw or cooked carrots, peas, or green beans
Green beans, then rice
Peas, carrots, and corn
Yam (green peas)
Baked potato, yam, or acorn squash w/butter
Carrots, raw or steamed (eggs or chicken)
Carrot juice, then peas and broccoli
Carrot juice, then oatmeal
Celery/romaine lettuce juice, then lima beans
Celery, parsley, and carrot juice (rice)

### Lunch
Salmon or swordfish and rice (peas)
Red snapper and broccoli (raw purple cabbage)
Mussels (rice and/or butter and/or kale)
Oysters and pasta (collard greens)
Shrimp, pasta, and peas (butter)
Corned beef and cabbage
Liver and onions and mustard greens, beet greens, or kale
Chicken, rice, and green beans, carrots, or broccoli
Cornish game hen and rice (spinach, kale, or mustard greens)

### Dinner
Salad of romaine lettuce, green onions, celery, and peas w/Hain creamy avocado dressing
Broccoli and rice, pasta, or mashed potato
Miso soup and broccoli, carrots, or squash
Carrots, peas, and rice or pasta
Basmati rice and mung bean sprouts
Rice or pasta (butter, broccoli, carrots, eggplant, and/or tomato sauce)
Soup—carrots, onions, broccoli, and barley in chicken broth
Pinto beans, rice, and/or corn tortilla
Yukon Gold potato and green beans

# Nervous System

*The Nervous System body type is symbolized by wires. Nerves are the "wires" that connect all parts of the body and keep the brain informed. Practical and efficient, Nervous System types are happiest when connecting with people and ideas.*

FAMOUS PEOPLE: Jim Carrey, Michelle Pfeiffer, Sandra Bullock, Don Knotts

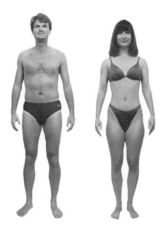

## NERVOUS SYSTEM
### Location and Function

The nervous system comprises the brain, the spinal cord, and all the nerves. It is the body's communication network, conveying nerve impulses from one part of the body to another.

## Psychological Profile

### Characteristic Traits

With their strong physical presence and mental focus, Nervous System body types are characterized and easily recognized by their direct, intense (often forceful), take-charge manner. They thrive on a lot of activity and love to get things moving. They derive most of their knowledge and stimulation from their interactions with others.

Although Nervous System types can at times be fairly reserved, they're typically gregarious and outgoing when they feel free to be themselves. Naturally curious, with excellent analytical abilities, they are interested in learning what other people know and how they do things. While they are quite conscientious about learning all that is necessary to use and integrate the information, they don't need to know every detail.

Nervous System types are happiest when they can collect knowledge from one person and bring it to another, like a bee going from flower to flower. Practical and efficient, they initially prefer the physical or concrete to the theoretical. Highly selective in what they like, most of their choices are ones that add meaning to their lives.

While they often appear to have a hard exterior, Nervous System types are quite sentimental. They are particularly good at helping or providing emotional support and encouragement to others. Well organized, logical, and persistent, they have the ability to determine what needs to be done in any situation and the physical stamina to follow projects through to completion, meeting their goals. Altruistically oriented, they often find a noble cause to serve.

### Motivation

Typically verbal with the ability to realistically synthesize and integrate information from a practical, grounded perspective, Nervous System types tend to assert their viewpoints forcefully. Strong-willed and determined, they can easily get too intense as their energy builds and they get excited or stressed. They express their emotions in their tone of voice, which unfortunately often comes across as abrasive. Not surprisingly, they often come from environments where they had to speak up forcefully to be heard. This forcefulness may then become their normal manner, making it easy for them to enter a situation, quickly size things up, and more or less take over.

Nervous System types tend to be perfectionists and to overdo, expending all their energy on duty and responsibility with little left for themselves. Because of their inherent strength, stamina, and clarity of direction, they tend to do things themselves rather than delegate, often taking on too much and spreading themselves too thin. Their belief is "I'm strong, I can handle it. It needs to be done, so I'll do it." People around them often feel intimidated by their expertise. Their intention is never to intimidate but simply to demonstrate that others can also do the task.

Movement is vital to their sense of well-being, so they thrive on a lot of activity and being constantly on the go. They have large quantities of energy, and if this energy is not used, they become nervous or sluggish. Using the energy through activities or exercise increases their sense of well-being. Because of their strong mental and physical connections, their energy is easily channeled productively. They abhor chaos and have even been known to clean someone else's house while paying a visit.

Adventure stimulates change for this body type. People often constitute the adventure, so they may travel simply to experience the people. They like activity, particularly activity that provides mental and emotional stimulation, which motivates them to participate in an activity just because it's a new experience. They don't like the restriction of rules and regulations and often do things differently to create change. Learning takes them to new places, and nature is a welcome teacher.

Because of the strength, depth, and intensity of their emotions, Nervous System types are fearful of expressing them. Their fear is that expression of the emotion, because of its strength, will upset things, even threaten their survival. This fear is reinforced by the frequent experience of having others leave them because they are not able to handle the intensity of the Nervous System type. Consequently they use their strong mental energies to block out or separate themselves from their feelings and redirect their attention to external things, such as physical activities or intellectual pursuits.

## "At Worst"

Blunt, outspoken, and abrasive, Nervous System types can control their environment and everyone around them. Intolerant, rigid, and inflexible, they demand that others follow their rules. Harsh, negative, and judgmental, they evaluate others by how well they follow these rules. Seeing everyone as inferior to themselves, Nervous System types believe that others are here to serve them, which justifies their using and draining others. Regardless of what others do, it's never enough.

When their abundance of energy is not properly channeled, Nervous System types become nervous themselves and/or make other people nervous. Being defensive, they often come across as offensive. Without sufficient emotional connection, their judgment is impaired, causing them to be too assertive in some situations and not assertive enough in others. To protect their egos, Nervous System types defend their rationalized viewpoints with a stubborn ferocity; yet afraid to jeopardize their relationships, they may hesitate to assert their legitimate interests. Because they are unable to deal with their own emotions and effectively express their anger without hurting those around them, they can't stand for others to express their emotions. When unable to resolve their negative feelings, they often become either moody or withdrawn.

By placing value on external appearances and making the outside world their reality, they try to control, becoming too mental and consequently too rigid. Their way is best, they feel, and everything has to be done according to their schedule, in a systematic fashion. Their networking and interactions with others are based on self-serving ulterior motives. Manipulative, they have a well-calculated agenda before they ask for what they want, and they make everyone miserable until they get it.

The more sensitive, responsible Nervous System types overextend themselves and take on too much rather than give adequate consideration to their own needs and limitations. As perfectionists, they often overdo and become too picky or exacting. By spending so much time and energy on duty and responsibility, they find they have little left for personal needs and become angry and resentful. Becoming very busy so they don't have to think about the problem or situation is a way of suppressing personal feelings.

## "At Best"

Nervous System body types connect things on all levels, which makes them excellent communicators, both verbally and in writing. Having a genuine interest in people, they know what others want and what motivates them. They are socially adept, gracious, polite, and charming. Elegant and meticulous about appearances, they love social situations and are exceptionally good at organizing them. They set the stage perfectly and make sure every detail is attended to with precision.

Gregarious and outgoing, Nervous System types are in their element at social gatherings where they can circulate and introduce people to one another. They love being the force that gets things moving. Motivated by their deep desire to help humanity, they tirelessly gather information and bring it to those who need it. Sensitive to the needs of other people, they are good at providing emotional support to friends and family. Giving compliments, reassurance, and encouragement comes naturally to Nervous System types at their best.

Born leaders, Nervous System types are energetic, determined, and achievement oriented, as well as logical, practical, and efficient. While mentally focused, they are flexible and spontaneous enough to let life flow. Accessing their creativity allows them to balance their strong masculine traits with the gentle, receptive feminine side that is best expressed through service. Since listening and service are synonymous for the Nervous System type, and creativity is best expressed when it involves other people, doing things for them such as organizing social events or doing social volunteer work makes their lives fulfilling.

Having found their inner peace and tranquillity by centering themselves and developing their spiritual connection, Nervous System types are highly intuitive and instinctive. Coupling their physical strengths of practicality and efficiency with their intuition allows them to express their full potential and purpose. Listening to emotions, their own as well as those of others, allows them to link emotions with experience and relay the lesson or message. Not only can they focus their energy productively, they can effectively communicate the message. By being a channel, or a messenger, they can be of great service to humanity.

---

### RECOMMENDED EXERCISE

Exercise is essential for Nervous System body types because it activates the immune system. It is also effective in releasing emotional stress and acting as a means of social interaction. At least 20 minutes of heavy exercise every other day is recommended. The best exercise varies with lifestyle changes. Common activities include weight lifting, all-over body movement such as yoga or swimming, and aerobic activity such as running, kick-boxing, biking, racquetball, rebounding or dance.

## Dietary Profile

### Main Focus

- Have a heavy breakfast with protein. Eat what is normally considered dinner for breakfast.
- Get adequate fat and protein.
- Eat raw vegetables for lunch and cooked or steamed vegetables for dinner. Reverse order when sensitive.
- Avoid fruit with dinner.
- External stimulation helps focus energy.

### Dietary Emphasis

- From 20 to 45 percent of your calories are to come from fats.
- Best fat sources: dense protein, Swiss cheese, butter, flaxseed oil, olive oil, sesame oil, nuts, and seeds.
- From 20 to 45 percent of your calories are to come from protein.
- From 10 to 30 percent of your calories are to come from dense protein.
- Best sources of the three amino acids threonine, isoleucine, and cystine: beef, tuna, and salmon.
- Caloric intake: 1,500 to 1,800 calories a day for women and 1,700 to 2,000 calories a day for men. If you are engaging in intense exercise (competition type) or hard labor, increase calories.
- Drink a minimum of 64 ounces of water a day. Drink water before and after meals, not with meals.
- Occasional desserts are best as an evening snack.
- Olive oil relieves constipation; potatoes support the lungs; whey aids digestion of carbohydrates.

### For Weight Loss

- Fat: 20 to 35 percent of daily calories.
- Protein: 20 to 40 percent of daily calories.
- Dense protein: 20 to 30 percent of daily calories.
- Weight loss will be inhibited if fats fall below 20 percent of calories.
- Reduce grains and sugars, including fruit.

### For Weight Gain

- Fat: 20 to 30 percent of daily calories.
- Protein: 30 to 45 percent of daily calories.
- Dense protein: 25 to 35 percent of daily calories.
- Eat 4 equally spaced meals per day.
- Follow healthy meal schedule.

## Healthy Foods List

There is no need to sacrifice delicious and filling foods to maintain a healthy Nervous System body type. The following lists will help you focus on foods that support your health, and avoid foods that can stress your system.

*You'll notice that some foods are printed in italics; these foods take more energy to assimilate and could be ones you will want to avoid when you are in a sensitive state due to any physical or emotional stresses.*

Be sure to read Chapter 3, "Implementing the Body Type Diet," for lots of important information about how to use these many foods to gain their full benefit.

### Ultra-Support Foods

Food to include in 3 to 7 meals a week, listed by category.

**Dense Protein:** beef, beef broth, beef liver, buffalo, lamb; chicken livers, Cornish game hen; bass, bonita, catfish, cod, flounder, haddock, halibut, herring, mackerel, mahimahi, perch, orange roughy, salmon, sardines, shark, red snapper, sole, swordfish, trout, tuna; calamari (squid), clams, eel, lobster, mussels, octopus, oysters, scallops, shrimp

**Vegetables:** asparagus, *avocado, broccoli,* carrots, cauliflower, corn, cucumbers, eggplant, potatoes (all varieties), seaweed (dulse, kelp, nori, wakame), spinach, *zucchini*

**Vegetable Juice:** carrot

**Fruit:** oranges

**Fruit Juice:** orange

**Sweetener:** stevia

**Beverages:** *coffee* with whipped cream or half-and-half; *Perrier water*

### Basic Support Foods

Foods to include in 1 to 2 meals a week.

**Dense Protein:** bacon, veal, venison, organ meats (heart, brain); chicken, chicken broth, duck, turkey; anchovy, lox; abalone, crab; eggs

**Dairy:** milk (whole, 2%, low fat, nonfat, raw, goat's), half-and-half, sour cream, sweet cream, kefir, plain or strawberry yogurt, frozen yogurt, ice cream (Ben & Jerry's, Dreyer's, Swensen's), butter

**Cheese:** American, blue, Brie, Camembert, cheddar, Colby, cottage, cream, Edam, feta, goat, Gouda, kefir, Limburger, Monterey Jack, mozzarella, Muenster, Parmesan, ricotta, Romano, Swiss

**Nuts and Seeds:** almonds, almond butter, Brazils, cashews, cashew butter, coconut, hazelnuts, macadamias, macadamia butter, peanuts, *peanut butter,* pecans, pine nuts, pistachios, walnuts (English, black), water chestnuts; seeds (caraway, pumpkin, sesame, sunflower), sesame seed butter, sunflower seed butter

**Legumes:** beans (adzuki, black, garbanzo, Great Northern, kidney, lima, navy, pinto, red, soy), lentils, black-eyed peas, split peas; hummus; miso, soy milk, tofu

**Grains:** amaranth, barley, buckwheat, corn, corn grits, corn tortillas, couscous, hominy grits, millet, oats, popcorn, quinoa, rice (brown or white basmati, long or short grain brown, Japanese, wild), rice bran, rice cakes, rye, triticale, whole wheat, wheat bran, wheat germ, refined wheat flour, flour tortillas, breads (corn, corn/rye, French, garlic, Italian, multigrain, oat, rice, rye, seven-grain, sourdough, sprouted grain, white, whole wheat), bagels, croissants, English muffins, crackers (oat, rye, saltines, wheat), pasta, udon noodles, Chinese rice noodles; cream of rice, cream of rye, cream of wheat

**Vegetables:** artichokes, *arugula,* bamboo shoots, beans (green, yellow wax), beets, bok choy, *broccoflower,* brussels sprouts, cabbage (green, napa, red), celery, cilantro, garlic, greens (beet, collard, mustard, turnip), jicama, kale, kohlrabi, leeks, lettuce (Boston, butter, endive, iceberg, red leaf, romaine), mushrooms, okra, olives (green, ripe), onions (chives, brown, green, red, Vidalia, white, yellow), parsley, parsnips, peas, snow pea pods, bell peppers (green, yellow, red), chili peppers, pimientos, pumpkin, radishes, daikon radishes, rutabaga, sauerkraut, seaweed (arame), shallots, spinach, sprouts (alfalfa, clover, mung bean, radish, sunflower), squash (acorn, banana, butternut, yellow [summer], spaghetti), sweet potatoes, Swiss chard, tomatoes, turnips, *watercress,* yams

**Vegetable Juices:** carrot/celery, celery, parsley, spinach, tomato, V-8

**Fruits:** apples (Golden or Red Delicious, Granny Smith, Jonathan, McIntosh, Pippin, Rome Beauty), apricots, bananas, berries (blackberries, blueberries, boysenberries, cranberries, gooseberries, raspberries, strawberries), cherries, dates, figs, grapes (black, green, red), guavas, kiwi, kumquats, lemons, limes, loquats, mangoes, melons (cantaloupe, casaba, Crenshaw, honeydew, watermelon), nectarines, papayas, peaches, pears, persimmons, pineapples, plums (black, purple, red), pomegranates, prunes, *raisins,* rhubarb, tangelos, tangerines

**Fruit Juices:** apple, apple cider, apple/apricot, apricot, red cherry, black cherry, cranapple, cranberry, grape (red, white, purple), grapefruit, guava, lemon, papaya, pear, pineapple, pineapple/coconut, prune, tangerine, watermelon

**Vegetable Oils:** all-blend, *almond,* avocado, *corn,* flaxseed, *peanut,* olive, *safflower,* sesame, *soy, sunflower*

**Sweeteners:** *fructose, honey, molasses, sorghum, sugar* (*brown, date, raw, refined cane*), *syrup* (*barley malt, brown rice, corn, maple*), *succonant*

**Condiments:** *horseradish, barbecue sauce, pesto sauce,* salsa, tahini, red wine vinegar, salt, sea salt, Vege-Sal

**Salad Dressings:** *blue cheese, French, ranch,* creamy Italian, *creamy avocado, Thousand Island,* vinegar and oil, lemon juice and oil; good substitute for mayonnaise: Hain creamy Italian dressing

**Desserts:** *custards, tapioca, puddings, pies, cakes, white chocolate, sherbet* (*orange, raspberry*)

**Chips:** bean, corn (blue, white, yellow), potato

**Beverages:** *coffee;* tea (*black,* green, herbal, Japanese, Chinese oolong); mineral water, sparkling water; *wine* (*red, white*), *sake, beer, barley malt liquor, hot apple cider and brandy, fruit juice and vodka, champagne, scotch, gin, vodka, whiskey; root beer*

## Stressful Foods

Have no more than once a month.

**Dense Protein:** *pork, ham, sausage*
**Dairy:** *buttermilk, most ice creams*
**Cheese:** *smoked*
**Grains:** *polished rice*
**Fruits:** *grapefruit*
**Vegetable Oil:** *canola*
**Sweeteners:** *saccharin, aspartame, Equal, Nutra-Sweet, Sweet'n Low*
**Condiments:** *catsup, mustard, mayonnaise, soy sauce, margarine*

**Desserts:** *dark chocolate, desserts containing dark chocolate*
**Beverages:** *diet sodas, regular sodas*

## Scheduling Meals

### Healthy

Nervous System body types can begin and end the day with heavy food intake—but take it easy at lunch. Schedule your meals as follows:

*Breakfast:* 6–8 A.M. Heavy, with protein, nuts, seeds, dairy, legumes, grain, vegetables, and/or fruit.
*Lunch:* 12–2 P.M. Light to moderate, with grain, legumes, dairy, nuts, seeds, raw vegetables, and/or fruit.
*Dinner:* 7–9 P.M. Moderate to heavy, with protein, nuts, seeds, dairy, legumes, cooked or steamed vegetables, and/or grain. Avoid fruit.

### Snacks (optional)
*Midmorning:* fruit, grain, protein, nuts, seeds, dairy, legumes, vegetables
*Midafternoon:* fruit, grain, nuts, seeds, dairy, vegetables, legumes, protein
*Evening:* (8 P.M.–2 A.M.) protein, vegetables, nuts, seeds, grain, legumes, dairy, fruit, sweets

### Sensitive

Adjust your intake as follows:

*Breakfast:* Light, with fruit.
*Lunch:* Heavy, with protein, nuts, seeds, dairy, legumes, grain, steamed vegetables (may also be raw for weight loss), and (occasionally) fruit.
*Dinner:* Moderate, with protein, dairy, legumes, raw vegetables, and (occasionally) nuts and seeds.

## Sample One-Week Menu

DAY 1
*Breakfast:* salmon, rice, and asparagus
*Lunch:* raw carrots, bell peppers, broccoli, and cauliflower w/blue cheese dip
*Snack:* (*bean dip with celery*)
*Dinner:* roast chicken, corn, and yam
*Snack:* (*sunflower seeds*)

DAY 2

*Breakfast:* steak, eggs, and potatoes
*Lunch:* salad of red leaf lettuce, carrots, cucumber, and red onion
*Snack: tomato tortilla with mango salsa*
*Dinner:* lamb and green beans
*Snack: green apple and cheddar cheese*

DAY 3

*Breakfast:* chicken, rice, onions, and green, yellow, and red bell peppers
*Lunch:* tuna, pasta primavera, and peas
*Snack: cashews or pistachios*
*Dinner:* barley lentil soup and spinach salad
*Snack: peach or nectarine*

DAY 4

*Breakfast:* lamb, cauliflower, broccoli, and carrots
*Lunch:* salad of romaine lettuce, feta cheese, cucumbers, avocado, and sunflower and sesame seeds w/Italian dressing
*Snack:* whey or egg protein powder with almond milk
*Dinner:* baked potato w/beef chili and cheese
*Snack:* hummus and cauliflower (raw)

DAY 5: CLEANSE

*Breakfast:* steamed squash or yam and green peas or baked potato
*Lunch:* raw jicama, carrots, bell pepper and/or tomatoes or juice of carrot/parsley, carrot/celery/spinach, (parsley)
*Dinner:* steamed asparagus, cauliflower, broccoli, (onions), squash or cabbage, onion, carrots and broccoli (puréed)

DAY 6

*Breakfast:* omelette w/buffalo or beef, mushrooms, onions, and avocado
*Lunch:* shrimp and/or scallops and rice
*Snack: carrots and/or celery and blue cheese dip*
*Dinner:* eggplant Parmesan, pasta, and red snapper
*Snack: almonds—unsalted*

DAY 7

*Breakfast:* Cornish game hen, acorn squash, and green beans

*Lunch:* salad of spinach, peas, cucumbers, and tomatoes w/lemon juice and oil (*sunflower seeds and/or hard-boiled egg*)
*Snack: protein bar with nuts*
*Dinner:* cod or flounder and broccoli
*Snack: grapes or strawberries*

## Alternative Menus

*(Foods in parentheses are optional.)*

Breakfast

Burrito—refried beans, Monterey Jack cheese, lettuce, and flour tortilla (rice, salsa, avocado)
Lamb, potato, cauliflower, and cheese
Protein powder with almond milk (fruit)
Nectarines, mangos, plums, or green or red grapes
Chicken livers, onions, and beets
Turkey, potato, and peas

Lunch

Calamari or mahimahi, pasta, and green salad
Hamburger or ground turkey, pasta and peas, green beans, cauliflower, or eggplant
Yogurt, cucumber, and raw vegetables
Shark or halibut, brown rice, and zucchini (tomato and/or onions)
Lamb chops and raw vegetables
Hard-boiled egg, tuna, and raw tomato (bread) (lettuce) (seeds)
Beef vegetable soup w/potato

Dinner

Chicken or bean burrito and rice
Almond chicken, rice, and peas
Sea bass, potato, and beets
Shrimp, linguini, and asparagus
Chicken, potato, cauliflower, and broccoli
Lamb chops, asparagus, and rice
Fish, rice, and green beans or broccoli and carrots
Orange roughy, rice, and raw salad

# Pancreas

*The Pancreas body type is symbolized by a champagne glass. Bubbly and joyful, Pancreas types love socializing, especially around food. With their genuine concern for people and their ability to use laughter to burst out of the most uncomfortable situations, they bring joy to their environment.*

FAMOUS PEOPLE: Roseanne Barr, Rosie O'Donnell, Dom DeLuise, John Goodman

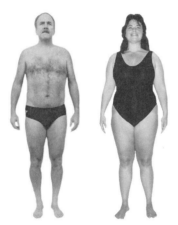

### PANCREAS
### Location and Function

The pancreas is located in the left upper abdomen behind the stomach, next to the spleen and duodenum. It secretes enzymes that aid in the digestion of proteins, carbohydrates, and fats. It also secretes insulin, which helps to control carbohydrate (sugar) metabolism.

## Psychological Profile

### Characteristic Traits

By nature, Pancreas body types are highly sociable, caring, considerate, and compassionate. They tend to maintain a joyous childlike quality that gives them a positive nature, full of laughter and lightness. With their delightful attitude, Pancreas types energetically transmit joy to those around them.

Food is a major issue for Pancreas types and is connected with having fun. Because food is usually present in positive social experiences, it's easy for Pancreas types to become pleasure eaters. Going out to eat is generally the basis of getting together with friends. So when they're alone, Pancreas types tend to be emotional eaters, using food to fill the void when they're feeling stressed, bored, or lonely. While they love to eat, they generally don't like to cook, so they tend to fall into a pattern of eating the same thing for several consecutive days. This stimulates their pancreas but also depletes it. Consequently, it's very easy for them to put on excess weight, particularly when they're not physically active.

Pancreas types like being with people and enjoy bringing delight to their surroundings. Physically expressive, they like to touch, nurture, and help others. They are good at using humor to alleviate stressful circumstances. While the last thing they want to do is offend, they are highly emotional and so enthusiastic that their spirited outbursts sometimes come across as pushy or overbearing.

### Motivation

While Pancreas types are socially oriented and genuinely like people, they often experience problems in their relationships due to limitations in their communication skills. Focused on accomplishing their agenda, they often come across as abrasive. They tend to need to talk a lot, using others as sounding boards to sort through their thoughts and feelings in order to clarify them and get necessary feedback. This is usually stream-of-consciousness speaking. Because of their inability to edit before they speak, they may make a request sound more like an order or demand.

Being extremely zealous and emotionally excitable, they tend to speak about things with such animation and force that they come across as curt, manipulative, abrasive, or controlling. Then they can't understand why others seem upset or angry. Once they learn to communicate effectively, they're very considerate and caring of others.

The childlike trusting nature of Pancreas types often sets them up for a rude awakening when someone they've put their faith in betrays their confidence. Because of their general innocence and lack of discernment, they may have difficulty evaluating the integrity of others, assuming an honesty that's just not there. When they are taken advantage of by those they believe in, they often experience deep hurt and disappointment that can cause them to close down and refuse to trust anyone.

Pancreas types fear scarcity, and this is reflected in the way their body processes food—hanging on to everything, getting the maximum benefit from every morsel. If the body is unable to process something it has taken in, it stores it as fat. This fear of scarcity is also reflected in the way Pancreas types need to have food around and keep their cupboards full and in the way they tend to hold on to things, resisting change and getting locked into patterns (like eating the same food for three or four days). Because food represents security, they often have a tendency to eat until their stomach hurts, especially when they are young. Excess weight is a way of holding on to energy, which represents security.

## "At Worst"

Needy and insecure, Pancreas types may play the victim by living off anyone who will give them a handout or may stay in codependent relationships and get locked into being a caretaker for someone else. In their desire for security in their relationships, they may neglect their own self-care. When they become overly stressed, they often withdraw into sleeping, bury themselves in a project, or go into hiding. Reluctant to make changes, they may set up and perpetuate a failure pattern, particularly when a significant initial effort is unsuccessful. Pancreas types get locked into patterns of behavior that keep them from realizing the fulfillment of their desires. Feeling insecure is the same as feeling powerless.

Pancreas types often have a fear of growing up, which may be associated with a fear of not being able to make it on their own. They have a feeling that too much is expected of them and a fear of not being successful. This is particularly true when their initial attempts to excel or achieve have failed, so further attempts to strike out their own are often delayed due to a fear of repeating the past. Men often get caught in the Peter Pan syndrome of wanting to stay in a safe spot, being taken care of forever. They may stay in codependent relationships until they evolve and learn to accept themselves. The fear of stepping out on their own often keeps them in bad situations too long.

When their insecurity levels are high, Pancreas types generally have no sense of control, so they need to have boundaries and rules, particularly around food. They can easily become emotional eaters, putting on a lot of extra weight, particularly when there is insufficient joy in their lives or a feeling of insecurity. For men, the extra weight is often a way of saying "I'm a big man and I have power." Their excess weight is generally insulation for an inferiority complex due to not fully realizing or implementing what they know to be true. This inferiority complex is often instilled at an early age, and the extra weight further confirms it.

Until Pancreas types feel secure, they don't like gray areas; they prefer to have everything black and white because it minimizes the chance of failure. They feel most comfortable when their jobs consist of tasks that are straightforward or well laid out for them. Projects that are ambiguous or overly complicated stir up feelings of inadequacy and fears of failure, bringing up past memories of personal defeat.

## "At Best"

Meticulous about learning new things, Pancreas types take great pleasure in teaching others what they have learned. Often acquiring knowledge through experience, they can be quite resourceful when it comes to applying their newly discovered information. Enthusiastic and dependable, they work well with others and are good team players. Having a responsible and take-charge attitude, they will conscientiously see a project through from start to finish.

Loyal, steadfast, and dependable, Pancreas types are good at routine or repetitive duties, successfully completing tasks that others may have abandoned as too tedious or humdrum. They generally excel in areas where their work is well defined. When a situation is clear-cut, they can apply new information and reliably complete the job.

Highly sociable, Pancreas types are at their best with others. Nothing gives them greater pleasure than bringing joy to their environment, which makes them extremely popular at social gatherings. Givers by nature, they are genuinely concerned with the welfare of others and are among the most altruistic of the body types.

## Dietary Profile

### Main Focus

- Rotation of foods is essential, ideally every 4 days to reduce pancreatic stress.
- Avoid dense protein for breakfast; minimize it at dinner.
- Make lunch with protein your main meal between 12 and 2 P.M.
- Have an early dinner, between 5 and 7 P.M.
- Limit fruit to breakfast and morning and evening snacks.
- Emphasize protein and vegetables.

### Dietary Emphasis

- From 25 to 35 percent of your calories are to come from fats.
- Best fat sources: olive oil, nuts, seeds, butter, cheese, and dense protein (chicken, turkey, and fish).
- From 20 to 35 percent of your calories are to come from protein.
- From 0 to 25 percent of your calories are to come from dense protein.
- Best sources of the three amino acids threonine, isoleucine, and cystine: sesame seeds and tuna.
- Caloric intake: 1,500 to 1,800 calories a day for women and 1,700 to 2,000 calories a day for men. If you are engaging in intense exercise (competition type) or hard labor, increase calories.
- Drink a minimum of 64 ounces of water a day. Drink water before and after meals, not with meals.
- Occasional desserts are best as an evening snack.
- Eat vegetables (mainly root type).
- Eat complex carbohydrates, like rice, potatoes, beans, and popcorn.
- Eat fruit, such as cherries, papayas, apples, and red grapefruit (with honey).
- Eat protein, particularly from fish and turkey or yogurt and cottage cheese.

### For Weight Loss

- Fat: 15 to 30 percent of daily calories.
- Weight gain will occur if fats fall below 10 percent of calories.
- Dense protein: 15 to 25 percent of daily calories.
- Rotate foods and vary them as much as possible.
- Exercise for at least 1 hour a day, 6 days a week.
- Get ample emotional support.
- Avoid bread, alcohol, caffeine, artificial sweeteners, and carbonated beverages.
- Reduce salt, sugar, and dairy.
- If you must have sweets, save for an evening snack.
- Emphasize low-glycemic foods (e.g., sweet potato is OK but not white potato).
- Pay attention to your body regarding quantity of food; avoid overeating. Stop when satisfied.
- Best to consume 60 percent of total food by 2 P.M. and, ideally, 100 percent by 7 P.M.

### For Weight Gain

- Fat: 25 to 40 percent of daily calories.
- Dense protein: 15 to 25 percent of daily calories.

## Healthy Foods List

There is no need to sacrifice delicious and filling foods to maintain a healthy Pancreas body type. The following lists will help you focus on foods that support your health, and avoid foods that can stress your system.

*You'll notice that some foods are printed in italics; these foods should be avoided when you are in a sensitive state due to any physical or emotional stresses.*

Be sure to read Chapter 3, "Implementing the Body Type Diet," for lots of important information about how to use these many foods to gain their full benefit.

## Ultra-Support Foods

Foods to include in 3 to 7 meals a week, listed by category.

**Dense Protein:** anchovy, *catfish,* cod, halibut, herring, mackerel, perch, red snapper, trout, water-packed tuna; calamari (squid), crab, eel, lobster, octopus, scallops

**Dairy:** *buttermilk,* pineapple kefir, plain yogurt, butter

**Cheese:** feta, Monterey Jack, mozzarella, Muenster, Parmesan, low-fat ricotta, Romano, Swiss

**Nuts and Seeds:** almond milk, water chestnuts; raw or roasted sesame seeds

**Legumes:** beans (garbanzo, Great Northern, pinto)

**Grains:** corn, corn tortillas, corn grits, hominy grits, popcorn, rice (brown or white basmati, Japanese), rice cakes, rye, durum wheat, breads (corn, corn/rye, pumpernickel, rye, sesame pita), rye or sesame crackers, pasta (all varieties), ramen noodles, cream of rice, cream of rye

**Vegetables:** basil, cooked celery, corn, cucumbers, hominy, jicama, snow pea pods, potatoes (red, White Rose), radishes, seaweed (dulse, kelp), squash (acorn, *banana,* butternut), sweet potatoes, *raw tomatoes,* yams

**Fruits:** apricots, cherries, grapefruit (red, white), guavas, papayas, *nectarines,* persimmons, pineapples

**Fruit Juices:** apricot, cranberry, grape (purple, red, white), pineapple

**Vegetable Oil:** olive oil

**Sweeteners:** honey, maple syrup, molasses, sorghum, stevia

**Condiments:** ginger, sea salt w/kelp

**Salad Dressing:** dill

**Beverages:** green tea; Calistoga berry water

## Basic Support Foods

Foods to include in 1 to 2 meals a week.

**Dense Protein:** beef, beef broth, beef liver, buffalo, lamb, veal, venison, organ meats (heart, brain); chicken, chicken broth, chicken livers, Cornish hen, duck, *turkey;* abalone, bass, bonita, flounder, haddock, mahimahi, orange roughy, salmon, sardines, *thresher shark,* sole, swordfish, tuna (ahi, yellowtail); clams, imitation crab, mussels, oysters, shrimp; eggs

**Dairy:** milk (whole, low fat, raw, *goat's*), half-and-half, sweet cream, *sour cream, kefir* (plain, peach, or strawberry), fruit-flavored yogurt, *ice cream* (Dreyer's, Swensen's), Ice Bean

**Cheese:** American, blue, Brie, Camembert, cheddar, Colby, low-fat or regular cottage, cream, Edam, Gouda, goat, kefir, Limburger, regular ricotta; all yellow cheeses

**Nuts and Seeds:** *almonds, almond butter,* Brazils, *cashews (raw or roasted),* cashew butter, cashew milk, coconut, hazelnuts, macadamias, macadamia butter, *peanuts,* peanut butter, pecans, pine nuts, pistachios, black or English walnuts; seeds (caraway, poppy, pumpkin, *sunflower*), sesame butter, *sunflower seed butter*

**Legumes:** beans (adzuki, black, kidney, lima, red, soy), lentils, black-eyed peas, split peas; hummus; miso, soy milk, tofu

**Grains:** amaranth, barley, buckwheat, couscous, millet, oats, quinoa, *rice (short or long grain brown, wild),* rice bran, triticale, refined wheat flour, wheat bran, wheat germ, sprouted wheat, flour tortillas, breads (French, Italian, oat, pita [plain, rye, or whole wheat], potato, sourdough, white), egg bagels, croissants, English muffins, *crackers (oat, saltine),* macaroni, udon noodles, cream of wheat

**Vegetables:** artichokes, *arugula,* asparagus, avocados, bamboo shoots, beans (green, yellow wax), beets, bok choy, broccoflower, broccoli, brussels sprouts, raw cabbage (green, napa, red), carrots, cauliflower, raw celery, cilantro, eggplant, garlic, greens (beet, collard, mustard, turnip), kale, kohlrabi, leeks, lettuce (Boston, butter, endive, *iceberg,* red leaf, romaine), mushrooms, okra, olives (*green, ripe*), onions (chives, brown, green, red, Vidalia, white), parsley, parsnips, peas, bell peppers (green, red, yellow), chili peppers, pimientos, potatoes (*russet,* Yukon Gold), pumpkin, daikon radishes, rutabaga, sauerkraut, seaweed (arame, nori, wakame), shallots, spinach, sprouts (alfalfa, clover, mung bean, radish, sunflower), squash (spaghetti, yellow [summer], zucchini), Swiss chard, cooked tomatoes, turnips, *watercress*

**Vegetable Juices:** carrot, carrot/celery, celery, parsley, spinach, tomato, V-8

**Fruits:** apples (Red and Golden Delicious, Granny Smith, Jonathan, McIntosh, Pippin, Rome Beauty), bananas, berries (blackberries, blueberries, boysen-berries, cranberries, gooseberries, raspberries, strawberries), frozen cherries, dates, figs, grapes (green, black, red), kiwi, kumquats, lemons, limes, loquats, mangoes, melons (cantaloupe, honeydew, watermelon), oranges, peaches, pears, plums (black, purple, red), pomegranates, prunes, raisins, rhubarb, *tangelos,* tangerines

**Fruit Juices:** apple, apple cider, apple/apricot, black cherry, cherry, cranapple, grapefruit, guava, lemon, orange, papaya, pear, pineapple/coconut, prune, tangerine

**Vegetable Oils:** *all-blend, almond, avocado, canola, corn, flaxseed, peanut, safflower, sesame, soy, sun-flower*

**Sweeteners:** sugar (date, *raw,* refined cane), syrup (barley malt, brown rice, corn), succonant

**Condiments:** *Dijon mustard, eggless mayonnaise, horseradish, barbecue sauce, pesto sauce, soy sauce,* salsa, tahini, *soy margarine,* vinegar, *Morton salt substitute,* sea salt

**Salad Dressings:** Marie's blue cheese, Hain avocado, Hain creamy Italian, French, *ranch,* Thousand Island

**Desserts:** *custards, tapioca, puddings, chocolate, desserts containing chocolate, sherbet (orange, rasp-berry)*

**Chips:** *bean,* corn (*blue, white, yellow*)

**Beverages:** tea (*black, herbal [mint, raspberry], Chinese oolong*); *mineral water, sparkling water;* wine (red, white), *beer, barley malt liquor, cham-pagne, gin, liqueurs, scotch, vodka, whiskey; regular sodas*

## Stressful Foods

Have no more than once a month.

**Dense Protein:** *pork, ham, sausage, bacon*
**Dairy:** *nonfat frozen yogurt, most ice creams*
**Grains:** *polished rice, whole wheat, cracked wheat, breads (multigrain, seven-grain, whole wheat), whole wheat crackers, whole wheat pasta*
**Fruits:** *casaba or Crenshaw melons*
**Sweeteners:** *fructose, brown sugar, saccharin, aspar-tame, Equal, NutraSweet, Sweet'n Low*
**Condiments:** *catsup, yellow mustard, mayonnaise, margarine*
**Beverages:** *coffee; Japanese tea; root beer, Pepsi, diet sodas*

## Scheduling Meals
### Healthy

Pancreas body types do not have to limit themselves to light meals. Schedule your meals as follows:

*Breakfast:* 8–9 A.M. Moderate, with grain, legumes, nuts, seeds, dairy, eggs, vegetables, and/or fruit. Avoid dense protein.
*Lunch:* 12–2 P.M. Heavy, with protein, legumes, nuts, seeds, dairy, vegetables, and/or grain. Avoid fruit.
*Dinner:* 5–7 P.M. Moderate, early, with vegetables, pro-tein, legumes, nuts, seeds, dairy, and/or grain. Avoid fruit.

### Snacks (optional)
*Midmorning:* grain, vegetables, nuts, seeds, protein, fruit
*Midafternoon:* (4 P.M.) grain, vegetables (no fruit for weight loss)
*Evening:* (9 P.M.–2 A.M.) sweets, fruit, vegetables, nuts, seeds, grain, protein, dairy

### Sensitive

*Breakfast:* Avoid fruit.
*Dinner:* Avoid dense protein.

## Sample One-Week Menu

DAY 1
*Breakfast:* banana and cottage cheese
*Lunch:* roast chicken and green beans
*Dinner:* garlic shrimp w/pasta

DAY 2
*Breakfast:* papaya or red grapefruit
*Lunch:* cod, sea bass, or sole, carrots, and broccoli
*Dinner:* Caesar salad

DAY 3
*Breakfast:* halibut
*Lunch:* roast turkey and a cucumber salad
*Dinner:* tuna (fillet, canned, or Japanese sashimi) and cucumber

DAY 4
*Breakfast:* oatmeal w/sesame seeds
*Lunch:* beef or vegetarian chili, avocado, and corn bread
*Dinner:* pasta w/steamed zucchini and pesto sauce

DAY 5: CLEANSE
*Breakfast:* watermelon or cantaloupe
*Lunch:* steamed cauliflower and/or squash and/or raw bell peppers, butter lettuce, carrots, celery and/or carrot/spinach juice
*Dinner:* steamed asparagus, broccoli, and/or squash and/or raw carrots, jicama and/or juice of carrot, carrot/celery

DAY 6
*Breakfast:* banana
*Lunch:* Cornish game hen, mashed rutabaga, and carrots
*Dinner:* Thai coconut milk soup or vegetable potato soup and a tossed green salad

DAY 7
*Breakfast:* yam and peas
*Lunch:* scallops, sea bass, or sole, white basmati rice or rice pilaf, and snow peas
*Dinner:* corn tortilla w/refried beans and salsa

## Alternative Menus

*(Foods in parentheses may be omitted.)*

### Breakfast
Green peas and white basmati rice
Corn grits or white basmati rice (w/small amount of butter)
Cream of wheat and pink grapefruit
Eggs and mushrooms
Hummus and carrots
Pasta w/olive oil, zucchini, broccoli, and mushrooms
Baked acorn or butternut squash (w/butter)
Papaya filled w/pineapple chunks
Banana or mango and sunflower seeds
Sausage patty

### Lunch
Chicken fajita, basmati rice, and steamed broccoli, cauliflower, and carrots
Baked chicken w/Thai peanut sauce and vegetables
Turkey sausage, brown rice, and green beans
Steak w/steak sauce and broccoli or green beans or salad of butter lettuce, celery, cucumbers, radishes with dill salad dressing
Pork chops and salad as above
Fish, rice, corn, and green beans or peas
Tuna, tomatoes, and pickle
Bean burrito (w/salsa)
Rice bowl of chicken, broccoli, carrots, onions, with soy sauce and ginger
Cobb salad w/eggs

### Dinner
Noodles w/broccoli, carrots, peas, and onions
White basmati rice, butternut squash, and carrots or peas
Pinto beans, white basmati rice, and corn bread or corn tortilla
Baked falafel, hummus, and tomato
Steamed potatoes, mushrooms, onions, and carrots
Grilled chicken, peas, and yams
Chicken and tomato
Sushi (peas)
Turkey or turkey ham and grits w/butter and black pepper
Tuna, spinach, and red onion
Feta cheese, cucumber, carrots, black olives, hummus, and jicama w/olive oil

# Pineal

*The Pineal body type is symbolized by the sun. Representing the intuition, the sun supplies light and awareness. Sunlight positively affects the emotional state of Pineal types, more so than any other body type.*

FAMOUS PEOPLE: Ron Howard, Barbara DeAngelis, Ph.D., Louise Hay

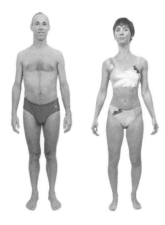

## PINEAL
### Location and Function

The pineal body (also called the pineal gland) is located in the center of the brain, above the brain stem and behind the thalamus. It synthesizes and releases melatonin, whose secretion is activated by sunlight. It is the key regulating factor in PMS irritability and mood swings.

## Psychological Profile

### Characteristic Traits

With their quick wit, strong active minds, and gift of verbal expression, Pineal body types often have trouble balancing their mental acuity with their intuition. Some shut down their intuition, ignore their insights, and try to live their lives from a purely mental perspective. While they may get by with it for a short time, closing down a part of themselves leads to problems, because self-realization is essential to their well-being.

The pineal gland is the body's "receiver" for intuition. Pineal types sense the emotional states of others. They may even absorb these emotions without realizing that the feelings are not their own. Natural givers, they have a strong tendency to be caretakers. In their desire to maintain a pleasant environment, they tend to blend in with the habits and patterns of those around them. They are highly sensitive to their environment, and beauty and nature are frequently essential to their attaining a quiet, peaceful state.

Having an abundance of valuable ideas, Pineal types often don't record or even remember them, and unless they can be communicated to someone else, the fruits of their imagination are lost forever. The challenge is to sort through them and translate their essence into practical terms. Pineal types frequently experience difficulty communicating ideas; consequently they tend to have a feeling of being different and misunderstood.

### Motivation

Personal intimacy is usually a challenge for Pineal types because their intellect tends to take precedence over their feelings, and this keeps them separated and alone. While they may be loved by many and have many friends, they find that true intimacy in a relationship can be elusive. Emotional issues are generally a challenge, as Pineal types often deny their feelings to avoid feeling weak or stupid. They then tend to emphasize their mental abilities and to overwork, particularly when they don't trust others to know as much as they do, and feel they need to handle everything. Sometimes, lacking a pragmatic approach to life, they may swing to the opposite extreme of doing nothing.

While they expect a lot from others, they expect superior abilities from themselves and are constantly striving to do greater and greater things in life.

Creative, expressive, and compassionate, they often have difficulty dealing with the harshness and practicalities of the physical world. They are independent thinkers and, except for directing and counseling others, like to work alone so they can focus on the task and let their intuition guide them.

Because Pineal types readily perceive things that are not apparent to others, they become impatient when others don't acknowledge or respond to their reality. They often have the ability to receive from other realms, and very few humans measure up to their standards, so they generally find it difficult to take orders or submit to others' leadership. If they're unhappy working within a conventional, hierarchical structure, they may (usually unconsciously) act to sabotage the system that stifles them. They prefer to plan, oversee, or supervise a project rather than do the work themselves. Their expertise often exists only in theory, and their lack of practical experience and know-how can sometimes cause problems.

## "At Worst"

Pineal types tend to be nervous and high-strung and can get so caught up in thinking about what they want to accomplish that they have a hard time getting started on a project. They can become trapped in their mental processes and fail to get things done, spending their time setting up rules and policies. With their strong mental focus, they can be very intense, staying with a subject until it's exhausted, sometimes getting caught in a mental loop or spacing out. Generally more dreamers than realists, they often have difficulty bringing their ideas to practical reality and can be very critical of themselves and others when things aren't accomplished according to their time frame. Some Pineal types take the opposite approach and become too impulsive and impatient, jumping in before they know what they are getting into.

Feeling superior, Pineal types like to be in control and think they have all the answers. Their tendency is to try to teach without recognizing when it's time to listen or be a student. Their feelings of superiority often coexist with feelings of inferiority, and they may try to avoid feeling weak or incompetent through denial. Insecure, they are easily triggered and readily jump to conclusions. Sensitive to subtle humor, they sometimes hear sarcasm where it was not intended. Though generally accommodating and considerate, they become assertive when they feel they are being belittled.

When stressed, Pineal types become highly emotional, hyperactive, and scattered, which can lead to an aggressive emotional reaction. Their lack of focus and clarity tends to be expressed as verbosity and abstractions. Emotionally insecure females often acquiesce to males. Another tendency is to panic, space out, or shift into fantasy and spend long periods of time staring off into space.

Impulsive behavior is often the underlying cause of their financial problems. Because beauty supplies a means of connecting with their spiritual center, Pineal types tend to look for beautiful things to enhance their environment. When their desire for beauty is coupled with impulsive behavior, they go on frivolous shopping sprees to lift their spirits.

## "At Best"

Being open-minded, quick, and bright, Pineal types are usually on the leading edge of new thought. With their intuitive awareness and clear mental focus, they are able to see how life's challenges allow them to find their own depth and understand life more fully. Acutely aware of the important role the mind and emotional states play in determining a person's reality, Pineal types are particularly effective counseling others. Combining their experience, intuitive awareness, and intense interest in people, they can successfully communicate their insights to others and become innovators in their chosen fields.

The Pineal types' greatest strength lies in their personal quest to reach self-realization and experience ultimate freedom. Inquisitive, free-thinking, and creative, they are idealists with high personal standards of excellence. Once they learn to connect their thoughts with their feelings, their intuition is free to come through, enabling them to express themselves from a centered place. From here they can connect with the physical world and translate their thoughts into practical terms. At this point, expressing their truth and sharing with others in a calm, relaxed manner is easy.

The Pineal types' greatest gift is their deep, intuitive universal connection. This allows them to access information from other dimensions, such as the collective unconscious or higher realms. They are then able to express these universal truths and bring this creative energy into physical form or practical manifestation. Listening to their intuition offers Pineal types a unique sense of freedom. While they still maintain and use their strong ability to analyze and understand deep or abstract concepts, it isn't necessary for them to have all possible information on a subject because they can act or respond according to their internal messages.

## Dietary Profile

### Main Focus

- Eat majority of protein at lunch between 11:30 A.M. and 2 P.M., although fish may be included at dinner, especially if protein deficient.
- Frequent small meals are often better than large; may include snacks.
- Rotation is important—no more than 2 consecutive days per food.

### Dietary Emphasis

- From 20 to 35 percent of your calories are to come from fats.
- Best fat sources: olive oil, nuts (roasted cashews, hazelnuts), seeds (sunflower and pumpkin), dense protein (fish, eggs, chicken, turkey), and cheese.
- From 25 to 40 percent of your calories are to come from protein.
- From 10 to 40 percent of your calories are to come from dense protein.
- Best sources of the three amino acids threonine, isoleucine, and cystine: tuna, sesame seeds, chicken, and salmon.
- Caloric Intake: 1,500 to 1,800 calories a day for women and 1,700 to 2,000 calories a day for men. If you are engaging in intense exercise (competition type) or heavy labor, increase calories.
- Drink a minimum of 64 ounces of water a day. Drink water before and after meals, not with meals.
- Occasional desserts are best as an evening snack.
- Breakfast is important.

- May have up to 3 eggs at each of 3 meals a week.
- May have potatoes every day, but limit each variety to 2 meals a week.
- Avoid eating potato or squash with dense protein.
- Avoid fruit for dinner.
- Eat most vegetables steamed or cooked. May have difficulty digesting raw vegetables, which are best eaten at lunch.
- Eat vegetables, particularly carrots and butter or red leaf lettuce, fresh fruits, fish, especially salmon, chicken, soups, and pasta with light sauce.
- Protein deficiencies are common when under prolonged stress.
- Make lunch the largest meal; emphasize protein.
- For dinner, minimize protein but may include fish.
- Sunlight is essential.

### For Weight Loss

- Dense protein: 20 to 35 percent of daily calories.
- May include snacks.
- Consume majority of food before 2 P.M.

### For Weight Gain

- Dense protein: 25 to 40 percent of daily calories.
- Fat: 25 to 40 percent of daily calories.
- Consume dense protein before 2 P.M.
- May experience weight loss from insufficient protein.

### Sensitive

- Increase protein at breakfast and lunch.
- Eliminate fruit at lunch.

## Healthy Foods List

There is no need to sacrifice delicious and filling foods to maintain a healthy Pineal body type. The following lists will help you focus on foods that support your health, and avoid foods that can stress your system.

*You'll notice that some foods are printed in italics; these foods should be avoided when you are in a sensitive state due to any physical or emotional stresses.*

Be sure to read Chapter 3, "Implementing the Body Type Diet," for lots of important information about how to use these many foods to gain their full benefit.

## Ultra-Support Foods

Foods to include in 3 to 7 meals a week, listed by category.

**Dense Protein:** *beef;* chicken (white), chicken broth, Cornish game hen; cod, halibut, mahimahi, orange roughy, salmon, *sardines, shark,* red snapper, *swordfish, trout,* tuna; *calamari (squid), clams, eel, lobster, scallops, shrimp*

**Dairy:** *half-and-half,* sweet cream, sour cream, butter

**Nuts and Seeds:** cashews, cashew butter, *coconut,* seeds (caraway, pumpkin, sesame, raw sunflower)

**Legumes:** beans (adzuki, garbanzo), *split peas;* hummus

**Grains:** barley, oats, oat bran, quinoa, white or brown basmati rice, rye, *flour tortillas,* breads (corn, corn/rye), pasta

**Vegetables:** *artichokes,* asparagus, yellow wax beans, beets, *red cabbage,* capers, carrots, *celery,* cilantro, *corn, cucumbers,* garlic, *beet greens,* jicama, *lettuce (butter, red leaf, romaine),* green onions, peas, bell peppers (green, red, yellow), radishes (daikon, red, white), rutabaga, *seaweed (arame, dulse, kelp, nori, wakame),* alfalfa sprouts, squash (acorn, banana, butternut, spaghetti, yellow [summer], *zucchini*), Swiss chard, taro root, yams

**Fruits:** *bananas,* berries (blueberries, raspberries), *lemons,* melons *(cantaloupe, honeydew, watermelon)*

**Sweeteners:** *honey, date sugar, brown rice syrup,* stevia

**Condiments:** basil, vanilla

**Beverages:** Good Earth tea, decaffeinated tea

## Basic Support Foods

Foods to include in 1 to 2 meals a week.

**Dense Protein:** beef broth, beef liver, buffalo, *ham, lamb,* veal, venison, organ meats (heart, brain); chicken (dark), chicken livers, duck, turkey; anchovy, bass, bonita, catfish, flounder, haddock, herring, mackerel, perch, sole, tuna (light chunk, yellowtail); abalone, *crab, mussels, octopus, oysters;* eggs

**Dairy:** milk *(whole, 2%, low fat,* nonfat, *raw goat's), buttermilk,* kefir, yogurt (low-fat or nonfat, plain, flavored), *frozen yogurt, ice cream* (Ben & Jerry's, Dreyer's, Swensen's)

**Cheese:** American, *blue,* Brie, Camembert, cheddar, Colby, cottage, cream, Edam, feta, *goat,* Gouda, kefir, Limburger, Monterey Jack, mozzarella, *Muenster, Parmesan,* ricotta, Romano, *Swiss*

**Nuts and Seeds:** Brazils, hazelnuts, macadamias (raw, roasted), macadamia butter, pecans, *pistachios, walnuts (black, English),* water chestnuts; flaxseed, sesame seed butter, sunflower seed butter

**Legumes:** beans (black, Great Northern, *kidney,* lima, pinto, red), lentils, black-eyed peas; miso, soy milk, *tofu*

**Grains:** *amaranth,* corn, blue corn, corn grits, corn tortillas, couscous, hominy grits, *millet,* popcorn, rice *(brown* or white long or short grain, Japanese, *wild),* rice cakes, *popcorn rice cakes,* rice bran, *whole wheat, wheat bran,* wheat germ, refined wheat flour, breads (French, garlic, Italian, *oat,* pita, raisin-nut, *rice, rye,* sourdough, *sprouted grain,* white, whole wheat), bagels, croissants, English muffins, crackers (oat, rye, saltines, *wheat thins*), udon noodles, Chinese rice noodles, cream of rice, cream of rye, cream of wheat

**Vegetables:** *arugula, avocados,* bamboo shoots, green beans, bok choy, broccoflower, broccoli, brussels sprouts, *cabbage (green, napa),* cauliflower, eggplant, greens (collard, mustard, turnip) kale, kohlrabi, leeks, *lettuce (Boston, endive),* mushrooms, okra, olives (green, ripe), onions (chives, brown, red, Vidalia, white, yellow), parsley, parsnips, snow peas, chili peppers, pimientos, potatoes *(red, russet,* White Rose, Yukon Gold), pumpkin, sauerkraut, shallots, spinach, sprouts (clover, mung bean, radish, sunflower), sweet potatoes, tomatoes, turnips, *watercress*

**Vegetable Juices:** carrot, carrot/celery, celery, parsley, spinach, tomato, V-8

**Fruits:** *apples (all varieties),* apricots (fresh or canned), berries (blackberries, *boysenberries,* cranberries, gooseberries, *strawberries), cherries,* fresh figs, black grapes, grapefruit, guavas, kiwi, kumquats, loquats, mangoes, melons (casaba, Crenshaw), nectarines, oranges, papayas, peaches, *pears,* persimmons, canned pineapples, *plums (black, red, purple),* rhubarb, tangelos, *tangerines*

**Fruit Juices:** *apple, apple cider,* apple/apricot, apricot, *black cherry, red cherry, cranapple, cranberry, cranberry concentrate,* grape (purple, red, white), guava, *lemon, orange, pear,* pineapple/coconut, *tangerine,* watermelon

**Vegetable Oils:** *all-blend, almond, avocado, cashew, coconut, corn, flaxseed,* olive, *peanut, safflower, sesame, soy, sunflower*

**Sweeteners:** *fructose,* sugar *(brown, raw, refined cane),* syrup *(barley malt, corn, maple), succonant*

**Condiments:** *mustard, mayonnaise, barbecue sauce, pesto sauce,* soy sauce, *brewer's yeast, tahini, vinegar, carob, Spike,* Veg-It, sea salt, Vege-Sal, Braggs Liquid Aminos, cinnamon

**Salad Dressings:** *blue cheese, French, ranch, creamy Italian, creamy avocado, Thousand Island,* vinegar and oil, lemon juice and oil

**Desserts:** *custards, tapioca, puddings, pies, cakes, sherbet (orange, raspberry)*

**Chips:** bean, corn (blue, white, yellow), potato

**Beverages:** tea *(black, green,* herbal *[peppermint],* Japanese, Chinese oolong); mineral water, sparkling water; *wine (red, white), sake, beer, barley malt liquor, champagne, gin, scotch, vodka, whiskey;* root beer, regular sodas

## Stressful Foods

Have no more than once a month.

**Dense Protein:** *pork, bacon, sausage*
**Dairy:** *most ice creams*
**Nuts and Seeds:** *almonds, almond butter, peanuts, peanut butter, pine nuts; roasted sunflower seeds*
**Legumes:** *navy beans, soybeans*
**Grains:** *buckwheat, multigrains, triticale, breads (multigrain, seven-grain), stoneground wheat crackers, seven-grain cereal*
**Fruits:** *red or green grapes, limes, pomegranates; dried apples, apricots, dates, Black Mission figs, pineapples, prunes, raisins*
**Fruit Juices:** *grapefruit, papaya, pineapple, prune*
**Vegetable Oil:** *canola*
**Sweeteners:** *molasses, sorghum, saccharin, aspartame, Equal, NutraSweet, Sweet'n Low*
**Condiments:** *catsup, horseradish, margarine, salt*

**Desserts:** *chocolate, desserts containing chocolate*
**Beverages:** *coffee; diet sodas*

## Scheduling Meals

### Healthy

Pineal body types should avoid heavy meals at the start and end of the day. Schedule your meals as follows:

*Breakfast:* 7–8 A.M. Moderate, with grain, dairy, nuts, seeds, vegetables, fruit, and/or protein.
*Lunch:* 11:30 A.M.–2 P.M. Moderate to heavy, with protein, dairy, nuts, seeds, grains, vegetables, legumes, and/or limited fruit. Need starch/grain with salad. Emphasize dense protein.
*Dinner:* 5–7 P.M. Light to moderate, early, with grain, vegetables, nuts, seeds, legumes, and/or dairy. Avoid fruit and protein.

#### Snacks (optional)
*Midmorning:* (10 A.M.) fruit, nuts, seeds, dairy, grain, or vegetables
*Midafternoon:* (3–4 P.M.) fruit, nuts, seeds, dairy, grain, or vegetables
*Evening:* (9 P.M.–2 A.M., at least 1 hour after dinner) sweets, grain, legumes, vegetables, protein, nuts, seeds, dairy, fruit

### Sensitive

Adjust your intake as follows:

*Breakfast:* Moderate, with protein, grain, vegetables, and/or fruit.
*Lunch:* Moderate to heavy, with protein, grain, and/or vegetables. Avoid fruit.
*Dinner:* Light to moderate, early, with grain, legumes or light protein, and/or vegetables.

## Sample One-Week Menu

DAY 1
*Breakfast:* corn grits w/butter
*Snack:* pistachios or raw sunflower seeds
*Lunch:* tuna, rice, and squash or green beans
*Snack:* celery w/cashew butter
*Dinner:* baked potato w/butter and chicken rice soup
*Snack:* yogurt

DAY 2

*Breakfast:* egg and kefir cheese omelet
*Snack:* blueberries and/or raspberries
*Lunch:* turkey, broccoli, carrots, and cauliflower
*Snack:* celery w/macadamia and cashew butter
*Dinner:* clam linguini

DAY 3

*Breakfast:* cream of rice w/butter and pecans
*Lunch:* salmon and yellow squash
*Dinner:* black beans, rice, and peas
*Snack:* avocado w/lemon and garlic on rice cakes

DAY 4

*Breakfast:* scrambled eggs w/onions
*Snack:* orange
*Lunch:* roasted chicken, couscous, and a salad of red leaf lettuce, broccoli, cauliflower, and raw sunflower seeds w/lemon juice
*Snack:* pecans
*Dinner:* red snapper, halibut, or tuna, and lettuce salad w/sesame seeds

DAY 5: CLEANSE

*Breakfast:* watermelon including seeds and white part of rind or papaya
*Lunch:* steamed globe artichoke, asparagus, beet, beet greens, zucchini, and/or raw cucumbers, jicama, and/or carrots
*Dinner:* steamed broccoli, cauliflower, carrots, onions, and/or squash and/or raw cucumbers, carrots, jicama, red or romaine lettuce, green peas and/or juice of carrot/celery (spinach)

DAY 6

*Breakfast:* cooked muesli w/rice milk and banana
*Snack:* carrots
*Lunch:* taco salad of shredded beef, romaine lettuce, tomatoes, cheddar cheese w/creamy avocado dressing
*Snack:* hazelnuts
*Dinner:* sushi and California roll (miso soup)

DAY 7

*Breakfast:* corn tortilla w/avocado and kefir cheese
*Snack:* banana
*Lunch:* Cornish game hen, wild rice, mushrooms, and onion and spinach salad
*Dinner:* stir-fried vegetables—peas, onions, peppers, bean sprouts, mushrooms, and bamboo shoots

## Alternative Menus

*(Foods in parentheses may be omitted.)*

### Breakfast

Cream of rice w/banana or cashews and sunflower or sesame butter
Fish, barley, and bok choy
Adzuki beans and avocado
Rice and black beans (eggs)
Rice, whey protein powder, and snow peas
Salmon, basmati rice, and broccoli
Millet and chicken broth
Yogurt w/cashews

### Lunch

Chicken, hard-boiled eggs, and a salad of spinach, carrots, celery, and raw sunflower seeds w/lemon juice
Turkey burrito, beans, rice, and salad of butter lettuce, red bell pepper w/ranch dressing
Chicken, beef, or bean burrito
Turkey and asparagus
Cashew chicken w/celery, bamboo shoots, and snow peas over rice
Teriyaki chicken or beef, bowl of white rice, broccoli, carrots, and snow pea pods
Chicken, broccoli, and cauliflower w/sesame tahini

### Dinner

Chicken vegetable soup
Lentil soup w/carrots and onions
Mushroom barley soup (sprouted wheat flour tortilla)
Artichokes w/butter and/or kefir cheese
Basmati rice and peas
Butternut squash (basmati rice)
Okra and rice or spelt
Salmon and basmati rice

# Pituitary

*The Pituitary body type is symbolized by a birthday cake. Happy and light, Pituitary types approach life with a childlike openness and wide-eyed innocence. Capable and responsible, they are stimulated by new ideas and concepts.*

FAMOUS PEOPLE: Sai Baba, John Gray, Lainie Kazan, Aretha Franklin

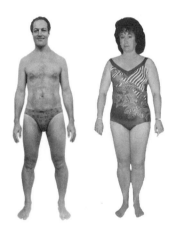

## PITUITARY
### Location and Function

The pituitary gland is located in the center of the forehead, half an inch above the eyebrows and two to three inches into the head. The pituitary gland governs the endocrine system, as directed by the hypothalamus; the anterior lobe secretes hormones regulating the function of the thyroid, gonads, and adrenal cortex (and is consequently of vital importance to growth, maturation, and reproduction); the posterior lobe regulates the kidneys through an antidiuretic hormone and activates cholesterol production to increase hormone levels.

## Psychological Profile

### Characteristic Traits

Pituitary body types are characterized by a childlike openness, curiosity, and creativity. Their bodies tend to have a soft, childlike look—a large head with a soft cushion of fat over the body, predominantly on the abdomen. Just as a baby learns more in the first six months than at any other time during its life, the Pituitary type exemplifies a grown-up version of that amazing mental acuity, curiosity, and stimulation, as well as exhibiting a young child's basic joy and love of life. Pituitary types can and must constantly learn and be stimulated by fresh new ideas and concepts to bring more joy and happiness into their environment and the world in general.

Their basic nature is kind, considerate, and compassionate. They easily connect with people and enjoy them. With good verbal skills, they readily communicate their thoughts and feelings. Sensitive to the feelings of others, they are extremely tactful and diplomatic, excelling at "people skills."

Pituitary types tend to take things in stride. They are not likely to get upset about circumstances beyond their control. Even in a tense situation they assume a philosophical detachment rather than reacting with anger or frustration. They are able to accept things as they are without feeling a strong need to manipulate or change them. Although analytical, they are rarely judgmental or critical of others and can see both sides of most situations.

Pituitary types have a high degree of mental acuity and clarity, which they balance through trusting their intuition. They are logical, analytical, and systematic, with a natural aptitude for computers as well as for the mental programming of the mind. There is a flexibility to their intellectual precision. Their soft, gentle exterior and cheerfulness often conceal a resilience and inner strength that generally only become apparent over time.

Most of the Pituitary types' energy is in their head, which is apparent by its physical size and their intellect. Balancing it requires moving energy down into the body through physical expression, including weight management. Physical exercise is a definite challenge for Pituitary types and requires much personal discipline.

### Motivation

External stimulation provides the motivation for Pituitary types to grow and change. Imaginative, with good reasoning abilities, they're stimulated by learning new things and have an excellent aptitude for mastering concepts and ideas. While mentally precise and adept at handling abstract details, they bring a lightness into learning by approaching it with childlike openness, curiosity, and creativity. Feeling happy gives them their greatest sense of satisfaction.

The Pituitary type's respect of others and of life in general is reflected in their altruistic attitude of helpfulness and harmony. Generous and giving, they often take on more than they can realistically handle and tend to spread themselves too thin until they learn to set appropriate limits. By being sociable and receptive, they foster an attitude of cooperation and agreement, making them quite successful at getting others to do what they want.

Dependable and reliable, Pituitary types keep their promises and do what they say they will to the best of their ability. They stay with a problem or project until they have successfully completed it. This persistence also applies to people and situations. They are very forgiving in relationships until they reach the point where they are finished. Once they have learned what they need to learn and feel complete with a relationship, it's over. Mentally focused and internally motivated, they are good at setting goals for themselves and then doing whatever is necessary to reach them.

Conflict makes Pituitary types feel vulnerable or uneasy, so they delay discussing things that may provoke others. Instead they are inclined to smooth things over to postpone confrontation. Even when they know that an unresolved conflict must eventually be faced, they still let a problem build up until it explodes or until they are otherwise forced to deal with it.

## "At Worst"

When their mental aspect becomes unbalanced, the power of the Pituitary types' determination can take on a headstrong or obstinate quality. Fear can make them domineering and controlling. They may develop a skeptical attitude or swing to the opposite extreme, of becoming weak or wishy-washy. In their desire to help or protect, they can become so focused on what they feel is right that they become picky and overly concerned with details.

Procrastination is common when Pituitary types have to make a decision or tackle something about which they are ambivalent. They tend to avoid doing things they perceive as unpleasant or difficult. Instead they'll

go for something fun such as eating creamy foods like ice cream, which stimulate the pituitary gland.

Feeling vulnerable or uneasy, Pituitary types suppress their emotions. Highly developed mentally, they have a tendency to live in their heads and escape into a world of make-believe, books, movies, television, or the computer. They may also use sleep, meditation, drugs, or alcohol as forms of escape. Needing to experience the physical world but often lacking stamina, Pituitary types are apt to experiment with recreational drugs. When they lack social skills, sexual addictions or fantasies are common. Food can also be a source of comfort, and there is a strong tendency toward obesity.

With low self-esteem, they can become trapped in addictive, codependent, or physically abusive relationships that keep them stifled. They can lose touch with reality and become irresponsible or self-centered, doing only what makes them feel happy in the moment. To support a habit, they may use their innocence to play on other people's sympathies. They can resort to lying, making promises they have no intention of keeping, or being a fair-weather friend.

## "At Best"

Pituitary types are happy and bring happiness to everyone they encounter. Their whole orientation to life is characterized by childlike openness, curiosity, and creativity. People love infants because of their connection with the spirit, and Pituitaries are able to retain this connection, bringing happiness into the adult world.

Maintaining a connection with their spiritual nature enables Pituitary types to express their divinity in the physical realm through their mind and body. They know they have the power to change and can accomplish whatever they desire, even though it may be difficult. They also know that others can achieve the same goals, and are able to communicate this awareness effectively.

Pituitary types have a positive attitude toward themselves and life in general, enabling them to bounce back from adversity. Displaying a basic joy and love of life, they are outgoing and gregarious, relaxed and easygoing. They balance their mental development with practical knowledge or common sense through physical activity and play. Relying on their intuition when dealing with unfamiliar information allows them to make the right decisions without lengthy deliberation.

Open to new concepts and ideas, Pituitary types possess a gentle quality, a freshness, and a receptivity, yet they are also prudent and practical. Reliable and dependable, with a good aptitude for detail and great integrity, they accomplish what they commit to do. They are self-motivated by their strong sense of wonder and curiosity. Finding new and challenging aspects of a situation, project, or relationship, they are able to fulfill their mission of bringing happiness to the world.

## Dietary Profile

### Main Focus

- Be happy.
- Get adequate protein at breakfast and lunch.
- Have a moderate to heavy breakfast and lunch, with the majority of calories by 2 P.M.
- Have a light early dinner without protein or grain.
- Minimize dairy; include cheese only up to 2 times a week.

### Dietary Emphasis

- From 20 to 30 percent of your calories are to come from fats.
- Best fat sources: dense protein (all), butter, coconut milk, and coconut.
- From 25 to 40 percent of your calories are to come from protein.
- From 0 to 30 percent of your calories are to come from dense protein.
- Best sources of the three amino acids threonine, isoleucine, and cystine: lean beef, chicken, and clams.
- Caloric intake: 1,500 to 1,800 calories a day for women and 1,700 to 2,000 calories a day for men. If you are engaging in intense exercise (competition type) or hard labor, increase calories.
- Drink a minimum of 64 ounces of water a day. Drink water before and after meals, not with meals.

- Get adequate protein—either from concentrated plant sources such as red algae and bee pollen or from animal protein prepared with as little fat as possible (beef, organ meat, chicken, fish).
- Include variety and rotate menus, particularly at breakfast.
- Eat red meat and/or exercise to stimulate adrenals.
- May include nuts 5 times a week.
- Eat carbohydrates in moderation (preferably whole grains).
- Eat abundant fruits and vegetables, balanced between cooked and raw, with more cooked than raw when sensitive.
- Protein at breakfast supplies more energy and decreases appetite later in the day; too little protein creates a craving for sweets later on.
- Occasional desserts are best as an evening snack.
- Best supporting foods are rice, chicken, and turkey.

### For Weight Loss

- Dense protein: 15 to 30 percent of daily calories.
- Reduce quantity of food.
- Restrict bread.
- Avoid late-night snacking.
- Eliminate all dairy except butter.
- Follow meal schedule by eating a substantial breakfast including meat or fish; wait 4 to 5 hours, then have a moderate lunch; wait 6 hours, then have a very light dinner.
- Exercise at least 3 times a week.

### For Weight Gain

- Fat: 20 to 35 percent of daily calories.
- Dense protein: 15 to 30 percent of daily calories.
- Increase food intake.
- Include snacks.

## Healthy Foods List

There is no need to sacrifice delicious and filling foods to maintain a healthy Pituitary body type. The following lists will help you focus on foods that support your health, and avoid foods that can stress your system.

*You'll notice that some foods are printed in italics; these foods take more energy to assimilate and could be ones you will want to avoid when you are in a sensitive state due to any physical or emotional stresses.*

Be sure to read Chapter 3, "Implementing the Body Type Diet," for lots of important information about how to use these many foods to gain their full benefit.

## Ultra-Support Foods

Foods to include in 3 to 7 meals a week, listed by category.

**Dense Protein:** beef with visible fat removed, beef broth, beef liver, buffalo, organ meats (heart, brain); chicken, chicken broth, chicken livers, turkey; halibut
**Dairy:** butter
**Cheese:** regular cottage, Swiss
**Legume:** hummus
**Grains:** corn, corn bread, corn grits, corn tortillas, oats, rice (all varieties), rice bran, rice cakes, cream of rice
**Vegetables:** green beans, carrots, grape leaves, jicama, sweet potatoes
**Fruits:** tart apples (Granny Smith, Pippin), bananas, cherries, green grapes, cantaloupes
**Sweetener:** stevia
**Condiments:** lite salt, *tahini*
**Beverages:** tea (herbal [chamomile, peppermint, rose hips, Good Earth herb blend], Green Magma)

## Basic Support Foods

Foods to include in 1 to 2 meals a week.

**Dense Protein:** lamb, pork, ham, bacon, sausage, veal, venison; Cornish game hen, duck; anchovy, bass, bonita, catfish, cod, flounder, haddock, herring, mahimahi, mackerel, perch, orange roughy, salmon, sardines, shark, red snapper, sole, swordfish, trout, tuna; abalone, calamari (squid), clams, crab, eel, lobster, mussels, octopus, oysters, scallops, shrimp; eggs
**Dairy:** *milk (whole, 2%, low fat, nonfat, raw),* flavored yogurt

**Cheese:** American, blue, Brie, Camembert, cheddar, Colby, cream, Edam, feta, Gouda, kefir, Limburger, *Monterey Jack,* mozzarella, Muenster, Parmesan, ricotta, Romano
**Nuts and Seeds:** almonds (raw, roasted), almond butter, Brazils, cashews (raw, roasted), cashew butter, *coconut,* hazelnuts, macadamias (raw, roasted), macadamia butter, peanuts (raw, roasted), peanut butter, pecans, pine nuts (raw, roasted), pistachios, walnuts (black, English), water chestnuts; raw or roasted seeds (caraway, pumpkin, sesame, sunflower), sesame seed butter, sunflower seed butter
**Legumes:** beans (adzuki, black, garbanzo, Great Northern, kidney, lima, navy, pinto, red, soy), lentils, black-eyed peas, split peas; miso, soy milk, tofu
**Grains:** amaranth, barley, buckwheat, *couscous,* hominy grits, millet, popcorn, quinoa, rye, triticale, flour tortillas, breads (corn/rye, garlic, oat, sesame pita, rice, rye, sourdough), crackers (oat, rye, saltines, wheat), *pasta, udon noodles,* rice noodles, fried rice of rice (any), carrots, green peas, celery, scrambled egg w/soy sauce; cream of rye
**Vegetables:** asparagus, artichokes, avocados, bamboo shoots, yellow wax beans, beets, bok choy, broccoflower, broccoli, brussels sprouts, cooked cabbage (green, napa, red), cauliflower, celery, cilantro, corn, cucumbers, eggplant, garlic, greens (beet, collard, mustard, turnip), hominy, kale, kohlrabi, leeks, lettuce (Boston, butter, endive, iceberg, red leaf, romaine), mushrooms, okra, olives (green, ripe), onions (chives, brown, green, red, Vidalia, white, yellow), parsnips, parsley, peas, snow pea pods, bell peppers (green, red, yellow), chili peppers, pimientos, potatoes (all varieties), pumpkin, radishes, daikon radishes, rutabaga, sauerkraut, seaweed (arame, dulse, kelp, nori, wakame), shallots, spinach, sprouts (alfalfa, clover, mung bean, radish, sunflower), squash (acorn, banana, butternut, spaghetti, yellow [summer], zucchini), Swiss chard, cooked tomatoes (canned, hothouse, vine-ripened), turnips, *watercress,* yams
**Fruits:** apples (Golden or Red Delicious, Jonathan, McIntosh, Rome Beauty), apricots, berries (blackberries, blueberries, boysenberries, cranberries, gooseberries, raspberries, strawberries), dates, figs (fresh, dried), grapes (black, red), grapefruit (white, red), guavas, kiwi, kumquats, lemons, limes, loquats, mangoes, nectarines, oranges, papayas, peaches, pears, persimmons, plums (black, purple, red), pomegranates, prunes, raisins, rhubarb, tangelos, tangerines

**Fruit Juices:** apple, apple cider, apple/apricot, apricot, black cherry, red cherry, cranapple, cranberry, grape (purple, red, white), orange, grapefruit, guava, lemon, papaya, pear, pineapple, pineapple/coconut, prune, raspberry, tangerine, watermelon

**Vegetable Oils:** all-blend, *almond, avocado, corn, flaxseed, olive, peanut, safflower, sesame, soy, sunflower*

**Sweeteners:** *fructose, honey, molasses, sorghum, sugar (brown, date, raw), syrup (barley malt, brown rice, corn, maple), saccharin, succonant*

**Condiments:** *curry, cinnamon, chili powder, horseradish, barbecue sauce, pesto sauce, salsa, tempeh, vinegar,* salt, sea salt, Vege-Sal

**Salad Dressings:** *blue cheese, French, ranch, creamy Italian, creamy avocado, Thousand Island, vinegar and oil,* lemon juice and oil

**Desserts:** *custards, tapioca, puddings, pies, cakes, sherbet (orange, raspberry)*

**Chips:** *bean, corn (blue, white, yellow), potato*

**Beverages:** *decaffeinated coffee;* tea (decaffeinated, Take-A-Break, Roastaroma, *Cafix);* Perrier water, Arrowhead carbonated water, mineral water; *wine (red, white), sake, beer, barley malt liquor, champagne, brandy, gin, scotch, vodka, whiskey*

## Stressful Foods

Have no more than once a month.

**Dairy:** *goat's milk, half-and-half, sweet cream, sour cream, buttermilk, kefir, plain yogurt, frozen yogurt, ice cream*

**Cheese:** *low-fat cottage, goat*

**Grains:** *whole wheat, wheat bran, wheat germ, sprouted wheat, refined wheat flour, breads (French, Italian, multigrain, seven-grain, sprouted grain, white, whole wheat), bagels (plain, sesame seed), croissants, English muffins, cream of wheat*

**Vegetables:** *arugula, raw cabbage (green, napa, red), raw tomatoes (canned, hothouse, vine-ripened)*

**Vegetable Juices:** *carrot, carrot/celery, celery, parsley, spinach, tomato, V-8*

**Fruits:** *melons (casaba, Crenshaw, honeydew, watermelon), pineapples*

**Vegetable Oil:** *canola*

**Sweeteners:** *refined cane sugar, aspartame, Equal, NutraSweet, Sweet'n Low*

**Condiments:** *catsup, mustard, mayonnaise, soy sauce, margarine*

**Desserts:** *chocolate, desserts containing chocolate*

**Beverages:** *coffee; tea (black, green, Japanese, Chinese oolong); root beer, diet sodas, regular sodas*

## Scheduling Meals

### Healthy

Pituitary types should begin the day with a heavy meal and then scale down to a light dinner. Schedule your meals as follows:

*Breakfast:* 7–8 A.M. Heavy, with main emphasis on protein, vegetables, grain, nuts, seeds, legumes, and/or fruit. Rotate varieties.

*Lunch:* 12–2 P.M. Moderate to heavy, with protein, vegetables, grain, nuts, seeds, legumes, dairy, and/or fruit. Salad is best after meat and grain.

*Dinner:* 5:30–6 P.M. (7 P.M. is OK if after a 4 P.M. fruit snack) Light to moderate, with vegetables, legumes, and/or fruit. Avoid protein and grain.

### Snacks (optional)

*Midmorning:* (10 A.M.) grain, vegetables

*Midafternoon:* (4 P.M.) fruit

*Evening:* (10–11 P.M.) fruit, vegetables, grain, nuts, seeds, sweets

### Sensitive

*Breakfast:* Moderate with emphasis on protein, vegetables, and grains. Rotate foods. (Lunch and Dinner are same as for healthy.)

## Sample One-Week Menu

DAY 1

*Breakfast:* turkey, sweet potato, and broccoli

*Lunch:* steamed clams, pasta, and mixed vegetables—squash, green beans, and peas

*Dinner:* beets and cucumber salad w/Italian dressing

DAY 2

*Breakfast:* chicken, eggs, potatoes, and corn tortilla

*Lunch:* ahi tuna and rice noodles w/bell peppers and jicama

*Dinner:* artichoke and raw carrot; or steamed or raw cauliflower

DAY 3

*Breakfast:* salmon and asparagus

*Lunch:* Cornish game hen stuffed w/long grain and wild rice, then cucumber and cold pea salad or mixed salad of red leaf lettuce, butter leaf, mush-rooms, chives w/blue cheese dressing

*Dinner:* cream of mushroom soup w/lentils

DAY 4

*Breakfast:* turkey and eggs

*Lunch:* broiled lamb chops and red potatoes, then a salad of romaine lettuce, grated carrots, parsley, green onion, and celery w/red wine vinegar

*Dinner:* sweet potato and green beans

DAY 5: CLEANSE

*Breakfast:* steamed broccoli, greens, spinach, and/or raw snow pea pods, carrots, celery

*Lunch:* steamed green cabbage w/onion, zucchini, and/or raw celery, carrots

*Dinner:* steamed asparagus, green cabbage, and/or raw bell pepper, jicama, carrots

DAY 6

*Breakfast:* halibut, carrots, and cauliflower

*Lunch:* turkey, mushrooms, onions, and salad of Boston lettuce, radishes, snow pea pods, alfalfa sprouts w/creamy avocado dressing

*Dinner:* wonton soup

DAY 7

*Breakfast:* steak, potato, onions, and green beans

*Lunch:* chicken burrito—flour tortilla, vegetables, chicken, and lettuce—w/rice and beans

*Dinner:* vegetable soup—tomato based, new potatoes, brown onions, green peas, carrots, zucchini, barley cooked in chicken broth, and a green salad

## Alternative Menus

*(Foods in parentheses may be omitted.)*

### Breakfast

Sausage and pancakes

Ham, Brazil nuts, and stir-fried zucchini, onions, squash, and mushrooms (orange juice)

### Breakfast or Lunch

Scrambled eggs and turkey sausage (fruit)

Corned beef hash and eggs

Ham and black beans

Turkey and sweet potatoes (peas)

Chicken, rice, and corn

Chicken breast, potato, and green beans

Deviled egg, chicken breast, and potato salad

Pork chops or sausage, peas, rice or potato, and onions, chilis, or garlic

Beef vegetable stew

Swordfish and sweet potatoes

Broiled sea bass, salmon, halibut, or shark w/lemon and rice

Tuna, pasta, and peas or green beans

Halibut, rice, and asparagus or green beans

Shark, sea bass, halibut, or salmon and baked potato w/butter and chives (steamed carrots)

Shark, rice, mixed vegetables, and asparagus or broccoli

Lamb chop, potato, asparagus, and/or beets and beet greens

### Lunch

Turkey, tomato, and buttered potato, cranberry, green beans

Sirloin tips, carrots, string beans, gravy, applesauce, and green salad

Shrimp, and salad of red leaf lettuce, avocados, carrots, celery, w/ranch dressing

### Dinner

Thai soup w/coconut milk and red or green curry

Dolmas and hummus

Baked apple and tahini

Smoothie—papaya juice, banana, and mango

Red potatoes, steamed broccoli, and carrots

Squash

Salad of romaine lettuce, finely diced cauliflower, broccoli, and cucumbers w/vinegar and olive oil

Salad of lettuce, garbanzo beans, green pepper, red pepper, and raw zucchini w/Caesar dressing

Apple, banana, cherries, or green peppers

# Skin

*The Skin body type is symbolized by a conch shell. The skin forms the body's shell, connecting it with the outside world. Sensitive to emotions, subtle energies, and vibrations, Skin body types communicate largely through their expanded sense of touch.*

FAMOUS PEOPLE: Luciano Pavarotti, Camryn Manheim, Sidney Poitier, Della Reese

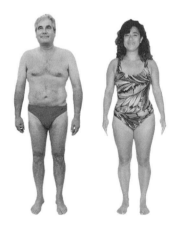

### SKIN
### Location and Function

The skin covers the entire body. Its function is to provide the body with borders and boundaries. It is the sensory organ of touch and the second-largest organ of elimination.

## Psychological Profile

### Characteristic Traits

The skin is a heightened sense organ that sends and receives feeling messages, making Skin body types extremely sensitive to vibrations and subtle energies. Being physically orientated, they have a strong, solid connection with the earth and nature, including the weather, which can often affect their moods. Many have an innate affinity for the Native American culture.

Sensual and romantic and with an enviable lust for life, Skin types like to experience their senses fully. They find satisfaction in natural, simple pleasures like the taste of foods, the sound of music, and the visual stimulation of bright colors and intriguing designs. Highly attuned to their sense of touch, they like the feel of things, particularly enjoying fabrics that have a pleasant texture, like silk, cashmere, or flannel.

Skin types are perceptive and visual (some even have a photographic memory). Schoolwork or formal learning is most appealing when they experience it in a visual way. They learn best when discovering the material directly or through multiple sensory perceptions.

Open and receptive, Skin types create a warm, nurturing environment where others feel safe and appreciated. Sociable in nature and extremely sensitive to other people, they are usually happiest when involved with others in a mutual undertaking. With their strong nurturing qualities, they are exceptionally good with children and particularly effective in service professions.

Their love and respect for life and all its creatures is often reflected in selflessness or altruism. With heightened empathic feeling, they have a tendency to take in and retain all they experience. If they're not careful, simply witnessing the emotional suffering of others can cause their own spirits to sink.

### Motivation

Being so responsive to the moods and feelings of those around them, as well as to their environment, Skin types often put on large amounts of weight to act as a protective buffer. Weight gain typically occurs following an accident, illness, personal violation, or other situation where energies are less than harmonious. Diet can also cause weight gain due to the Skin types' inability to process refined sugar and the resulting loss of muscle mass.

Being inordinately sensitive, Skin types tend to take the responses of others too seriously. This sensitivity can often leave them feeling vulnerable, with a need to defend themselves. They then disconnect and direct their attention elsewhere. The energy shift can be so dramatic that the others can feel they have been abandoned or that the Skin type is angry with them.

Being so sensitive to others' disapproval and rejection, Skin types are often reluctant to share their knowledge and ideas. Unfortunately, this not only deprives others of the Skin type's insights, but severely limits the Skin types themselves because discovery and social interaction are so important to them.

While Skin types are good at receiving ideas, they can have difficulty following through on their ideas and plans. Anything that is overly mundane, mechanical, or conventional can leave them feeling bored or frustrated. When a project no longer requires creativity, lacks excitement, or becomes routine, they need to move on because their life path is to experience and stretch, moving physically and/or mentally. Consequently they may lack direction in life and are often late bloomers, not discovering their true life's work until after the age of forty.

## "At Worst"

Skin types can be reluctant to share information and knowledge when their environment doesn't feel safe, usually due to someone's disapproval, rejection, or anger. They can also swing to the opposite extreme and express themselves in an aggressive manner. Some are able to see pictures and receive insights that they shared when it wasn't appropriate, only to experience the painful repercussions of their lack of discretion.

When dealing with an emotional situation, Skin types may either deny its existence or immerse themselves in it. Once they get involved, they don't know how to let it go, even if they can't solve the problem. Feeling more secure when they know what will happen, they attempt to control circumstances and situations by becoming caretakers and taking on others' responsibilities. They have a tendency to take on the problems of those around them to a degree that can interfere with their ability to nurture themselves adequately.

The Skin types' desire to hide can come from not wanting to stand out or be noticed. They may abruptly retreat from relationships and become inaccessible, leaving others feeling offended or abandoned. When

stressed, Skin types close down; they become lazy and depressed, disconnect mentally, and feel sorry for themselves. These problems arise when they become indulgent, using food as a stimulant. Overeating then causes a loss of self-esteem and self-acceptance, which triggers the cycle of using food, particularly sweets, for self-nurturing. Other common methods of escape include alcohol and drugs. Because their bodies do not process refined sugar well, it is easy for them to become addicted to alcohol or chocolate.

Skin types can set unrealistic expectations for themselves. They then move into a pattern of self-doubt where they do not accept themselves and compensate by setting unrealistic expectations for others. Their self-doubt continues to build until it hinders every other aspect of their lives. To break the cycle, they need to move a giant step forward; doing something feels good and helps them move through the fear of not being perfect.

## "At Best"

With a flair for life, Skin types are light and romantic, open to new experiences and discovery. They are artistic and imaginative, and clever original ideas come to them easily. They are very intuitive yet well grounded. Being especially visual, they tend to see images, which can then be translated into usable information. Highly social, they enjoy people and life in general. They approach life with respect and a sense of altruism.

Extremely receptive, Skin types are able to sense what is going on and allow energy to flow around and through them without absorbing it. Physical activity that doesn't require thought, such as stretching, gardening, or going for a walk, can move blocked energy. Emotionally detaching allows them to go with the flow and accept whatever is happening. They are then able to use their sensitivity to feel safe in the world. Nature helps them rebalance and get reconnected with God. The key is to connect with spirit by going through the body, as in an active meditation or by taking time to be by themselves.

Receptive and intuitive, the Skin types' special strength lies in receiving information rather than directing or controlling it. This is how new discoveries are made. The first step is to release the need to control the outcome and be truly comfortable regardless of which way it goes. Once they get their direction, they can proceed in a practical, competent, and reliable manner.

Having developed self-confidence, Skin types are able to express their inner truth and essence without fear of rejection. They are able to share when appropriate without taking other people's responses personally. They can feel safe even in a harsh or insensitive world. When connected with their spiritual side, they often receive information and can be excellent channels, using the information for counseling or healing.

## Dietary Profile

### Main Focus

- Back to nature: If you can hunt it, pick it, catch it, or grow it, you can eat it. If processed, forget it.
- You are extremely sensitive to foods that have been altered (e.g., microwaved, engineered).
- Avoid refined sugar because it can cause muscle degeneration and weight gain.
- Include fruit (but avoid it with dinner and as a midafternoon snack).
- Occasional desserts are best as an evening snack.
- Eat vegetables; keep foods and meals simple.
- Let go of the need to use weight as a protection; identify and clear emotional stress.

### Dietary Emphasis

- From 15 to 35 percent of your calories are to come from fats.
- Best fat sources: almonds, sunflower and sesame seeds, tahini, avocados, olive oil, fish, meat, and poultry.
- From 25 to 40 percent of your calories are to come from protein.
- From 0 to 35 percent of your calories are to come from dense protein.

- Best sources of the three amino acids threonine, isoleucine, and cystine: almonds, pumpkin seeds, and sunflower seeds.
- Caloric intake: 1,500 to 1,800 calories a day for women and 1,700 to 2,000 calories a day for men. If you are engaging in intense exercise (competition type) or hard labor, increase calories.
- Drink a minimum of 64 ounces of water a day. Drink water before and after meals, not with meals.
- Dairy foods often interfere with memory; especially avoid them for dinner.
- Follow these food-combining rules:
  Avoid combining meat and breads (as in sandwiches).
  Avoid combining dense protein and fruit.
  Avoid combining two proteins (meat and milk or cream sauce).
  Avoid combining acids and grains (vinegar and rice).
- Concentrated herbal products and rice powders (in water) are often effective in rebuilding body.
- Eat melons alone.
- Most vegetables combine well with protein and with grains.
- Eat brown or wild rice with vegetables.

### For Weight Loss

- Fat: 15 to 30 percent of daily calories.
- Dense protein: 15 to 35 percent of daily calories.
- Eliminate refined sugar, alcohol, dairy, and breads (because of yeast and sweetener).
- Reduce salt.
- Avoid snacks; if you need to snack, an evening snack is best.
- Eat potatoes (different varieties) 4 to 6 times a week.
- Eat grains 4 to 6 times a week.
- Rotate foods.
- Stretch at least 15 minutes a day.

## For Weight Gain

▸ Increase food consumption, focusing on best sources.

# Healthy Foods List

There is no need to sacrifice delicious and filling foods to maintain a healthy Skin body type. The following lists will help you focus on foods that support your health, and avoid foods that can stress your system.

*You'll notice that some foods are printed in italics; these foods should be avoided when you are in a sensitive state due to any physical or emotional stresses.*

Be sure to read Chapter 3, "Implementing the Body Type Diet," for lots of important information about how to use these many foods to gain their full benefit.

## Ultra-Support Foods

Foods to include in 3 to 7 meals a week, listed by category.

**Dense Protein:** game meats (buffalo, pheasant, rabbit, venison); Cornish game hen, duck; flounder, haddock, halibut, herring, mackerel, mahimahi, perch, red snapper
**Dairy:** butter
**Nuts and Seeds:** almonds (raw, roasted), almond butter, cashews (roasted), cashew butter; raw or roasted seeds (caraway, pumpkin, sesame, sunflower), sesame seed butter, sunflower seed butter
**Legumes:** beans (*garbanzo,* lima); miso
**Grains:** corn, corn grits, oats, rice (all varieties), rice bran, rice cakes, Swedish crisp bread, pasta (durum, semolina), udon noodles, rice noodles, cream of rice
**Vegetables:** asparagus, avocados, green beans, beets, broccoli, napa cabbage, carrots, cauliflower, celery, cilantro, corn, garlic, mustard greens, shiitake mushrooms, onions (all varieties), peas, *bell peppers* (*green, red, yellow*), chili peppers, *potatoes* (*all varieties*), pumpkin, *daikon radishes,* spinach, sprouts (alfalfa, clover, radish, sunflower), squash (banana, yellow [summer]), sweet potatoes, turnips, *yams*
**Fruits:** bananas, berries (blackberries, blueberries, boysenberries, cranberries, gooseberries, strawber-

ries), figs (fresh, dried), green grapes, melons (cantaloupe, honeydew, watermelon), oranges
**Sweetener:** stevia
**Condiments:** *salsa,* tahini
**Beverages:** Arrowhead flavored carbonated water (cherry, lemon, lime, orange)

## Basic Support Foods

Foods to include in 1 to 2 meals a week.

**Dense Protein:** *beef,* beef broth, beef liver, lamb, pork, bacon, ham, sausage, veal, organ meats (heart, brain); chicken, chicken broth, chicken livers, turkey; anchovy, bass, bonita, catfish, *cod,* orange roughy, salmon, sardines, shark, sole, swordfish, trout, tuna; abalone, calamari (squid), clams, crab, eel, lobsters, mussels, octopus, oysters, scallops, shrimp; eggs in foods (e.g., with rice, broccoli)
**Dairy:** half-and-half, sweet cream, sour cream, yogurt (regular and low-fat plain, *nonfat plain and flavored*), ice cream (Baskin 31 Robbins, Ben & Jerry's, Dreyer's, Swensen's)
**Cheese:** American, blue, Brie, Camembert, cheddar, Colby, *cottage, cream,* Edam, feta, Gouda, kefir, Limburger, Monterey Jack, mozzarella, Muenster, Parmesan, ricotta, Romano, Swiss
**Nuts and Seeds:** Brazils, raw cashews, coconut, hazelnuts, macadamias (raw, roasted), macadamia butter, peanuts (raw, roasted), peanut butter, pecans, pine nuts (raw, roasted), pistachios, walnuts (black, English), water chestnuts
**Legumes:** beans (adzuki, black, Great Northern, kidney, lima, mung, navy, pinto, red, soy), lentils, black-eyed peas, split peas; hummus; soy milk, *tofu*
**Grains:** amaranth, barley, *buckwheat,* corn tortillas, couscous, hominy grits, millet, popcorn, quinoa, rye, triticale, *whole wheat,* wheat bran, wheat germ, refined wheat flour, flour tortillas, breads (corn, corn/rye, French, garlic, Italian, multigrain, oat, rice, rye, seven-grain, sourdough, sprouted grain, white, whole wheat), bagels, croissants, English muffins, crackers (oat, rye, saltines, wheat), unsalted pretzels, cream of rye, *cream of wheat*
**Vegetables:** artichokes, *arugula,* yellow wax beans, bamboo shoots, bok choy, broccoflower, brussels sprouts, cabbage (green, red), cucumbers, eggplant, greens (beet, collard, turnip), hominy, jicama, kale, kohlrabi, leeks, lettuce (Boston, butter, endive, *iceberg,* red leaf, romaine), mushrooms, okra, olives (green, ripe), parsley, parsnips, snow pea pods,

pimientos, radishes (red, white), rutabaga, sauerkraut, seaweed (arame, dulse, kelp, nori, wakame), shallots, squash (acorn, butternut, spaghetti, *zucchini*), mung bean sprouts, Swiss chard, *tomatoes* (*canned, hothouse, vine-ripened*), *watercress*

**Vegetable Juices:** carrot, carrot/celery, celery, parsley, spinach, tomato, V-8

**Fruits:** apples (Gala, Golden or Red Delicious, *Granny Smith,* Jonathan, McIntosh, *Pippin,* Rome Beauty), *apricots,* cherries, dates, grapes (black, Concord, red), guavas, *kiwi,* kumquats, lemons, limes, loquats, melons (casaba, Crenshaw), mangoes, nectarines, papayas, peaches, pears, persimmons, pineapples, plums (black, purple, red, umeboshi), pomegranates, prunes, raisins, raspberries, rhubarb, tangerines, tangelos

**Fruit Juices:** apple, apple cider, apple/apricot, apricot, black cherry, red cherry, cranapple, cranberry, grape (purple, red, white), *grapefruit,* guava, lemon, orange, papaya, pear, pineapple, pineapple/coconut, prune, tangerine, watermelon

**Vegetable Oils:** *all-blend, almond, avocado, corn, flaxseed,* olive, *peanut, safflower, sesame, soy, sunflower*

**Sweeteners:** *fructose, molasses, sorghum, date sugar, syrup* (*barley malt, brown rice, corn, maple*), *succonant*

**Condiments:** *catsup, mustard, horseradish, barbecue sauce, pesto sauce,* soy sauce, vinegar, dill pickles, pickle relish, regular salt, sea salt, Vege-Sal, Spike, Braggs Liquid Aminos

**Salad Dressings:** *Blue cheese, French, ranch, creamy Italian, creamy avocado, Thousand Island,* vinegar and oil, lemon juice and oil

**Desserts:** *custards, tapioca, puddings, pies, cakes, sherbet* (*orange, raspberry*), carob squares

**Chips:** bean, corn (blue, white, yellow), potato

**Beverages:** tea (*black, green,* herbal [chamomile], Ignatia, Japanese, Chinese oolong); mineral water, sparkling water; *wine* (*red, white*), *sake, beer, barley malt liquor, champagne, gin, scotch, vodka, whiskey; root beer, regular sodas*

## Stressful Foods

Have no more than once a month.

**Dense Protein:** *eggs* (alone)
**Dairy:** *milk* (*whole, 2%, low fat, nonfat, raw, goat's*), *buttermilk, kefir, frozen yogurt, ice cream*
**Cheese:** goat

**Fruits:** *grapefruit* (*white, red*)
**Vegetable Oil:** canola
**Sweeteners:** *honey, sugar* (*brown, raw, refined cane*), *saccharin, aspartame, Equal, NutraSweet, Sweet'n Low*
**Condiments:** *mayonnaise, margarine*
**Desserts:** *chocolate, desserts containing chocolate*
**Beverages:** *caffeinated beverages* (*coffee, diet sodas*)

## Scheduling Meals

Schedule your meals as follows:

*Breakfast:* 7–8 A.M. Light, with grain, vegetables, nuts, seeds, and/or fruit.
*Lunch:* 12–2 P.M. Moderate to heavy, with vegetables, grain, nuts, seeds, legumes, protein, fruit, and/or dairy.
*Dinner:* Early, by 6 P.M. Light to moderate, with protein, grains, vegetables, nuts, seeds, and/or legumes. Avoid fruit and dairy.

### Snacks (optional)
*Midmorning:* grain, alone or with nut butter and/or fruit
*Midafternoon:* nuts, seeds, grain, vegetables
*Evening:* (10 P.M.–midnight) protein, vegetables, grain, fruit, nuts, seeds

## Sample One-Week Menu

DAY 1
*Breakfast:* avocado and corn tortilla
*Lunch:* turkey breast, rice, and yellow squash
*Dinner:* salad of baby greens, shrimp or tuna, corn, jicama, and tomatoes w/balsamic dressing
*Snack:* sunflower seeds

DAY 2
*Breakfast:* yam
*Lunch:* pork or chicken or beef lo mein
*Dinner:* miso soup w/scallions, rice, and vegetables such as broccoli, bok choy, greens, onions, celery, and/or carrots
*Snack:* dates and cream cheese

DAY 3
*Breakfast:* pumpkin seeds or watermelon
*Lunch:* almond chicken

*Dinner:* sea bass, salmon, or steamed clams, napa cabbage, and a salad of mustard greens, onions, mushrooms, sunflower sprouts, and sunflower seeds w/avocado dressing

## DAY 4
*Breakfast:* oatmeal w/banana and butter
*Lunch:* brown rice and vegetables—broccoli, peas, cabbage, bok choy
*Dinner:* salmon fillet and Swiss chard
*Snack:* cherries (fresh or frozen)

## DAY 5: CLEANSE
*Breakfast:* Watermelon including seeds and white part of rind
*Lunch:* steamed asparagus, green beans, and/or raw carrots, celery, spinach, bell peppers, and/or carrot/celery juice
*Dinner:* steamed cauliflower, squash, kale, and/or raw broccoli, celery, cucumbers

## DAY 6
*Breakfast:* apple w/almond butter
*Lunch:* chili relleno—rice, beans, salsa, and/or avocado
*Dinner:* baked potato, snow pea pods, yellow wax beans, and red bell peppers
*Snack:* almonds

## DAY 7
*Breakfast:* beans
*Lunch:* roasted duck and wild rice w/shiitake mushrooms
*Dinner:* noodle soup w/vegetables—cabbage, carrots, pea pods, and leeks

## Alternative Menus

The following meals may be eaten for breakfast by those who are sensitive or protein deficient. Otherwise they may also be eaten for lunch or dinner. Foods in parentheses are optional.

Red snapper and asparagus
Perch and lima beans
Flounder and asparagus
Beef and brussels sprouts
Chopped liver and celery

Tuna w/olive oil, chopped green onion, and mustard
Salad of salmon, romaine lettuce, tomatoes, and jicama
Cornish game hen and carrots
Chicken or chicken livers and coleslaw w/rice vinegar
Eggs and broccoli, spinach, onions, bell pepper, and tomato
Eggs with onions and broccoli

### Breakfast
Blueberries or boysenberries and sunflower seeds
Blackberries, blueberries, or boysenberries and hazelnuts
Almonds and banana
Amaranth and pumpkin or sesame seeds

### Lunch
Baked potato and broccoli (w/butter)
Steak, potato, and broccoli
Amaranth and vegetables—broccoli, peas, cabbage, bok choy
Beef steak and broccoli
Broccoli and couscous
Lamb and green beans
Green beans and rice
Chicken and peas

### Lunch or Dinner
Roasted chicken and a salad of spinach, carrots, onions, and radishes w/ranch dressing, (brown rice)
Halibut and steamed or stir-fried squash, zucchini, broccoli, onions, and carrots
Lamb w/garlic, onion, potato, rice, or amaranth, and carrots
Chicken, rice, onions, bell pepper, broccoli, and cauliflower
Turkey and corn tortilla w/olive oil and salsa (salad of iceberg lettuce, bell peppers, cilantro, and celery w/creamy avocado dressing)
Split pea soup

### Dinner
Mushroom barley soup
Cornish game hen and a salad of spinach and artichoke w/sunflower oil and lemon juice
Orange roughy and broccoli
Halibut or snapper and a green salad w/sprouts and seeds
Salad of spinach, beets, sunflower seeds, and green or red onions w/balsamic vinegar

# Spleen

*The Spleen body type is symbolized by a horseshoe magnet. The spleen reclaims the iron from red blood cells and disseminates energy as needed. Tenacious, Spleen body types provide the sustaining energy needed to get a job done right.*

FAMOUS PEOPLE: Jack LaLanne, Drew Carey, Christina Onassis, Maria Callas

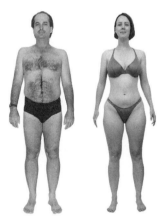

## SPLEEN
### Location and Function

The spleen is located in the upper left abdomen between the stomach and the diaphragm. As the largest organ in the lymphatic system (a major part of the immune system), the spleen serves several important functions, including the removal of iron from old red blood cells.

## Psychological Profile

### Characteristic Traits

Basically social and naturally outgoing, Spleen body types are personable and thrive on helping others. Social interaction gives them a sense of fulfillment, particularly when they can be the authority or center of attention. Spleen types are generally good organizers and like to do things in a big way, such as being involved in organizing huge social events.

Intense and forceful by nature, they tend to be passionate in their ideas and convictions and may express their enthusiasm so forcefully that they overwhelm people and may be perceived as aggressive. They love to present new ideas or viewpoints and find introducing others to nontraditional or alternative ways of seeing or doing things especially rewarding. Passionate about their ideas regarding change and reform, they often express them with such emotional fervor that other people feel uncomfortable.

Spleen types are tenacious. Whatever their focus, they stay with it until they get the results they desire. They may get so focused on a particular detail that they keep a conversation or project at a standstill until it is resolved. They derive a sense of security from detail clarification and a solid, organized structure.

### Motivation

Spleen types love being achievers regardless of the area, and will persist in a task, giving it their best. When they don't succeed in everything they set out to do, however, they feel like total failures and blame themselves. So if they have any doubt about their ability to succeed, they procrastinate by finding excuses and diversions as an acceptable means of avoidance.

Spleen types love to eat and are often excellent cooks. It's easy for them to put on and carry excess weight because their bodies are so strong that they rarely get indigestion or a bloated feeling from overindulgence or dietary indiscretions. Deriving a great deal of sensual pleasure from food, they find it easy to rationalize and bend the rules to get the treats they want. Consequently food and diet suggestions need to be very clear, including specific quantities, or they interpret moderation to fit their desires, which for them can mean unlimited quantities. While losing weight may be important, the sacrifice is often too great unless there is sufficient social support.

More people- than task-oriented, Spleen types are

better working with others than independently. Working with someone provides the motivation that is difficult to find on their own, particularly for activities such as exercise. Unless they have evolved to the point of being self-motivated, they put off activities that require discipline unless they can find a partner. Personal motivation is inherently low, so emotional support and structure are essential for follow-through in areas that require consistency.

## "At Worst"

The tenacity of Spleen types can be a liability when it comes to resolving conflict. Being exceedingly fixed and dogmatic in their beliefs, once their minds are made up, that is the end of the subject, and they show little if any flexibility. Domineering, bossy, and controlling, they tend to think that their way is the only way and are not open to listening to or learning from others.

Defensive, stubborn, and inflexible, Spleen types can be deadly when confronted with an opposing point of view, particularly when their personal interest is at stake. They may go after the person with the opposing view, rather than just the view, and overpower the opposition through personal harassment and character assassination. Direct and to the point, their written words can be lethal. Verbally adept, they can kill with well-chosen words. They often display an adversarial attitude and are out to win at any cost.

The need for security, both financial and emotional, motivates Spleen types. It's easy for them to overfocus on career at the expense of their family or personal health. When aggressive, they can be ruthless in their business dealings and charm and seduce people in an effort to enhance their image. To ensure that people need them, they may make themselves indispensable in some way or set themselves up in controlling positions to make others dependent upon them. They often make big promises, playing on others' hopes and dreams, but then never quite follow through.

When feeling insecure, Spleen types often resort to food for comfort and put on large amounts of excess weight. Just as they tend to hang on to their dogmatic beliefs, they tend to hang on to their weight until they learn to let go and be flexible in other areas of their lives. Prone to obsessive/compulsive behavior, they can swing to the opposite extreme of losing weight when their security is threatened or when they feel abandoned.

## "At Best"

The tenacity of Spleen types allows them to see a job through, staying with a problem until they have reached a viable solution. With a strong mental focus, they are good at figuring things out and resolving challenging tasks, especially when the task is viewed by others as being nearly impossible. Spleen types enjoy helping their friends and will consistently be there whenever the need arises. By truly giving from their hearts, they connect with their spiritual side and experience a true sense of security.

Spleen types are most effective when they can first gain a good mental understanding of something, whether it be how something is physically put together, what motivates others, the various aspects of themselves, or life in general. Allowing themselves to be flexible by detaching their focus from structure and detail, they are free to see the greater picture. Feeling secure, they are comfortable opening their hearts and sharing their emotions, integrating all aspects of themselves.

Once Spleen types have learned to integrate their feelings by connecting their head and heart through their spiritual nature, they are able to embody energy and powerfully disseminate it into the world. Being able to see the big picture, they can accurately forecast change, including market trends, which allows them to succeed in enterprises of major proportions. They are highly effective in spearheading social reforms, bringing new awareness to humanity and continually supplying the necessary energy until change is fully accomplished.

## Dietary Profile

### Main Focus

- ▶ Rotate foods.
- ▶ Make lunch your heaviest meal.

### RECOMMENDED EXERCISE

Exercise releases stress. While it is not necessary to lose weight, it is good for muscle tone. Mornings are the best time, ideally 1 hour before breakfast, 4 times a week, getting the heart rate up to 120 for a minimum of 30 minutes. Exercise that provides mental, physical, and emotional integration is best. Examples include low-impact aerobics, walking, Callanetics, and dance such as swing and jitterbug.

▸ Eat a light early dinner.

▸ Focus on vegetables but not vegetable juices.

## Dietary Emphasis

▸ From 25 to 30 percent of your calories are to come from fat.

▸ Best fat sources: nuts, seeds, oils (especially sunflower seed oil), and low-fat yogurt.

▸ From 20 to 30 percent of your calories are to come from protein.

▸ From 10 to 25 percent of your calories are to come from dense protein.

▸ Best sources of the three amino acids threonine, isoleucine, and cystine: chicken, ricotta cheese, turkey, and catfish.

▸ Caloric intake: 1,500 to 1,800 calories a day for women and 1,700 to 2,000 calories a day for men. If you are engaging in intense exercise (competition type) or hard labor, increase calories.

▸ Drink a minimum of 64 ounces of water a day. Drink water before and after meals, not with meals.

▸ Occasional desserts are best as an evening snack.

▸ Avoid eating potato or squash with dense protein.

▸ Eat vegetables, especially green beans.

▸ Eat fish at 2 meals a week; rotate type.

▸ Blueberries strengthen white blood cells.

▸ Have spices, especially curry, up to 4 times a week. Curry strengthens red and white blood cells and capillaries. Cayenne pepper stimulates the lymphatics.

## For Weight Loss

▸ Make lunch your largest meal.

▸ Have a light, early dinner, ideally between 5 and 6 P.M.

▸ Limit sugar, including fruit, to twice a week.

▸ Limit bread to no more than 3 times a week.

▸ Avoid snacks, especially late-night snacking.

## For Weight Gain

▸ Dense protein: 20 to 25 percent of daily calories.

▸ Include snacks.

## Healthy Foods List

There is no need to sacrifice delicious and filling foods to maintain a healthy Spleen body type. The following

lists will help you focus on foods that support your health, and avoid foods that can stress your system.

*You'll notice that some foods are printed in italics; these foods should be avoided when you are in a sensitive state due to any physical or emotional stresses.*

Be sure to read Chapter 3, "Implementing the Body Type Diet," for lots of important information about how to use these many foods to gain their full benefit.

## Ultra-Support Foods

Foods to include in 3 to 7 meals a week, listed by category.

**Dense Protein:** beef broth, beef liver, buffalo, veal; chicken, chicken broth, chicken livers, Cornish game hen, duck, turkey; bass, orange roughy, trout

**Dairy:** yogurt (low-fat, nonfat, plain, flavored), butter

**Cheese:** raw goat's milk feta, ricotta

**Nuts and Seeds:** natural peanut butter, walnuts (black, English); roasted, unsalted seeds (pumpkin, sesame, sunflower), caraway seeds

**Legumes:** beans (black, garbanzo, lima, pinto, red, soy), black-eyed peas, split peas; hummus

**Grains:** amaranth, barley, buckwheat, corn tortillas, oats, oat bran, oatmeal, popcorn, white basmati rice, rye, breads (oat, rye), crackers (oat, rye)

**Vegetables:** artichokes, asparagus, avocados, bamboo shoots, beans (green, Italian green, yellow wax), beets, bok choy, broccoflower, broccoli, brussels sprouts, cabbage (green, napa, red), carrots, cauliflower, cilantro, corn, cucumbers, *eggplant, garlic,* lettuce (endive, red leaf, romaine), pumpkin, spinach, Swiss chard

**Fruits:** apples (Golden or Red Delicious, Granny Smith, Jonathan, McIntosh, Pippin), apricots, berries (blackberries, blueberries, boysenberries, cranberries, gooseberries, raspberries), dates, grapes (green, red), melons (casaba, Crenshaw, honeydew, watermelon), raisins

**Fruit Juices:** lime in water, orange

**Vegetable Oils:** all-blend, almond, avocado, corn, *flaxseed, olive, peanut,* safflower, *sesame,* soy, sunflower

**Sweeteners:** fructose, honey, barley malt syrup, stevia

**Condiments:** salsa, especially nutmeg, Spike

**Beverages:** tea (Take-A-Break Roastaroma, Orange Spice, licorice)

## Basic Support Foods

Foods to include in 1 to 2 meals a week.

**Dense Protein:** beef, bacon, lamb, venison, organ meats (heart, brain); anchovy, bonita, catfish, cod, flounder, haddock, halibut, herring, mackerel, mahimahi, perch, *salmon,* sardines, shark, *snapper,* sole, swordfish, tuna; abalone, calamari (squid), clams, crab, eel, lobsters, mussels, octopus, oysters, scallops, shrimp; eggs

**Dairy:** milk (whole, 2%, low fat, nonfat, raw, goat's), half-and-half, sweet cream, sour cream, buttermilk, kefir, regular yogurt, Dreyer's imitation yogurt, *ice cream* (Ben & Jerry's, Dreyer's, Swensen's)

**Cheese:** American, blue, Brie, Camembert, cheddar, Colby, cottage, cream, Edam, pasteurized feta, goat, Gouda, kefir, Limburger, low-fat Monterey Jack, mozzarella, Muenster, Parmesan, Romano, Swiss

**Nuts and Seeds:** almonds, almond butter, Brazils, *cashews,* cashew butter, coconut, hazelnuts, macadamias, macadamia butter, peanuts, pecans, pine nuts, pistachios, steamed or cooked water chestnuts; sesame seed butter, sunflower seed butter

**Legumes:** beans (adzuki, kidney, Great Northern, navy), lentils; miso, soy milk, soy protein, tofu

**Grains:** *corn, corn grits,* couscous, hominy grits, millet, quinoa, rice (brown basmati, long or short grain brown, Japanese, wild), rice bran, rice cakes, triticale, whole wheat, wheat bran, wheat germ, refined wheat flour, flour tortillas, breads (*corn,* corn/rye, French, garlic, Italian, multigrain, pita, rice, seven-grain, sourdough, sprouted grain, white, whole wheat), bagels, croissants, English muffins, crackers (saltines, whole wheat), pasta, udon noodles, Chinese rice noodles, cream of rice, cream of rye, cream of wheat

**Vegetables:** *arugula, celery,* greens (beet, collard, mustard, turnip), hominy, jicama, kale, kohlrabi, leeks, lettuce (Boston, butter, iceberg), mushrooms, okra, olives (green, ripe), onions (chives, brown, green, red, Vidalia, white, yellow), parsley, parsnips, peas, snow pea pods, bell peppers (green, red, yellow), chili peppers, pimientos, potatoes (all varieties), radishes, daikon radishes, rutabaga, sauerkraut, seaweed (arame, dulse, kelp, nori, wakame), shallots, sprouts (alfalfa, clover, mung bean, radish, sunflower), squash (acorn, banana, butternut, spaghetti, yellow [summer], zucchini), sweet potatoes, tomatoes, turnips, *watercress,* yams

**Vegetable Juices:** *carrot, celery, carrot/celery, parsley, spinach, tomato, V-8*

**Fruits:** Rome Beauty apples, bananas, *strawberries,* cantaloupes, cherries, figs, black grapes, guavas, kiwi, kumquats, lemons, limes, loquats, mangoes, nectarines, oranges, papayas, peaches, pears, persimmons, pineapples, plums (black, red, purple), pomegranates, prunes, rhubarb, tangelos, tangerines

**Fruit Juices:** *apple, apple cider, apple/apricot, apricot, black cherry, red cherry, cranapple, cranberry, grape (red, purple, white), grapefruit, guava, lemon, papaya, pear, pineapple, pineapple/coconut, prune, raspberry, tangerine, watermelon*

**Sweeteners:** *fructose, molasses, sorghum, sugar (brown, date, raw, refined cane), syrup (barley malt, brown rice, corn, maple), saccharin, succonant*

**Condiments:** *horseradish, barbecue sauce, pesto sauce, soy sauce, spaghetti sauce, tomato sauce,* tahini, vinegar, *halva, carob,* salt, sea salt, Vege-Sal

**Salad Dressings:** *blue cheese, French, ranch, creamy Italian, creamy avocado, Thousand Island,* vinegar and oil, lemon juice and oil

**Desserts:** *custards, tapioca, puddings, pies, cakes, chocolate, desserts containing chocolate, raspberry sherbet*

**Chips:** *bean, corn (blue, white, yellow), potato*

**Beverages:** tea (*black,* Calli with stevia, *green,* herbal, Japanese, Chinese oolong); mineral water, sparkling water; *wine (red, white), sake, beer, barley malt liquor, champagne, gin, scotch, vodka, whiskey;* root beer, regular sodas

## Stressful Foods

Have no more than once a month.

**Dense Protein:** *pork, ham, sausage*
**Dairy:** *frozen yogurt, most ice creams*
**Nuts:** *commercial peanut butter*
**Grain:** *polished rice*
**Fruit:** *grapefruit*

**Vegetable Oil:** *canola*
**Sweeteners:** *saccharin, aspartame, Equal, NutraSweet, Sweet'n Low*
**Condiments:** *catsup, mustard, mayonnaise, margarine*
**Beverages:** *any drink with caffeine; diet sodas*

## Scheduling Meals

Heavy meals are never best for Spleen body types. Schedule your meals as follows:

*Breakfast:* 7–9 A.M. Light to moderate, with protein, vegetables, grain, fruit, nuts, seeds, legumes, and/or dairy. May have coffee with grain twice a week.
*Lunch:* 12–2 P.M. Moderate to heavy, with protein, vegetables, grain, fruit, nuts, seeds, legumes, and/or dairy.
*Dinner:* 5–6 P.M. Light, with protein, vegetables, grain, fruit, nuts, seeds, legumes, and/or dairy.

### Snacks (optional)
*Evening:* (9–10 P.M., 4 hours after dinner) light with fruit, vegetables, grain, protein, nuts, seeds, legumes, dairy, and/or sweets.

## Sample One-Week Menu

DAY 1
*Breakfast:* low-fat or nonfat plain or flavored yogurt
*Lunch:* angel-hair pasta w/ground turkey, peas, leeks, and tomato sauce
*Dinner:* orange roughy and green beans

DAY 2
*Breakfast:* eggs w/salsa, broccoli, and rice
*Lunch:* salmon, rice, water chestnuts, and green beans
*Dinner:* salad of spinach, bok choy, broccoli, mushrooms, and steamed new baby potatoes w/poppy seed or creamy avocado dressing

DAY 3
*Breakfast:* cottage cheese
*Lunch:* lamb, couscous, and eggplant
*Dinner:* fish tacos

DAY 4
*Breakfast:* baked potato
*Lunch:* roast chicken burritos—shredded chicken, vegetarian refried beans, cheese, red leaf lettuce, and salsa in flour tortilla

*Dinner:* baked potato and asparagus w/butter

DAY 5: CLEANSE (NO JUICE)
*Breakfast:* steamed asparagus, squash, (all) and/or raw carrots, celery
*Lunch:* steamed green beans, chard, kale, snow peas, and/or raw cabbage (any), cucumbers, celery, spinach
*Dinner:* steamed broccoli, cauliflower, spinach, and/or raw bell peppers (any), tomato

DAY 6
*Breakfast:* sunflower seeds
*Lunch:* beef chili (spicy), celery, and carrots
*Dinner:* French onion soup, vegetable soup, or lentil soup

DAY 7
*Breakfast:* mushrooms and stir-fried vegetables w/green onions, bamboo shoots, broccoli, carrots, bok choy, and bell pepper
*Lunch:* Cornish game hen, brown and wild rice, and a salad of butter lettuce and celery w/ranch dressing
*Dinner:* sweet potato and green beans

## Alternative Menus

*(Foods in parentheses are optional.)*

### Breakfast
Apple, orange, banana, or blueberries
Peanut butter and apple or banana
Cottage cheese w/pineapple
Oatmeal w/banana or apple, and sunflower seeds
Shredded wheat w/milk
Rice and broccoli
Lentils and broccoli
Eggs and low-fat Monterey Jack cheese

### Lunch
Salad of tuna, onion, celery, and eggs w/creamy Italian dressing on pumpernickel bread
Shrimp, pasta, and a salad of spinach and tomato w/sesame oil
Shrimp fried rice w/egg, mixed vegetables, and soy sauce
Trout and eggplant fried in olive oil and garlic
Chicken breast and spaghetti
Chicken, rice, and green beans
Chef's salad w/chicken—no dressing

Lamb, carrots, and green beans

Lasagna—w/ricotta cheese only—and Italian green beans

Fish chowder—white fish, tomato, and basil

## Lunch or Dinner

Chicken, baked potato, and red onions

Chicken marinated in white wine, garlic, ginger, pepper, and onion; bok choy, squash, and onions

Salad of lettuce, mushrooms, hard-boiled egg, chicken breast, and Cajun spices w/oil or herb dressing (apple for dessert)

Salad of shrimp, leaf lettuce, carrots, onions, and bok choy w/low-fat ranch or low-fat Italian dressing

Eggs, low-fat Monterey Jack cheese, and rice

Steamed yellow crookneck squash w/butter

Lamb stew and potatoes

## Dinner

Tuna, celery, romaine lettuce, and rice

Fillet of halibut, rice, and broccoli

California roll—crab, avocado, and rice wrapped in seaweed

Turkey, pasta w/butter, green beans, and carrots

Chicken or turkey, oriental rice noodles, and mixed vegetables

Sesame chicken, rice, and broccoli

Beef, squash, and beets

Mashed sweet potato w/orange juice (cinnamon)

Lentils w/rice and broccoli (artichoke hearts)

# Stomach

*The Stomach body type is symbolized by fire. Digestion requires heat, which is focused energy. Focusing their attention on what's at hand allows Stomach types to ignite their passion, enjoy the moment, and accomplish their goals.*

FAMOUS PEOPLE: Elizabeth Taylor, John Wayne, Richard Burton, Julia Roberts

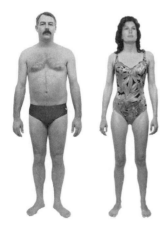

## STOMACH
### Location and Function

The stomach is located in the upper abdomen on the left side, immediately below the diaphragm and between the liver and the spleen. It functions in the process of digestion, particularly of protein.

## Psychological Profile

### Characteristic Traits

Stomach body types have a strong mental orientation to reality. Although they prefer to develop an intellectual grasp of a situation before taking action, they can be impulsive, relying on their heart or gut feelings. Once they have assimilated significant material, they'll simplify and organize it in a manner that is clear and easy to teach and understand.

In their communication, Stomach types are articulate and precise and project strength by the way they express themselves, causing people to listen when they speak. Trusting their intellect over their feelings and their own opinions over those of others can make them skeptical of new ideas and opposing beliefs. Balance comes once they have learned to listen and trust their intuition.

Stomach types have a unique way of dealing with people, tasks, and situations. They focus their total attention on them as though they were engulfing them within their energy field. This allows them to ignite their own passion and experience things more intensely. This approach is particularly apparent in the way they make love.

Fun and creativity are integral parts of the Stomach types' makeup. No matter how difficult or routine the task, Stomach types can figure out a way to make it light and enjoyable.

### Motivation

A challenge often serves to motivate Stomach types to succeed at difficult or seemingly impossible tasks. Being basically social in nature, Stomach types enjoy the public recognition that their accomplishments can bring.

Stomach types have a strong desire to please others; the responses of those around them are crucial to their sense of self-worth. They pay close attention to others' behavior and often push themselves to do something because of the way they think others will respond. Women often link their personal identity and value with their physical attractiveness.

Male Stomach types, generally, truly love women. They are inherently attracted to them but don't know how to deal with them when conflict arises. Many would prefer to leave, then come back when the stress has dissipated. Female Stomach types are generally much better at learning how to handle conflict. Men often have the need to experience many women as a way of learning about their own feminine side, particularly if they have a strong macho pattern. Women are more likely than men to commit to a relationship and stay committed, because family and particularly children are a high priority for them. While family is also a high priority for men, unless it's their main focus they do not allow it to interfere with their current goal.

## "At Worst"

Stomach types need to be in control, which can include controlling a situation to prevent anyone from being upset. The more insecure they are, the stronger the need. When others don't do what they wish, they can become impatient, irritable, or angry. Insecurity can lead to behavior that is self-centered and manipulative and to the need to be right. Strong-minded, with a strong will and definite beliefs, they can easily be forceful, stubborn, or dogmatic, skeptical of change or of new ideas that can't be physically verified.

In an attempt to lighten or release their suppressed feelings, they are apt to rely on humor or to play the role of a trickster. Unresolved emotional issues are often underneath their poking fun at people or excessive teasing.

Dealing with conflict is difficult for Stomach types; they either blame themselves or deny any responsibility whatsoever. Their tendency is to avoid the issue by becoming evasive, burying themselves in work, leaving relationships, or going where they can be alone, often comforting or nurturing themselves in a destructive manner. They are prone to filling themselves with food, drugs, or alcohol to insulate against feelings of emptiness and deprivation. Not being able to "stomach" conflict, they link emotional fulfillment with feeling full.

Passionate by nature, Stomach types often use sex as a way of validating themselves, associating their ability to attract the opposite sex with their self-worth. Their insecurities often lead to problems with jealousy.

When their self-esteem is low, Stomach types can be quite critical of themselves and often rate their performance lower than deserved. Being perfectionists, they are never satisfied with their own achievements, particularly when their sense of self-worth is dependent on the way they think others perceive them.

## "At Best"

Stomach types have a unique ability to encompass someone with their attention. Being the center of their attention gives others the feeling of being unconditionally loved. Coupled with their sensitivity and desire to please, this ability makes Stomach types ideal friends or lovers. With a good sense of humor and a gregarious nature, they can be fun to be around.

When they direct their passion, strong will, determination, and effort, they have a winning combination. This is particularly apparent when expressed onstage in music or dance. Because they also have the ability to activate others' passion and appreciation, they make excellent speakers or performers.

When wholeheartedly devoting themselves to their endeavors, Stomach types can be imaginative and enterprising. When they feel universally supported, they are open to new experiences, ideas, and emotions and able to adapt to whatever life brings. This is particularly evident when dealing with confrontation, as they handle it in a positive, constructive manner through discussion and respect (especially with the opposite sex).

Once Stomach types have learned to listen to everything around them (including their own inner voice, God, their feelings, their body, and both their masculine and their feminine sides), they develop inner strength, validate themselves, and become secure within themselves. From here they can evaluate a situation according to their inner truth rather than relying on outside appearances, partial information, or assumptions. This is when they are able to enjoy the

---

### RECOMMENDED EXERCISE

Aerobic exercise enhances feelings of well-being for Stomach body types. Emotionally beneficial, it releases stress, lifts depression, and can be a means of personal expression. Stomach types are naturally excellent dancers. Water skiing, surfing, swimming, in-line skating, bicycling, walking, Callanetics, rebounding, kick-boxing, and weight lifting are some exercises that are good for the vascular system. This body type easily builds muscle and responds well to heavy exercise, especially when balanced with flexibility exercise like stretching and yoga.

moment completely, giving it their all while staying in balance. This is the essence of abundance.

## Dietary Profile

### Main Focus

- Focus on protein and vegetables.
- Avoid fruit in the morning.
- Exercise can release stress as long as it is fun.

### Dietary Emphasis

- From 25 to 35 percent of your calories are to come from fat.
- Best fat sources: all dense protein, including fish (especially tuna) and eggs, and butter.
- From 25 to 40 percent of your calories are to come from protein.
- From 25 to 35 percent of your calories are to come from dense protein.
- Best sources of the three amino acids threonine, isoleucine, and cystine: turkey, chicken, and eggs.
- Caloric intake: 1,500 to 1,800 calories a day for women and 1,700 to 2,000 calories a day for men. If you are engaging in intense exercise (competition type) or hard labor, increase calories.
- Drink a minimum of 64 ounces of water a day. Drink water before and after meals, not with meals.
- Occasional desserts are best as an evening snack.
- Avoid spicy foods when your digestive system is stressed or sensitive.
- Salads are best at dinner, before or with the main course.
- Have a light breakfast.
- Have a moderate lunch, emphasizing fish and vegetables.
- Have a heavier dinner.

### For Weight Loss

- Fat: 20 to 30 percent of daily calories.
- When fat intake falls below 20 percent, weight loss is inhibited.
- Dense protein: 25 to 35 percent of daily calories.
- Avoid fruit.
- Restrict bread.
- Potatoes are good as long as you rotate varieties.

- Reduce dairy products.
- Eliminate caffeine.
- Avoid alcohol; it inhibits weight loss.
- Avoid snacking.
- Exercise daily.
- Be sure to eat adequately during the day.

### For Weight Gain

- Fat: 25 to 40 percent of daily calories.
- Dense protein: 25 to 35 percent of daily calories.
- Increase food quantity.

## Healthy Foods List

There is no need to sacrifice delicious and filling foods to maintain a healthy Stomach body type. The following lists will help you focus on foods that support your health, and avoid foods that can stress your system.

*You'll notice that some foods are printed in italics; these foods take more energy to assimilate and could be ones you will want to avoid when you are in a sensitive state due to any physical or emotional stresses.*

Be sure to read Chapter 3, "Implementing the Body Type Diet," for lots of important information about how to use these many foods to gain their full benefit.

### Ultra-Support Foods

Foods to include in 3 to 7 meals a week, listed by category.

**Dense Protein:** beef, beef broth, beef liver, buffalo, lamb, *pork,* bacon, *ham, sausage;* chicken, chicken broth, chicken livers, Cornish game hen, duck, turkey; anchovy, bass, bonita, cod, flounder, haddock, halibut, herring, mahimahi, perch, orange roughy, salmon, sardines, shark, red snapper, sole,

---

**RECOMMENDED CUISINE**

Home-style cooking, Italian, Mexican, Moroccan, Chinese, Irish, Hungarian.

swordfish, tuna; abalone, eel, lobster, mussels, octo-pus, scallops, shrimp; eggs

**Dairy:** milk (whole, 2%, low fat, nonfat, raw), butter

**Cheese:** ricotta

**Grains:** barley, corn, corn grits, corn tortillas, cous-cous, popcorn, wild rice, *whole wheat, wheat bran, wheat germ,* shredded wheat, breads (corn, *whole wheat*), whole wheat crackers, pasta, udon noodles, Chinese rice noodles, *cream of wheat*

**Vegetables:** *artichokes,* avocados, cilantro, peas, snow pea pods, radishes (red, white), spinach, tomatoes, zucchini

**Fruits:** *bananas,* grapes (black, green, red), papayas, pineapples, plums (black, purple, red), raspberries, watermelons

**Sweetener:** stevia

**Condiments:** mustard, salt, sea salt

**Beverages:** (caffeine once a day) tea (*black, green,* herbal, Japanese, Chinese oolong); mineral water, sparkling water; *root beer*

## Basic Support Foods

Foods to include in 1 to 2 meals a week.

**Dense Protein:** veal, venison, organ meats (heart, brain); catfish, mackerel, trout; calamari (squid), clams, crab, oysters

**Dairy:** goat's milk, half-and-half, sweet cream, sour cream, kefir, plain or flavored yogurt, *frozen yogurt,* ice cream (Ben & Jerry's, Dreyer's, Swensen's)

**Cheese:** American, blue, Brie, Camembert, cheddar, Colby, cottage, cream, Edam, feta, goat, Gouda, kefir, Limburger, Monterey Jack, mozzarella, Muenster, Parmesan, Romano, Swiss

**Nuts and Seeds:** almonds, almond butter, Brazils, cashews, cashew butter, hazelnuts, macadamias, macadamia butter, peanuts, peanut butter, pecans, pine nuts, pistachios, walnuts (black, English), water chestnuts; seeds (caraway, pumpkin, sesame, sunflower), sesame seed butter, sunflower seed but-ter

**Legumes:** beans (adzuki, black, garbanzo, kidney, Great Northern, lima, navy, pinto, red, soy), lentils, black-eyed peas, split peas; hummus; miso, soy milk, tofu

**Grains:** amaranth, buckwheat, hominy grits, millet, *oats, oat bran, oat bran flakes,* quinoa, rice (brown or white basmati, long or short grain brown, Japanese), rice bran, rice cakes, rye, triticale, refined wheat flour, flour tortillas, breads (corn/rye, French, garlic, Italian, *multigrain, oat,* rice, rye, *seven-grain,* sourdough, sprouted grain, white), bagels, croissants, English muffins, crackers (*oat,* rye, saltines), cream of rice, cream of rye

**Vegetables:** *arugula, asparagus,* bamboo shoots, beans (green, yellow wax), beets, bok choy, broc-coflower, broccoli, brussels sprouts, cabbage (green, napa, red), carrots, cauliflower, celery, corn, cucumbers, eggplant, *garlic,* greens (beet, collard, mustard, turnip), hominy, jicama, kale, kohlrabi, leeks, lettuce (Boston, butter, endive, iceberg, red leaf, romaine), mushrooms, okra, olives, onions (chives, brown, green, red, Vidalia, white, yellow), parsnips, bell peppers, chili peppers, pimientos, potatoes (purple, red, russet, White Rose, Yukon Gold), pumpkins, daikon radishes, rutabaga, sauer-kraut, seaweed (arame, dulse, nori, wakame), shal-lots, sprouts (alfalfa, clover, mung bean, radish, sunflower), squash (acorn, banana, butternut, yel-low [summer], spaghetti), sweet potatoes, Swiss chard, turnips, *watercress,* yams

**Vegetable Juices:** carrot, carrot/celery, celery, spinach, tomato, V-8

**Fruits:** apples (Golden or Red Delicious, Granny Smith, Jonathan, McIntosh, Pippin, Rome Beauty), apricots, berries (blackberries, blueberries, boysen-berries, cranberries, gooseberries, strawberries), dates, figs, grapefruit (white, red), guavas, kiwi, kumquats, lemons, limes, loquats, mangoes, melons (cantaloupe, *casaba, Crenshaw, honeydew*), nec-tarines, oranges, peaches, pears, persimmons, pomegranates, prunes, raisins, rhubarb, tangelos, tangerines

**Fruit Juices:** apple, apple cider, apple/apricot, apri-cot, black cherry, red cherry, cranapple, cranberry, grape (red, purple, white), grapefruit, guava, lemon, orange, papaya, pear, pineapple, pineap-ple/coconut, prune, tangerine, watermelon

**Vegetable Oils:** *all-blend, almond, avocado, corn, flaxseed, olive, peanut, safflower,* sesame, *sunflower*

**Sweeteners:** *fructose, honey, molasses, sorghum, sugar (brown, date, raw, refined cane), syrup (bar-ley malt, brown rice, corn, maple), saccharin, suc-conant*

**Condiments:** *catsup (cinnamon, mint), horseradish, barbecue sauce, pesto sauce, soy sauce, salsa, tahini, vinegar,* Vege-Sal

**Salad Dressings:** *blue cheese, French, ranch, creamy Italian, creamy avocado, Thousand Island,* vinegar and oil, lemon juice and oil

**Desserts:** *custards, tapioca, puddings, pies, cakes,*

*chocolate, desserts containing chocolate, sherbet (orange, raspberry)*
**Chips:** bean, corn (blue, white, yellow), potato
**Beverages:** *coffee (decaffeinated, regular); wine (red, white), sake, beer, barley malt liquor, champagne, gin, scotch, vodka, whiskey; regular sodas*

## Stressful Foods

Have no more than once a month.

**Dairy:** *buttermilk, most ice creams*
**Vegetables:** *kelp, parsley*
**Vegetable Juices:** *parsley*
**Fruits:** *cherries, coconut*
**Vegetable Oils:** *canola, soy*
**Sweeteners:** *aspartame, Equal, NutraSweet, Sweet'n Low*
**Condiments:** *mayonnaise, margarine*
**Beverages:** *diet sodas*

## Scheduling Meals

### Healthy

Schedule your meals as follows:

*Breakfast:* 5–9 A.M. Light to moderate, with protein and/or grain. May include dairy, nuts, seeds, legumes, and/or vegetables. Avoid fruit.
*Lunch:* 11 A.M.–2 P.M. Moderate to heavy, with protein, grain, vegetables, legumes, dairy, nuts, seeds, and/or fruit.
*Dinner:* 5–9 P.M. Moderate to heavy, with protein, grain, vegetables, legumes, dairy, nuts, seeds, and/or fruit.

### Snacks (optional)
*Midmorning:* (10:30 A.M.) protein, grain, vegetables
*Midafternoon:* fruit, vegetables, grain, protein, dairy, nuts, seeds, sweets
*Evening:* (10 P.M.–2 A.M.) fruit, grain, vegetables, protein, nuts, seeds, dairy, sweets

### Sensitive

You may have sugar with a large meal that includes quality protein at either lunch or dinner but not at both meals in the same day. You can handle sugar twice a week but not for an evening snack. Avoid fruits for lunch and dinner.

## Sample One-Week Menu

DAY 1
*Breakfast:* plain yogurt
*Lunch:* salmon and asparagus
*Dinner:* Roasted chicken, baked russet potato, and a salad of endive, butter lettuce, radishes, and bell peppers

DAY 2
*Breakfast:* eggs and sourdough toast
*Lunch:* tuna fillet, broccoli, and zucchini
*Dinner:* chicken, rice, and a green salad w/avocado and sunflower seeds

DAY 3
*Breakfast:* corn flakes w/milk or soy milk
*Lunch:* turkey, White Rose potato w/gravy, and corn
*Dinner:* orange roughy, pasta, olive oil, broccoli, and a spinach salad

DAY 4
*Breakfast:* carrots or carrot juice
*Lunch:* beef stew
*Dinner:* halibut or red snapper and green beans

DAY 5: CLEANSE
*Breakfast:* steamed asparagus or zucchini or raw carrots and celery and/or juice of carrot/celery/(spinach)
*Lunch:* steamed beets, cauliflower, chard, greens (beet, collard, mustard, turnip) sweet potato or squash (all), and/or raw green salad with cooked beets, carrots, and/or juice of carrot/celery/spinach, and/or apple, pear, pineapple
*Dinner:* steamed green beans, broccoli, cauliflower, asparagus, zucchini, and/or raw celery, cucumbers, jicama, lettuce, spinach, tomato and/or apple, pear, cantaloupe, watermelon, and/or juice of carrot/celery (spinach)

DAY 6
*Breakfast:* omelette w/avocado
*Lunch:* turkey vegetable soup
*Dinner:* Cornish game hen and wild rice w/almonds, mushrooms, and onions

DAY 7
*Breakfast:* corn tortilla w/avocado
*Lunch:* fish taco—mackerel or whitefish, onions, tomatoes, and romaine lettuce

*Dinner:* rack of lamb or lamb roast, red potato, and peas

## Alternative Menus

*(Foods in parentheses are optional.)*

### Breakfast
Bran cereal w/milk
Eggs and hash browns
Cream of wheat w/milk
Cream of rice w/milk
Amaranth and corn flakes or quinoa
Rye and rice cereal and ground flaxseed
Oat bran muffin w/wheat flakes and low-fat milk
Brown rice and beans
Rice and chicken
Scrambled eggs w/spinach

### Lunch
Chinese stir-fry with snow pea pods, asparagus, bamboo shoots, bok choy, carrots, celery, and green onions
Eggs and broccoli
Lentils, rice, spinach, and onions
Steamed clams, kale, basmati rice, and cooked spinach
Tuna and avocado (rye toast or crackers)
Lamb and cooked or raw carrots
Beef and zucchini

Chicken breast, steamed carrots, and broccoli or potato
Steamed greens, broccoli, and a salad of lettuce w/flaxseed oil

### Lunch or Dinner
Crab on romaine lettuce and steamed vegetables
Steak and new red potatoes
Trout and zucchini (yellow squash)
Salmon and asparagus (rice)
Chicken primavera
Ham, potato, and green beans
Rack of lamb or lamb roast, red potato, carrots, and broccoli
Spinach salad w/eggs
Split pea soup w/ham

### Dinner
Salmon, lima beans, and carrots
Halibut, kale, and collards
Chicken, broccoli, and cauliflower
Almond chicken
Turkey, chicken, or fish, green beans, zucchini, and/or mushrooms
Beef tamales
Roast beef, potatoes, and broccoli (green beans and/or squash and/or cauliflower)
Pasta w/tomato sauce and broccoli, zucchini, and/or peppers

# Thalamus

*The Thalamus body type is symbolized by a satellite dish. Collecting and evaluating information before passing it on, Thalamus types are open to new ideas and sensitive to vibrations. Music is essential to them and can readily shift their mood.*

FAMOUS PEOPLE: Prince Charles, Nicole Kidman, Helen Hunt, Patrick Swayze

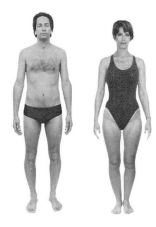

## THALAMUS
### Location and Function

The thalamus is located in the center of the brain base, between the hypothalamus and the pineal glands. It is a relay center passing sensory impulses to the cerebral cortex.

## Psychological Profile

### Characteristic Traits

Thalamus types are characterized by sensitivity to and awareness of their physical and emotional surroundings. They listen intently to what is going on around them and notice things that others miss, often simply storing the information in their well-organized memory banks.

Their superb organizational skills are reflected in their surroundings. They may even go so far as to have a filing cabinet in their bedroom to keep track of personal papers, articles, and reference material that could be needed at some future date.

Oriented to reality through the mind, they deliberate carefully before arriving at a clear decision about how to solve a problem. They learn easily and enjoy studying subjects that interest them. Investigative and analytical, they possess a high degree of intellectual curiosity and enjoy conversations that allow them to express the depth of their thoughts.

Curious and observant, Thalamus types are fairly adventurous and intrigued by the prospect of exploring new horizons. However, their daring is tempered by caution, and they have a "look before you leap" attitude. They are generally people of substance and depth who feel it's important to select activities and endeavors that are worthwhile; this produces their greatest high and most rewarding experiences.

### Motivation

Thalamus types have strong, active, inquiring minds and relate to life by understanding how things work and why they are the way they are. Their ability to evaluate information and their highly developed powers of observation are their greatest strengths. They have an innate feeling that if they know what is going on and why, they will be safe and can feel secure.

Initially Thalamus types are open and receptive, freely taking in new information without judging or censoring it. The next stage is a thorough, skeptical mental analysis, and then the decision. When they rely too heavily on their mind, they judge and categorize everything as black or white, the skeptical side begins to dominate, and they get caught in the mental process or in overanalysis. It's when they are not in touch with their feelings or do not trust their intuition that the decision process can become blocked. The greater their insecurity, the greater their need to gather every possible piece of information, evaluate and reevaluate all the data, constantly question, and even repeatedly ask the same question to make sure everything that is done is done perfectly. They procrastinate when they have a need for clarity, particularly when situations are vague or complicated.

Thalamus types are extremely sensitive to vibrations, particularly sound, and their hearing is often unusually acute. Music is particularly important, as it provides a direct link to their emotions. When stressed, Thalamus types disconnect emotionally, and music is generally the quickest way for them to reconnect and let go of stress. Music allows them to shift their strong mental focus to more relaxing, nurturing, or creative modes. Music can not only calm and balance them, but also stimulate or energize them.

## "At Worst"

When Thalamus types get too caught up in details, they become mentally tense and can be effectively immobilized (paralysis of analysis) or just lose their ability to progress at a satisfactory rate. Carried to the extreme, their caution and attentiveness become nitpicky. Sometimes they swing to the opposite extreme and throw caution to the wind, becoming impatient and inattentive or even impulsive and reckless. When they hold back from saying something that needs to be said (because they are wary of the consequences), they usually wind up having an outburst later from having stifled their emotions.

Thalamus types can disconnect from their body, emotions, and/or inner knowing by ignoring pain, pushing their body, failing to heed warning signs, or not paying attention to where they are going. Getting sidetracked or circling around the problem without ever directly dealing with it is a way of not listening to themselves and their inner knowing. Another form of escape is to get caught in fantasy, going over and over every possible scenario, despite realizing that this is a waste of time and energy.

Supercritical of themselves, Thalamus types struggle with low self-esteem and are very susceptible to the "I'm not good enough" syndrome. Their lack of self-confidence can cause paralysis to the point where they don't feel comfortable making major decisions or taking action, so they simply procrastinate, letting life or others set their course.

At their worst, Thalamus types rely so heavily on the judgment and opinions of others, particularly authority figures, that they become immobilized. Fear of failure and lack of courage can cause them to spend so much time in research that they lose their effectiveness and never quite accomplish what they set out to achieve. Constantly seeking reassurance and support, they can become demanding and draining to those around them.

## "At Best"

Thalamus types are attentive to details and can handle technical work competently. They have excellent organizational skills, strive for excellence, and work well independently, preferring to work at their own pace. They examine a new pursuit carefully before actually embarking on it. They are dependable, and once a project is started, they maintain good momentum and can sustain their energy until the job is successfully completed.

Thalamus types are basically responsible and reliable, with a strong sense of loyalty. They have a sensitive nature and are relatively mild-mannered and easygoing, tending to internalize anger rather than express it directly. In relationships they are gentle, giving, and nurturing. Having a strong social nature, they tend to be patient, compassionate, tactful, and sympathetic to others, placing a higher value on people than on tasks.

When in tune with themselves, Thalamus types are self-reliant and take excellent care of themselves. They are generally aware of their dietary and exercise needs and have the motivation and discipline to follow through on an appropriate health program.

Thoughtful and observant of the world around them, Thalamus types are also reflective about themselves. The more they've learned to accept and respect

---

### RECOMMENDED EXERCISE

Exercise is beneficial to Thalamus types because it calms the mind. Ideally, they should get some exercise daily, even if only for a few minutes scattered throughout the day. Best activities include walking, tennis, swimming, and Pilates. Almost all other exercise, including dance, racquetball, and volleyball, is acceptable. Jogging and running are poor choices. Being out in nature provides a sense of freedom. Music allows for connection with body and emotions.

themselves through personal growth, the more they are willing to confront their own mistakes, take responsibility for some of the difficult situations they find themselves in, and make the changes they need to make. Being open-minded and adaptable, they are able to challenge their own behavior and beliefs and change what no longer serves them.

## Dietary Profile

### Main Focus

- ▶ Eat seeds, beans, vegetables, and protein.
- ▶ Get adequate protein and fats to maintain energy.
- ▶ Include fruit only at breakfast and as an evening snack.
- ▶ Frequent meals support energy.

### Dietary Emphasis

- ▶ From 20 to 35 percent of your calories are to come from fats.
- ▶ Best fat sources: seeds (sunflower, pumpkin, and sesame, including sesame tahini), dense protein (chicken, turkey, eggs, fish, and beef), and butter.
- ▶ From 20 to 40 percent of your calories are to come from protein.
- ▶ From 10 to 30 percent of your calories are to come from dense protein.
- ▶ Best sources of the three amino acids threonine, isoleucine, and cystine: beef and sesame, sunflower, and pumpkin seeds.
- ▶ Caloric intake: 1,500 to 1,800 calories a day for women and 1,700 to 2,000 calories a day for men. If you are engaging in intense exercise (competition type) or hard labor, increase calories.
- ▶ Drink a minimum of 64 ounces of water a day. Drink water before and after meals, not with meals.
- ▶ Occasional desserts are best as an evening snack.
- ▶ Avoid eating potato or squash with dense protein.
- ▶ Eat more cooked than raw vegetables.

### For Weight Loss

- ▶ Fat: 25 to 40 percent of daily calories.
- ▶ When fat intake falls below 15 percent, weight loss is inhibited.
- ▶ Dense protein: 20 to 30 percent of daily calories.
- ▶ Eliminate refined sugar, alcohol, honey, and all artificial sweeteners.

---

> **RECOMMENDED CUISINE**
>
> Frequently: Mexican, Thai, seafood. Moderately: Italian, Middle Eastern, Chinese.

- ▶ Avoid fruit juice.
- ▶ Minimize breads and butter.
- ▶ Midmorning and midafternoon snacks may be included.

### For Weight Gain

- ▶ Fat: 25 to 40 percent of daily calories.
- ▶ Dense protein: 25 to 30 percent of daily calories.
- ▶ Increase food intake.
- ▶ Include snacks.

## Healthy Foods List

There is no need to sacrifice delicious and filling foods to maintain a healthy Thalamus body type. The following lists will help you focus on foods that support your health, and avoid foods that can stress your system.

*You'll notice that some foods are printed in italics; these foods should be avoided when you are in a sensitive state due to any physical or emotional stresses.*

Be sure to read Chapter 3, "Implementing the Body Type Diet," for lots of important information about how to use these many foods to gain their full benefit.

### Ultra-Support Foods

Foods to include in 3 to 7 meals a week, listed by category.

**Dense Protein:** beef, beef broth, beef liver, buffalo; chicken, chicken broth, chicken livers, Cornish game hen, turkey; anchovy, bonita, catfish, flounder, haddock, herring, perch, trout; clams, eel, lobsters, octopus, shrimp

**Dairy:** goat's milk, buttermilk, yogurt (all), butter

**Cheese:** Colby, Monterey Jack, Muenster, Romano, Swiss

**Nuts and Seeds:** Brazils, cashews (raw, roasted), cashew butter, macadamia/cashew butter, hazelnuts, *peanuts* (*raw, roasted*), pine nuts (raw, roasted), walnuts (black, English), water chestnuts, nut milks; raw or roasted seeds (caraway, pumpkin, sesame, sunflower), sesame seed butter, sunflower seed butter

**Legumes:** beans (adzuki, black, garbanzo, Great Northern, kidney, *lima,* navy, pinto, red, soy), black-eyed peas, split peas

**Grains:** blue corn, blue corn tortilla, oats, oat muffins, oat pancakes, rice (white or brown basmati, Japanese), rye, sprouted grains, breads (oat, rye [without wheat], sprouted rye, sprouted wheat), granola

**Vegetables:** artichokes, bamboo shoots, beans (green, yellow wax), bok choy, *broccoli,* brussels sprouts, cabbage (green, napa, red), carrots, cauliflower, celery, eggplant, *garlic,* peas, pumpkin, *spinach,* squash (acorn, banana, butternut, spaghetti, zucchini), Swiss chard, tomatoes (canned, hothouse, vine-ripened), turnips

**Fruits:** bananas, berries (blackberries, raspberries, strawberries), grapes (black, green, red), kiwi, oranges, peaches

**Fruit Juices:** cranapple, pineapple/coconut

**Vegetable Oils:** almond, avocado, canola, corn, olive, safflower, sesame, soy, sunflower

**Sweetener:** stevia

**Condiments:** mustard, Hain safflower mayonnaise, garlic powder

**Chips:** blue corn

**Beverage:** Constant Comment tea

## Basic Support Foods

Foods to include in 1 to 2 meals a week.

**Dense Protein:** ham, pork, lamb, veal, venison, organ meats (heart, brain); duck; bass, cod, halibut, mackerel, mahimahi, orange roughy, salmon, *sardines,* shark, red snapper, sole, swordfish, tuna; abalone, *calamari* (*squid*), crab, mussels, scallops; eggs

**Dairy:** raw milk, half-and-half, sweet cream, sour cream, kefir, frozen yogurt, *ice cream* (Ben & Jerry's, Dreyer's, Swensen's)

**Cheese:** American, blue, Brie, Camembert, cheddar, cottage, *cream,* Edam, feta, Gouda, kefir, Limburger, mozarella, Parmesan, ricotta

**Nuts and Seeds:** coconut, macadamias (raw, roasted), macadamia butter, pecans, pistachios, *peanut butter*

**Legumes:** hummus; *miso,* soy milk, tofu

**Grains:** amaranth, barley, buckwheat, corn, corn grits, corn tortillas, couscous, hominy grits, millet, popcorn, quinoa, rice (long or short grain brown, wild), rice bran, rice cakes, triticale, whole wheat, wheat bran, wheat germ, refined wheat flour, flour tortillas, breads (corn, corn/rye, *French,* garlic, *Italian,* kamut, *multigrain,* potato, Poulsbo, rice, *seven-grain, sourdough,* sprouted grain, *white, whole wheat*), bagels, croissants, English muffins, crackers (oat, rye, saltines, wheat), pretzels, pasta, udon noodles, Chinese rice noodles, cream of rice, cream of rye, cream of wheat

**Vegetables:** *arugula,* asparagus, *avocados,* beets, broccoflower, cilantro, *corn, cucumbers,* greens (beet, collard, mustard, turnip), hominy, jicama, kale, kohlrabi, leeks, lettuce (Boston, butter, endive, iceberg, red leaf, romaine), mushrooms, okra, olives (green, ripe), onions (chives, brown, green, red, Vidalia, white, yellow), parsley, parsnips, snow pea pods, bell peppers (green, red, yellow), mild chili peppers, pimientos, potatoes (purple, red, *russet,* White Rose, Yukon Gold), radishes, daikon radishes, rutabaga, sauerkraut, seaweed (arame, dulse, kelp, nori, wakame), shallots, yellow (summer) squash, sprouts (alfalfa, clover, mung bean, radish, sunflower), sweet potatoes, *watercress,* yams

**Vegetable Juices:** carrot, carrot/celery, celery, parsley, spinach, tomato, V-8

**Fruits:** apples (Golden or Red Delicious, Granny Smith, Jonathan, McIntosh, Pippin, Rome Beauty), apricots, berries (blueberries, boysenberries, cranberries, gooseberries), cherries, dates, figs (fresh, dried), grapefruit (white, red), guavas, kumquats, lemons, limes, loquats, mangoes, melons (cantaloupe, casaba, Crenshaw, honeydew, watermelon), nectarines, papayas, pears, persimmons, pineapples, plums (black, purple, red), pomegranates, prunes, raisins, rhubarb, tangelos, tangerines

**Fruit Juices:** apple, apple cider, apple/apricot, apricot, black cherry, red cherry, cranberry, grape (purple, red, white), grapefruit, guava, *lemon,* orange, papaya, pear, pineapple, prune, raspberry, tangerine, watermelon

**Vegetable Oils:** all-blend, flaxseed, peanut

**Sweeteners:** *fructose, honey, molasses, sorghum, sugar* (*brown, date, raw, refined cane*), *syrup* (*barley malt, brown rice, corn, maple*), *saccharin, aspartame, Equal, NutraSweet, Sweet'n Low, succonant*

**Condiments:** *horseradish, barbecue sauce, pesto sauce, soy sauce,* salsa, tahini, *tamari,* vinegar, salt, sea salt, Vege-Sal, curry, Italian seasoning

**Salad Dressings:** *blue cheese, French, ranch, creamy Italian, creamy avocado, Thousand Island,* vinegar and oil, lemon juice and oil

**Desserts:** custards, tapioca, puddings, pies, cakes, chocolate, desserts containing chocolate, sherbet (orange, raspberry)

**Chips:** bean, corn (white, yellow), potato

**Beverages:** *coffee;* tea (*black, green,* herbal, Japanese, Chinese oolong); mineral water, sparkling water, lemonade; *red wine, sake, barley malt liquor, champagne, gin, scotch, vodka, whiskey; root beer, regular sodas*

## Stressful Foods

Have no more than once a month.

**Dense Protein:** *bacon, sausage; oysters*

**Dairy:** *pasteurized milk (whole, 2%, low fat, nonfat), most ice creams*

**Nuts and Seeds:** *almonds (raw, roasted), almond butter*

**Legumes:** *lentils*

**Grains:** *almond croissant*

**Condiments:** *catsup, mayonnaise, margarine, hot chili peppers*

**Beverages:** *white wine, diet soda*

# Scheduling Meals

Thalamus body types can enjoy a varied food intake throughout the day. Schedule your meals as follows:

*Breakfast:* 8–9 A.M. Light to moderate, with light protein such as eggs, fruit, grain, nuts, seeds, dairy, vegetables, and/or legumes.

*Lunch:* 12–2 P.M. Moderate to heavy, with protein, vegetables, legumes, nuts, seeds, grain, and/or dairy. Avoid fruit.

*Dinner:* 6–8 P.M. Moderate, with protein, vegetables, grain, legumes, nuts, seeds, and/or dairy. Avoid fruit.

## Snacks (optional)

*Midmorning:* (10:30–11 A.M.) nuts, seeds, grain, dairy, vegetables

*Midafternoon:* (4–5 P.M.) protein, grain, vegetables, nuts, seeds, dairy

*Evening:* (9–12 P.M.) fruit, protein, grain, vegetables, nuts, seeds, dairy, legumes, sweets

# Sample One-Week Menu

DAY 1

*Breakfast:* roasted sunflower seeds or blueberries
*Lunch:* chicken breast, Spanish rice, and green beans
*Snack:* celery w/cashew butter
*Dinner:* kefir cheese

DAY 2

*Breakfast:* oatmeal w/bananas or peaches
*Lunch:* beef steak, jicama, and globe artichoke
*Dinner:* sushi, fillet of halibut, or snapper and green salad w/sprouts and seeds

DAY 3

*Breakfast:* scrambled eggs w/onions
*Snack:* celery w/sesame seed butter
*Lunch:* lamb, green beans, and rice
*Snack:* walnuts
*Dinner:* salad of spinach, beets, sunflower seeds, and green or red onions w/balsamic dressing

DAY 4

*Breakfast:* Granny Smith apple and hazelnuts
*Lunch:* green pepper stuffed w/rice and beef, lamb, chicken, or turkey
*Snack:* popcorn
*Dinner:* orange roughy, rice, and broccoli

DAY 5: CLEANSE

*Breakfast:* (ginger tea) (peppermint in water) soaked pumpkin seeds
*Lunch:* steamed kale, Swiss chard, yellow squash, spinach, and/or raw carrots, celery, spinach, and/or juice of carrots/celery/spinach
*Dinner:* steamed broccoli, cauliflower, (onions) and/or kale, carrots, and/or juice of carrot/celery/spinach

DAY 6

*Breakfast:* acorn or banana squash w/butter
*Snack:* pumpkin seeds
*Lunch:* turkey, rice, cranberry sauce, and broccoli
*Dinner:* mushroom barley soup, rice, and carrots

DAY 7

*Breakfast:* split pea soup
*Snack:* sunflower seeds
*Lunch:* sea bass or red snapper, rice, and asparagus
*Dinner:* Cornish game hen, spinach, and artichoke salad w/ranch dressing

## Alternative Menus

*(Foods in parentheses may be omitted.)*

### Breakfast
Banana or peaches
Strawberries and rice—any variety
Plantains (tahini)
Mango and kiwi
Papaya and pecan
Papaya and kefir cheese
Eggs, rice, and peas
Egg drop soup, snow pea pods, and steamed rice
Steamed spinach, carrots, and tofu
Yams and black walnuts

### Lunch
Beef steak, broccoli, and couscous
Baked chicken, carrots, celery, onions, and rice
Chicken, rice, and coleslaw or brussels sprouts, asparagus, or peas
Tuna, pasta, and peas
Stir-fried broccoli, bamboo shoots, green beans, bok choy, carrots, celery, and green onions, and basmati rice w/soy sauce
Cashew chicken and steamed rice

### Dinner
Lentil soup
Split pea soup
Potato, eggplant, cilantro, and kefir cheese
Chicken and baked beans or lima beans
Lamb, parsnips, and broccoli
Fish and cauliflower (rice or pasta)
Tuna, noodles, and zucchini or green beans
Broccoli, yellow squash, okra, and onion
Spinach and artichoke noodles (tofu)
Turkey and asparagus (spinach salad, pasta, or celery)

# Thymus

*The Thymus body type is symbolized by a shield. Shielded from forces that could cause change, protected environments are stable and constant. Resisting change of any kind, Thymus types are loyal and responsible, committed to keeping their environment constant.*

FAMOUS PEOPLE: Clint Eastwood, Sharon Stone, Jerry Hall, Matthew Perry

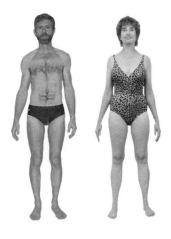

## THYMUS
### Location and Function

The thymus is located in the upper middle of the chest, below the thyroid gland and above the heart. It produces lymphocytes and antibodies for the immune system.

## Psychological Profile

### Characteristic Traits

Thymus body types are particularly strong-willed, forceful, and determined. Being very practical, they like things they can see and touch and that preferably have been proven over time. Thymus types are most comfortable when their lives are steady and constant, the only changes being those they instigate.

Even though Thymus types tend to view things more from their heads than their hearts, they are not especially analytical in their approach to problem solving. Their tendency is to take a broad overview, dive into a project, and deal with any difficulties as they arise—generally by trying to bulldoze their way through. Their basic attitude toward work is to take things as they come and delegate the details whenever possible.

Known for having particularly high standards and high expectations, especially of themselves, Thymus types are often idealistic perfectionists. They like to be in charge, and often control through their energy or presence. Generally tall, their size alone is often intimidating to people. Most have an extraordinarily strong desire to be the center of attention and expect people to accommodate them automatically.

### Motivation

The primary concern of Thymus body types is to protect themselves and those they care about. In their pursuit of self-protection, they strongly embrace the tried and true and the well established. They tend to see everything as either black or white, one way or the other, with little consideration for in-betweens, degrees, shades, probabilities, or compromises.

They can be very firm about seeing or doing things one way, and that is usually their way. Because of their single-minded intensity, giving up their own preferences or compromising can sometimes be very challenging. Thinking things through requires an effort, so they often bypass the process once they have dichotomized something as right or wrong and put anything similar into these categories.

Thymus types usually respond to anything new in a negative way, at least initially, as they feel threatened by proposed changes. Their motivation for change is primarily physical pain, and because they are inclined to suppress their emotions, they often realize a change is needed only because of their physical condition.

Since their nature is to be in control, they feel they should be able to handle everything. When things don't work as they had planned, their tendency is to blame others. Being more aware of their outside environment than their internal feelings, they find it difficult to understand themselves and others. Relationships are challenging, as they have a strong need to control in order to feel secure.

Emotional stimulation produces a sense of power (even if destructive), heightening the feeling of being alive and allowing for a greater energy flow. Manifestation of energy in a negative manner, however, makes them prone to mistakes. Unresolved emotional turmoil causes increasing irritability, intensifies areas of negativity, and results in anything from inadvertent self-inflicted injury to self-sabotage.

## "At Worst"

Thymus types are the epitome of judgment, control, prejudice, and rigidity. Their judgments are quick and fixed, and the ones they judge most harshly are themselves. Their thinking is extremely rigid with a lot of "shoulds" and expectations of an ideal world. With a strong need to be the best, Thymus types expect perfection in themselves and everything and everyone around them. Demanding perfection in this lifetime, and feeling they know best, they usually react with anger or defensiveness when things don't go their way. When there's nothing more that can be done, they internalize their anger and pout or become depressed.

Thymus types are caught in a double bind through judging everyone as better or less than themselves. If they judge a person as better than themselves, they feel inferior and either beat themselves up or tear down the other person. If they judge a person as less than themselves, they expect that person to serve them. Since they cannot relate to anyone on an equal basis, their expectations are never met and they drive people away, reinforcing their deep-seated abandonment issues.

More demanding than giving of attention, they usually want to be center stage. If an activity or event is not their show, they usually don't want to play. Thymus men, more than Thymus women, often demand attention, and if they don't get what they want, they withdraw and pout or become even more forceful and direct and take over the situation. Thymus women tend to be more subtle and control their environment by trying to control others' lives in

the guise of "this is what is best for you" or by blocking their own emotions.

## "At Best"

Thymus types are stable, loyal, and dependable and can be trusted to accomplish what they agree to do. They are rule-abiding to the extent that the rules are their own or support their purposes, but otherwise they don't let rules interfere with their way of doing things. Thymuses are steady, consistent, and responsible and have the stamina to fulfill their duties and honor their commitments, sometimes taking a well-deserved sense of pride in their self-control.

Thymus types have good leadership qualities, a natural take-charge attitude, and are able to meet challenges and direct others to effective action. Their ability to control allows them to give others the external support they might need while gratifying their own need for stability and protection. Change often comes slowly, but once committed to something, Thymus types usually stay with it. Their pronounced sense of loyalty makes them very loving and protective toward those they care about. As they become more secure within themselves, they are able to identify with the feelings of others.

Motivated by succeeding at a personal challenge, Thymus types experience true success when they have genuine regard for themselves and others. This comes when they can allow latitude for others' feelings rather than needing to make the world perfect. Rather than expecting and taking, they aquire an attitude of allowing and giving, realizing that all is perfect and that what appear to be mistakes are merely learn-

### RECOMMENDED EXERCISE

Exercise is essential for Thymus body types because it activates the immune system. They should exercise for at least 15 minutes daily, at any time of day. The Thymus body type needs sunlight, so outdoor activity is especially beneficial. The best forms of exercise include swimming, basketball, running, jogging, walking, low-impact aerobics, and tai chi. Also recommended are stationary bicycling or cross-country training. Weight lifting strengthens and helps build muscle. The most efficient exercise is Callanetics.

ing experiences. They take total responsibility for what is going on in their life by realizing that what they experience is what they have attracted and that if they don't like the experience they need to determine why, so they can clear the old belief structures or learn the lesson.

The ultimate for Thymus types is manifesting unconditional love for themselves and others, essentially reaching perfection in this lifetime. When they are able to release the judgments that keep them separate and to resolve conflict through connecting with another's essence, they are able to integrate power and love. This is when they can be the most powerful and influential of all the types.

## Dietary Profile

### Main Focus

- Eat protein, ideally at breakfast and lunch.
- May have 4 eggs a day, 7 days per week.
- Lamb and rye support the thymus gland.

### Dietary Emphasis

- From 25 to 35 percent of your calories are to come from fats.
- Best fat sources: dense protein, all seeds, nuts (almonds, Brazils, peanuts, pine nuts), olive oil, and kefir.
- From 25 to 40 percent of your calories are to come from protein.
- From 10 to 35 percent of your calories are to come from dense protein.
- Best sources of the three amino acids threonine, isoleucine, and cystine: chicken, swordfish, and sea bass.
- Caloric intake: 1,500 to 1,800 calories a day for women and 1,700 to 2,000 calories a day for men. If you are engaging in intense exercise (competition type) or hard labor, increase calories.
- Drink a minimum of 64 ounces of water a day. Drink water before and after meals, not with meals.
- Occasional desserts are best as an evening snack.
- Avoid sugar, as it stresses the immune system.
- Include rye, seeds, nuts, vegetables, and olive oil.

### For Weight Loss

- Fat: 25 to 30 percent of daily calories.
- Dense protein: 20 to 30 percent of daily calories.

- Eat dense protein for breakfast and lunch.
- Eliminate refined sugar, particularly sugary desserts and sweet drinks, including fruit juices and alcohol.
- Minimize bread.
- Avoid all dairy products except butter.

### For Weight Gain

- Increase fat intake to 35 percent of daily calories.
- Increase dense protein intake to 20 to 35 percent of daily calories.
- Include snacks.
- Exercise daily.

## Healthy Foods List

There is no need to sacrifice delicious and filling foods to maintain a healthy Thymus body type. The following lists will help you focus on foods that support your health, and avoid foods that can stress your system.

*You'll notice that some foods are printed in italics; these foods take more energy to assimilate and could be ones you will want to avoid when you are in a sensitive state due to any physical or emotional stresses.*

Be sure to read Chapter 3, "Implementing the Body Type Diet," for lots of important information about how to use these many foods to gain their full benefit.

### Ultra-Support Foods

Foods to include in 3 to 7 meals a week, listed by category.

**Dense Protein:** beef, beef broth, beef liver, buffalo, lamb, pork, ham, bacon, sausage, venison, organ meats (heart, brain); game meats (all); chicken, chicken broth, chicken livers; bass, bonita, catfish, cod, flounder, haddock, mackerel, mahimahi,

---

**RECOMMENDED CUISINE**

Frequently: Chinese, Thai, Greek. Moderately: Mexican, Italian, Japanese, seafood, and pizza.

perch, orange roughy, sardines, shark, red snapper, sole, swordfish, tuna (Chicken of the Sea, yellowtail); clams, eel, mussels, octopus, oysters; eggs

**Dairy:** *milk (whole, 2%, low fat, nonfat, raw, goat's),* plain kefir, butter

**Cheese:** *cheddar, Colby,* pineapple cottage, *Monterey Jack, Muenster*

**Nuts and Seeds:** cashew butter, cashew milk, coconut, macadamias, macadamia/cashew butter, peanuts, pine nuts, walnuts (black, English); seeds (pumpkin, sesame, sunflower), sesame butter

**Legumes:** beans (black, garbanzo, *kidney,* lima, soy), black-eyed peas; hummus; miso, soy milk, tofu

**Grains:** couscous, oats, quinoa, rice (brown or white basmati, *long or short grain brown,* Japanese, wild), rice cakes, rye, breads (oat, oat bran, *rye, rye/pumpernickel*), *wheat/pumpernickel bagels,* crackers (*graham,* oat, rye, Ry-Krisp), pasta, udon noodles, Chinese rice noodles, cream of rice, cream of rye

**Vegetables:** artichokes, asparagus, bamboo shoots, basil, yellow wax beans, bok choy, broccoli, brussels sprouts, carrots, cauliflower, celery, white corn, greens (beet, collard, mustard, turnip), kale, shiitake mushrooms, onions (chives, green, Vidalia, white, yellow), parsley, parsnips, peas, snow pea pods, red potatoes, radishes, rutabaga, seaweed (arame, dulse, kelp, nori, wakame), spinach, sprouts (alfalfa, clover, mung bean, radish, sunflower), squash (acorn, banana, butternut, spaghetti, yellow [summer], zucchini), pumpkin, red Swiss chard, stewed tomatoes, turnips

**Vegetable Juices:** carrot, tomato, V-8

**Fruits:** apples (Red or Golden Delicious, Granny Smith, Jonathan, McIntosh, Pippin, Rome Beauty), bananas, berries (blackberries, boysenberries, blueberries, cranberries, gooseberries, raspberries), cherries, dates, green grapes, *white grapefruit,* kiwi, nectarines, oranges, *lemons, limes,* papayas, peaches, pineapples, pomegranates, prunes, rhubarb, watermelons

**Fruit Juices:** apple (raw, unfiltered), apple cider, apricot, apple/apricot, black cherry, red cherry, cranapple, cranberry, grape (purple, red, white), grapefruit, lemon, orange, papaya, pineapple, pineapple/coconut, prune, raspberry, watermelon

**Vegetable Oils:** *all-blend,* almond, *avocado, corn, flaxseed,* olive, *peanut, safflower, sesame, soy, sunflower*

**Sweetener:** stevia

**Condiments:** medium or hot salsa, Tabasco

**Beverages:** flavored or plain mineral water, soda water

## Basic Support Foods

Foods to include in 1 to 2 meals a week.

**Dense Protein:** veal; Cornish game hen, duck, turkey; anchovy, halibut, herring, salmon, trout, *tuna;* abalone, calamari (squid), crab, lobster, scallops, shrimp

**Dairy:** Lact-Aid milk, half-and-half, sweet cream, sour cream, *buttermilk,* flavored kefir, *plain or flavored yogurt, ice cream* (Ben & Jerry's, Dreyer's, Swensen's)

**Cheese:** *American, blue, Brie, Camembert, cottage, cream, Edam, feta, goat, Gouda,* kefir, *Limburger, mozzarella, Parmesan, ricotta,* Romano, *Swiss*

**Nuts and Seeds:** almonds, almond butter, Brazils, cashews, hazelnuts, macadamia butter, peanut butter, pecans, pistachios, water chestnuts; seeds (caraway, poppy), sunflower seed butter

**Legumes:** beans (*adzuki, Great Northern, navy, pinto, red*), lentils, split green peas, split yellow peas

**Grains:** amaranth, barley, buckwheat, corn, corn grits, corn tortillas, hominy grits, millet, popcorn, rice bran, triticale, whole wheat, wheat bran, wheat germ, refined wheat flour, flour tortillas, breads (corn, corn/rye, *French, garlic, Italian, multigrain,* rice, *seven-grain, sourdough, sprouted wheat, white, whole wheat*), bagels, croissants, English muffins, crackers (saltines, wheat), cream of wheat

**Vegetables:** *arugula,* avocados, *green beans,* beets, cabbage (green, napa, red), capers, cilantro, yellow corn, cucumbers, eggplant, garlic, hominy, jicama, kohlrabi, leeks, lettuce (Boston, butter, endive, iceberg, red leaf, romaine), mushrooms, okra, olives (green, ripe), brown or red onions, peppers (green, red, yellow bell; jalapeño), pimientos, *potatoes (purple, russet, White Rose, Yukon Gold),* daikon radishes, sauerkraut, shallots, sweet potatoes, *raw tomatoes, watercress,* yams

**Vegetable Juices:** carrot/celery, celery, parsley, spinach

**Fruits:** apricots, figs, grapes (black, red), pink grapefruit, guava, kumquats, loquats, mangoes, melons (cantaloupe, casaba, *Crenshaw,* honeydew), oranges, pears, Fuyu persimmons, plums (black, purple, red), raisins, strawberries, tangelos, tangerines

**Fruit Juices:** apple juice/water, guava, pear, tangerine

**Sweeteners:** *fructose, honey, molasses, sorghum,*

*sugar (brown, date, raw, refined cane), syrup (barley malt, brown rice, corn, maple), succonant*

**Condiments:** *mayonnaise, horseradish, barbecue sauce, pesto sauce, soy sauce,* tahini, rice vinegar, salt, sea salt, Vege-Sal

**Salad Dressings:** *blue cheese, French, ranch, creamy Italian, creamy avocado, Thousand Island,* vinegar and oil, lemon juice and oil

**Desserts:** *custards, tapioca, puddings, pies, cakes, chocolate, desserts containing chocolate, sherbet (orange, raspberry)*

**Chips:** *bean, corn (blue, white, yellow), potato*

**Beverages:** *tea (black, green,* herbal, *Japanese, Chinese oolong);* sparkling water, sparkling cider; *wine (white, red), sake, champagne, beer, barley malt liquor, vodka, scotch, gin, whiskey; root beer, regular sodas*

## Stressful Foods

Have no more than once a month.

**Dairy:** *frozen yogurt, most ice creams*
**Vegetable:** *broccoflower*
**Vegetable Oil:** *canola*
**Sweeteners:** *saccharin, aspartame, Equal, NutraSweet, Sweet'n Low*
**Condiments:** *catsup, mustard, margarine*
**Beverages:** *coffee; diet sodas*

## Scheduling Meals

Thymus body types should begin with a heavy meal and end the day with a light one. Schedule your meals as follows:

*Breakfast:* 7–8 A.M. Heavy, with protein, grain, vegetables, nuts, seeds, dairy, and/or legumes.
*Lunch:* 11:30 A.M.–2:30 P.M. Moderate to heavy, with protein, grain, nuts, seeds, dairy, legumes, and/or vegetables.
*Dinner:* 6–9 P.M. Light to moderate, with legumes, grain, vegetables, fruit, nuts, seeds, eggs, dairy, and/or protein.

Alternatively, if breakfast is light, compensate by eating a heavy lunch and/or dinner, although not preferred. Bulk of protein can be consumed at dinner if necessary. Avoid having fruit at both breakfast and lunch or breakfast and dinner.

### Snacks (optional)

*Snack:* (10 A.M. or 4 P.M.) vegetables, dairy, nuts, seeds, grain
*Midafternoon:* (4 P.M.) fruit, vegetables, dairy, nuts, seeds, grain
*Evening:* (10 P.M.–1 A.M.) fruit, protein, vegetables, grain, nuts, seeds, dairy, sweets

## Sample One-Week Menu

**DAY 1**
*Breakfast:* chicken and eggs
*Lunch:* lamb, red potatoes, and peas
*Dinner:* cauliflower, broccoli, carrots, almonds, and cashews
*Snack:* cashews

**DAY 2**
*Breakfast:* chicken and red potato
*Lunch:* red snapper, green beans, and rice
*Dinner:* split pea soup and a salad of romaine lettuce and tomatoes w/avocado dressing or Italian dressing

**DAY 3**
*Breakfast:* cream of rye w/butter and vegetables
*Lunch:* lamb and basmati rice
*Dinner:* tuna, rice noodles, and green beans

**DAY 4**
*Breakfast:* turkey, yellow corn, and sourdough bread
*Lunch:* roast chicken, red potatoes, and asparagus
*Dinner:* pinto beans, rice, and corn tortilla w/guacamole

**DAY 5: CLEANSE**
*Breakfast:* juice of carrot/celery/parsley, (cucumber), (spinach)
*Lunch:* steamed broccoli or squash (any) or raw carrots, celery, cucumbers, jicama, and/or juice of carrot/celery/parsley/(cucumber)/(spinach)
*Dinner:* steamed squash and/or raw cucumbers, and/or juice of carrot/celery/parsley/spinach

**DAY 6**
*Breakfast:* eggs, chicken, mushrooms, and onions
*Lunch:* Cornish game hen and rice
*Dinner:* apple w/cashew butter

DAY 7
*Breakfast:* cream of rye w/sesame seeds and eggs
*Lunch:* roast duck over wild rice w/mushrooms, green
beans, and onions
*Dinner:* baked yam w/butter and peas

## Alternative Menus

*(Foods in parentheses may be omitted.)*

### Breakfast, Lunch, or Dinner
Chicken and asparagus (potatoes or rice)

### Breakfast
Chicken and white basmati rice
Red snapper, eggs, and rice
Eggs, Monterey Jack cheese, and hamburger
Omelette w/avocado or spicy beef
Omelette w/tomatoes, onions, and bell pepper (zuc-
chini)
Beef and cream of rye
Cream of rice w/butter (almonds, cashews, pecans,
walnuts, or peanuts)
Granola
Oatmeal w/butter and eggs
Hamburger and spinach (carrots, sourdough rye bread)
Chicken, mashed potatoes, and green beans

### Lunch
Chicken, turkey, or lamb, and pasta
Chicken, baked potato, peas, and onions

Oriental chicken, beef, or shrimp, broccoli, and white
basmati rice
Salad of chicken, hummus, black bean chips, and carrots

### Lunch or Dinner
Turkey or chicken, pasta, mushrooms, carrots, bell
peppers, onions, and butter
Thai chicken w/red or yellow curry, bamboo shoots,
eggplant, and rice
Lamb gyros and green and/or red bell pepper
Moussaka—lamb, beef, cabbage, eggplant, and cheese
Steak, potatoes, mushrooms, and brussels sprouts
Steak, potatoes, cauliflower, broccoli, and carrots

### Dinner
Turkey soup
Plain pasta w/basil pesto or marinara sauce and arti-
chokes (parsley)
Pasta primavera
Rye or rice cereal w/butter (egg)
Corn grits (egg)
Chicken noodle soup and Ry-Krisp (orange)
Clam chowder, then apple
Cucumber roll and vegetable tempura
Vegetable beef soup and rye crackers (apple)
Spaghetti w/tomato sauce and salad of romaine let-
tuce, cucumbers, jicama, red bell pepper with
creamy Italian dressing
Scallops and pasta w/white sauce

# Thyroid

*The Thyroid body type is symbolized by gears. Synchronized movement is essential to getting things done. Bridging the gap between the theoretical and practical, Thyroid body types thrive on doing things that are worthwhile.*

FAMOUS PEOPLE: Hillary Rodham-Clinton, Richard Chamberlain, Katharine Hepburn, Leonard Nimoy

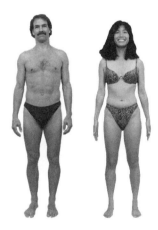

## THYROID
### Location and Function

The thyroid is located in the front center of the throat. It secretes hormones that regulate metabolism, particularly those that cause rapid mobilization of fats. It also controls basal metabolic rate and during childhood affects growth. It is activated by the anterior pituitary gland.

## Psychological Profile

### Characteristic Traits

The sensitivity of Thyroid types is often apparent in their eyes, which are bright and reveal an openness and availability. Thyroid types characteristically have a strong compassion and empathy for others. With a multifaceted nature, they are capable of understanding and relating to all the other body types.

Being intimately connected to both head and body, Thyroid types can bridge the gap between the mental and the sensuous. Many have an intense interest in gaining knowledge, as their whole orientation to life is intellectual, while at the same time they have a keen awareness of their body and sensory perceptions. Their senses are very finely tuned, with a heightened sense of touch. They frequently demonstrate an intense interest in things aesthetic, whether it be music, theater, or fine art.

Thyroid types can be quite sociable and gregarious, fitting in well with others and enjoying their company. Though talkative, open, and receptive, they generally give a sense that there's still a whole lot more that's not being expressed. Being exceptionally self-contained, they can also be soft-spoken and reserved, to the point of appearing aloof, secretive, or withdrawn. Internalizing rather than assertively expressing their feelings and attitudes, they have a definite sense of privacy and independence about them.

### Motivation

Motivated by their desire for self-realization, Thyroid types seek personal growth and deal with what's not working in their lives on an ongoing basis. Because of their intensity and lack of fear when exploring spiritual and emotional realms, they can access areas that most people around them don't understand. Consequently, they generally have less of a need to share what's going on in their lives than most other body types.

Typically Thyroid types were aware of being different and misunderstood as children, so they learned to be emotionally self-sufficient and responsible for themselves. Generally in touch with their feelings, they can also be quite aware of the feelings of others. Not wanting to do anything to hurt someone else's feelings or to suffer from being belittled, betrayed, or misunderstood, Thyroid types often exercise restraint in expressing themselves, controlling their emotions and evading areas of potential conflict.

Sensitive to the emotional environment around them and not wanting to upset their equilibrium or the harmony they value with others, Thyroid types are likely to avoid dealing with conflict and disharmony. Having discovered as children that directly speaking their truth was difficult for those around them to handle, and not having the skills to solve the problem, Thyroid types tend to stifle their feelings. By not discussing areas of conflict, preferring to smooth things over or let them slide, they often hold back communication that could be valuable. When they do have to face conflict, they tend to do so gingerly and indirectly.

Mentally adept and able to see both sides of a question, Thyroid types have the ability to dive in, identify a problem and its cause, formulate a viable solution or theory, and speak clearly and directly.

## "At Worst"

It's easy for Thyroid types to fall into a pattern of self-denial, putting other things and people first, taking things too seriously, and taking on too much. Seeing themselves as capable and responsible, they often get caught in helping others so much that they deplete own their energy or overextend themselves to the point where there's not enough time left for their own needs.

Thyroid types can become irritable or depressed and withdrawn when they don't feel they are doing something worthwhile or that their efforts are making any real difference in the world. Needing to be productively engaged in something meaningful, they may become obsessed with trying to fulfill this deeply felt need, which is closely related to their self-nurturing and fulfillment.

By nature one of the most reserved types, they can come across as cold, unfeeling, distant, or detached. Being overly focused on one of their various mental pursuits, they can close themselves off to others and become almost oblivious to their emotional concerns. They can become mentally rigid, particularly once they've reached a decision on something, making it very difficult for them to consider anyone else's viewpoint.

Mental rigidity occurs when they become overly linear and bogged down by details, losing touch with their spiritual connection. Dogmatism, self-righteousness, and victimhood may appear when they let themselves become plagued by worry and self-doubt.

## "At Best"

Thyroid types become truly empowered when they connect with their feelings and verbally communicate in a manner others can relate to, hear, and accept. Maintaining their inner peace, Thyroid types excel when they're doing something that is worthwhile. Hardworking, strong-willed, and idealistic about their chosen pursuits, once they make up their mind to do something, they do whatever it takes to accomplish the goal, persevering long after others would have given up. They have a sense of dedication that almost guarantees success in whatever they choose to undertake.

There's a quiet passion in the way Thyroid types operate that reflects their unconditional commitment to doing whatever it takes to accomplish their mission, whether it be self-realization or assisting someone else. By balancing their mental acuity with their spiritual connection and creative expression, Thyroid types are able to be successful in whatever they undertake and make significant contributions to the world. Using their ability to connect the theoretical with the practical, their talent for formulating and implementing theories, and their flexibility to adjust the results as needed, Thyroid types are able to transform ideas into reality, bringing peace and understanding to the world.

## Dietary Profile

### Main Focus

- ▶ Emphasize protein and vegetables.
- ▶ Eat almonds, raw soaked or roasted unsalted.
- ▶ Restrict breads and dairy.
- ▶ Restrict sugar, choosing tart rather than sweet fruit.

### RECOMMENDED EXERCISE

Exercise offers Thyroid body types the physical benefits of muscle tone, figure control, and mind-body connection. Activities such as Callanetics, dance, kick-boxing, yoga, and hiking develop endurance, stamina, and muscular strength. Aerobic exercise such as walking or using a rebounder or trampoline is good for developing muscle. Abdominal exercise stimulates bowel function.

## Dietary Emphasis

- From 20 to 35 percent of your calories are to come from fats.
- Best fat sources: almonds and dense protein (chicken, turkey, eggs, fish).
- From 20 to 40 percent of your calories are to come from protein.
- From 10 to 35 percent of your calories are to come from dense protein.
- Best sources of the three amino acids threonine, isoleucine, and cystine: turkey, chicken, and eggs.
- Caloric intake: 1,500 to 1,800 calories a day for women and 1,700 to 2,000 calories a day for men. If you are engaging in intense exercise (competition type) or hard labor, increase calories.
- Drink a minimum of 64 ounces of water a day. Drink water before and after meals, not with meals.
- Occasional desserts are best as an evening snack.
- Avoid eating potato or squash with dense protein.
- Consume more cooked than raw vegetables.
- Beets and/or beet greens cleanse the liver and stimulate bowel function.
- Asparagus aids the liver.
- Fruit or fruit juice after protein often assists digestion.
- Limit sweet fruit because it contains too much thyroid-stimulating simple sugar.

## For Weight Loss

- Fat: 20 to 30 percent of daily calories.
- Dense protein: 20 to 30 percent of daily calories.
- Limit fruit, other than lemon, to 2 meals a week.
- Avoid bread, refined sugar, and dairy (except butter).
- Limit snacks to midafternoon or evening.
- Focus more attention on the body.

## For Weight Gain

- Protein: 30 to 40 percent of daily calories.
- Dense protein: 25 to 35 percent of daily calories.
- May include fruit twice a day.

---

### RECOMMENDED CUISINE

Thai, Chinese, seafood; simple foods and combinations with mild to moderate seasonings.

---

# Healthy Foods List

There is no need to sacrifice delicious and filling foods to maintain a healthy Thyroid body type. The following lists will help you focus on foods that support your health, and avoid foods that can stress your system.

*You'll notice that some foods are printed in italics; these foods take more energy to assimilate and could be ones you will want to avoid when you are in a sensitive state due to any physical or emotional stresses.*

Be sure to read Chapter 3, "Implementing the Body Type Diet," for lots of important information about how to use these many foods to gain their full benefit.

## Ultra-Support Foods

Foods to include in 3 to 7 meals a week, listed by category.

**Dense Protein:** chicken, chicken broth, chicken livers, Cornish game hen, turkey; bonita, flounder, haddock, halibut, perch, orange roughy, salmon, sardines, shark, red snapper, sole, swordfish, tuna; abalone, calamari (squid), crab, clams, eel, mussels, octopus, scallops; eggs

**Dairy:** butter

**Nuts and Seeds:** almonds (roasted unsalted or raw soaked), almond butter

**Grains:** oats, popcorn, rice (white or brown basmati, short grain brown), brown rice flour, rice cakes, oat flour, oat crackers

**Vegetables:** artichokes, asparagus, bamboo shoots, beets, steamed broccoli, carrots, green peas, snow pea pods, bell peppers (green, red, *yellow*), nori seaweed

**Fruits:** apples (Granny Smith, Jonathan, Pippin), apricots (fresh or unsulfured), berries (cranberries, gooseberries, raspberries), cherries, lemons, mangoes, *persimmons, pomegranates*

**Fruit Juices:** *apple,* apple/apricot, black cherry, cherry cider, *cranberry,* pineapple/coconut, *raspberry*

**Sweetener:** stevia

**Beverage:** herbal tea

## Basic Support Foods

Foods to include in 1 to 2 meals a week.

**Dense Protein:** beef broth, *beef liver,* buffalo, lamb, *veal,* venison, organ meats (heart, brain); duck; *anchovy,* bass, catfish, cod, herring, mackerel, mahimahi, trout; lobster, oysters, shrimp

**Dairy:** *milk (whole, 2%, low fat, nonfat, raw, goat's), half-and-half, sour cream, kefir, plain or flavored yogurt, ice cream* (Ben & Jerry's, Dreyer's, Swensen's)

**Cheese:** *American, blue, Brie, Camembert, cheddar, Colby, cream, cottage, Edam, feta, goat, Gouda, kefir, Limburger, Monterey Jack, mozzarella, Muenster, Parmesan, ricotta, Romano, Swiss*

**Nuts and Seeds:** Brazils, cashews, cashew butter, coconut, coconut milk, hazelnuts, macadamias, macadamia butter, macadamia/cashew butter, *peanuts, peanut butter,* pecans, pine nuts, pistachios, *walnuts (black, English),* water chestnuts; *seeds (caraway, pumpkin, sesame, sunflower), sesame seed butter, sunflower seed butter*

**Legumes:** *beans (adzuki, black, garbanzo, Great Northern, kidney, lima, navy, pinto, red, soy), lentils,* split peas, *black-eyed peas; hummus; miso, soy milk*

**Grains:** *amaranth with chicken broth,* barley, corn, corn grits, corn tortillas, couscous, *hominy grits, millet,* quinoa, rice (*long grain brown,* Japanese, wild), rice bran, rye, *triticale, wheat bran, refined wheat flour, flour tortillas,* breads (corn, corn/rye, French, garlic, Italian, oat, rice, rye, sourdough, sprouted grain, white), *bagels, croissants, English muffins, crackers* (oat, rye, saltines), pasta (semolina, sesame), udon noodles, Chinese rice noodles, cream of rice, cream of rye, *cream of wheat*

**Vegetables:** *arugula,* avocados, beans (green, *yellow wax*), bok choy, *broccoflower, raw broccoli, brussels sprouts,* cabbage (*green, napa, red*) *cauliflower,* celery, *cilantro, corn,* cucumbers, eggplant, garlic, greens (beet, collard, mustard, turnip), lettuce (romaine, red leaf), jicama, kale, kohlrabi, leeks, okra, mushrooms, *olives (green or ripe),* onions (*chives,* brown, *green,* red, Vidalia, white, yellow), parsley, parsnips, *chili peppers,* pimientos, potatoes (all varieties), pumpkin, *radishes,* daikon radishes, *rutabaga, sauerkraut,* seaweed (arame, dulse, kelp, wakame), shallots, spinach, *sprouts (alfalfa, sunflower, clover), squash (acorn, banana, butternut, yellow [summer], spaghetti),* Swiss chard, *turnips, watercress,* yams

**Vegetable Juices:** carrot, carrot/beet/celery, carrot/celery/parsley/spinach, *tomato,* V-8

**Fruits:** *apples (Golden or Red Delicious, McIntosh, Rome Beauty),* canned apricots, *bananas,* berries (blackberries, *blueberries,* boysenberries, *strawberries), dates, figs,* grapes (*black, green, red*), grapefruit (white, red), *guavas, kiwi, kumquats, limes, loquats, melons (cantaloupe, Crenshaw, honeydew, watermelon),* nectarines, oranges, papayas, peaches, pears, pineapples, plums (*black, purple, red), prunes, raisins, rhubarb, tangelos, tangerines*

**Fruit Juices:** apple cider, apricot, red cherry, *cranapple,* grape (*purple, red, white*), grapefruit, guava, lemon, *orange, papaya, pear,* pineapple, *prune, tangerine, watermelon*

**Vegetable Oils:** *all-blend, almond, avocado, corn, flaxseed, olive, peanut, safflower, sesame, soy, sunflower*

**Sweeteners:** *fructose, honey, molasses, sorghum, sugar (brown, date, raw), syrup (barley malt, brown rice, corn, maple), saccharin, succonant*

**Condiments:** *mustard, horseradish, barbecue sauce, pesto sauce, soy sauce, paprika, salsa, tahini, vinegar, Morton's Lite salt, sea salt, Vege-Sal*

**Salad Dressings:** *blue cheese, French, ranch, creamy Italian, creamy avocado, Thousand Island,* vinegar and oil, lemon juice and oil

**Desserts:** *custards, tapioca, puddings, pies, cakes, chocolate, desserts containing chocolate, sherbet (orange, raspberry)*

**Chips:** *bean, corn (blue, white, yellow), potato*

**Beverages:** *coffee;* tea (*black, green,* Japanese, *Chinese oolong); Cafix;* mineral water, sparkling water; *wine (red, white), sake, gin, vodka; root beer, regular sodas*

## Stressful Foods

Have no more than once a month.

**Dense Protein:** *beef, pork, ham, bacon, sausage*

**Dairy:** *sweet cream, buttermilk, frozen yogurt, most ice creams*

**Legumes:** *tofu*

**Grains:** *buckwheat, whole wheat, wheat germ, breads (multigrain, seven-grain, whole wheat), whole wheat crackers, seven-grain cereal*

**Vegetables:** *lettuce (all varieties except romaine and red leaf), sprouts (mung bean, radish), sweet potatoes, tomatoes, zucchini*

**Fruit:** *casaba melons*

**Vegetable Oil:** *canola*

**Sweeteners:** *refined cane sugar, aspartame, Equal, NutraSweet, Sweet'n Low*

**Condiments:** *catsup, mayonnaise, margarine*

**Beverages:** *beer, barley malt liquor, champagne, scotch, whiskey; diet sodas*

## Scheduling Meals

### Healthy

Schedule your meals as follows:

*Breakfast* (7–8 A.M.), *Lunch* (12–2 P.M.), *and Dinner* (7–9 P.M.): Light to heavy, with protein, nuts, seeds, grain, vegetables, legumes, dairy, and/or fruit. Keep combinations simple. Size and number of meals are flexible depending on lifestyle and the day's activities. Avoid dairy for lunch and dinner.

### Snacks (optional)

*Midmorning:* (10–11 A.M.) vegetables, nuts, protein
*Midafternoon:* (4–5 P.M.) fruit or fruit juices, vegetables, grain, nuts
*Evening:* (optional) fruit, fruit juice, or sweets, nuts, grain, dairy, vegetables

### Sensitive

Adjust your intake as follows:

*Breakfast:* Moderate, with protein, grain, vegetables, and/or fruit. Avoid dairy.
*Lunch:* Light to moderate, with protein, nuts, vegetables, grain, and/or fruit.
*Dinner:* Light to heavy, with protein, grain, vegetables, and/or fruit.

## Sample One-Week Menu

### DAY 1
*Breakfast:* scrambled eggs w/broccoli
*Lunch:* turkey, cranberry sauce, romaine lettuce, and carrots
*Dinner:* scallops, pasta, and raw red bell pepper

### DAY 2
*Breakfast:* chicken and green beans
*Lunch:* sautéed Jerusalem artichokes and spinach salad w/almonds
*Dinner:* lamb and peas

### DAY 3
*Breakfast:* turkey and asparagus

*Lunch:* sushi or California roll—crab, avocado, rice, and nori seaweed—w/cucumber salad
*Dinner:* baked potato w/butter, carrots, and green bell pepper

### DAY 4
*Breakfast:* oatmeal w/butter and almonds
*Lunch:* orange roughy or sole, rice, and broccoli
*Dinner:* calamari and a salad of red leaf lettuce, celery, red cabbage, lemon juice, and avocado

### DAY 5: CLEANSE
*Breakfast:* watermelon including seeds and white part of rind or juice of carrot/celery/spinach
*Lunch:* steamed asparagus, beets and/or beet greens, broccoli, and/or raw bell peppers, cucumbers and/or juice of carrot/beet/celery, carrot/celery/parsley/spinach
*Dinner:* steamed globe artichoke or green beans, (onions) and/or raw cucumbers and/or bell peppers and/or juice of carrot/beet/celery, carrot/celery/parsley, (spinach) (carrot tops)

### DAY 6
*Breakfast:* yam and peas
*Lunch:* stir-fried shrimp, bok choy, mushrooms, pea pods, bamboo shoots, and onions
*Dinner:* salmon and green beans

### DAY 7
*Breakfast:* Granny Smith or Pippin apple w/almond butter
*Lunch:* Cornish game hen, rice, and broccoli
*Dinner:* Japanese noodle soup

## Alternative Menus

*(Foods in parentheses can be omitted.)*

### Breakfast
Corn grits w/butter
Pineapple/coconut juice
Rice and green peas
Calamari sautéed in butter (parsley) and white basmati rice
Cornish game hen and peas
Basmati or short grain brown rice, chicken, and mushrooms in chicken broth

### Lunch or Dinner
Thai coconut milk soup w/shrimp, scallops, and/or calamari (rice)

Thai scallops and vegetables

Scallops, broccoli, carrots, and onions

Turkey and oriental vegetables

Salmon and spinach soufflé

Buffalo patty w/lettuce (carrots)

Mushroom barley soup

Roasted almonds, raw bell pepper, and/or carrot

Stir-fried scallops or calamari, bamboo shoots, mushrooms, and napa cabbage (carrots, onions, snow pea pods, rice)

Oriental almond chicken w/snow pea pods, bell peppers, shiitake mushrooms, and basmati rice

Chicken and wild rice (asparagus)

Shrimp, green onions, and rice w/ginger

Chicken and a salad of romaine lettuce, carrots, jicama, and green bell pepper

Butternut squash and couscous (w/butter, seasoning, and/or onions)

Artichokes, rice, peas, onions, and carrots

# Resources

Abravanel, Elliot D., M.D. *Dr. Abravanel's Body Type and Lifetime Nutritional Plan*. New York: Bantam Doubleday Dell, 1983.

Blaylock, Russell. *Excitotoxins: The Taste That Kills*. Santa Fe: Health Press, 1996.

Breler, Henry G., M.D. *Food Is Your Best Medicine*. New York: Random House, 1965.

Grudermeyer, David, Ph.D., Rebecca Grudermeyer, Psy.D., and Lerissa Nancy Patrick. *Sensible Self-Help: The First Road Map for the Healing Journey*. San Diego: Willingness Works Press, 1996.

Mein, Carolyn L., D.C., *Releasing Emotional Patterns with Essential Oils*. San Diego: Vision Ware Press, 1998.

Web sites with more information on aspartame:
http://www.aspartamekills.com   http://www.doorway.com

## The Carolyn L. Mein, D.C., Educational Center

A resource center founded by Dr. Carolyn L. Mein to provide supportive programs to assist people in reaching their goals. The programs include Body Typing, Weight Loss, Exercise and Movement, Emotional Clearing, and Aromatherapy.

Training and certification are available to professionals interested in incorporating these programs into their practices. Call 1-888-269-8973 for more information.

*Core Fitness Video* by Carolyn L. Mein, D.C., and Beth Levy. This video focuses on effectively strengthening the abdominal muscles with Pilates-based exercises using a Fitness Ball. The weakest point of the body is the pelvis, and this can cause weakness of the lower abdominal muscles and lower back pain. Sitting on the ball forces you to use your pelvic and lower abdominal muscles. This improves posture, reduces wrist problems, and stimulates cerebrospinal fluid movement, resulting in increased alertness and mental clarity. The 60-minute video includes a 40-minute workout on the Fitness Ball, a mini workout that targets your weakest areas, and exercises that can be done at your desk while sitting on the ball. Call 1-858-756-3704 for more information.

For ongoing body type information and e-newsletter, visit web site at http://www.bodytype.com

# Index

# About the Author

**Dr. Carolyn L. Mein** began her private practice using applied kinesiology in 1974, and is a charter member diplomate of the International College of Applied Kinesiology. In addition to her chiropractic degree, she holds a B.A. in Bio-Nutrition, is certified in acupuncture, and is a Fellow of the American Council of Applied Clinical Nutrition.

Research-oriented, Dr. Mein's focus has been to optimize a person's health and vitality in the most effective and efficient ways possible. Realizing that optimal health and happiness requires balance, support, and integration of all areas, Dr. Mein developed a technique known as Transpersonal Physiology to correct and stabilize the structure, neuroemotional reprogramming, and a body typing system.

Studying the vast field of nutrition, Dr. Mein quickly became aware of the apparent contradictions in the information. While there are general principles that are true for everyone, she found too many questions that needed to be answered on an individual basis. Fortunately, her research led her to discover a common ground—body typing. Having 25 different types answered the question of how people could be so different, yet also explained why certain people had a unique similarity.

In her desire to make a worthwhile contribution to the world by improving the quality of the lives of individuals, Dr. Mein put together "The 25 Body Type System." It is designed to provide people with the specific information and the essence of what they need to know about themselves to be personally responsible for their own health, growth, and well-being.

Dedicated to the betterment of mankind, Dr. Mein lectures, writes, and maintains an active practice in Rancho Santa Fe, California.